Roger A. MacKinnon, M.D.

Professor of Clinical Psychiatry, Columbia University, College of Physicians and Surgeons; Training and Supervising Analyst, Columbia University Center for Psychoanalytic Training and Research, New York, New York

Robert Michels, M.D.

Barklie McKee Henry Professor and Chairman, Department of Psychiatry, Cornell University Medical College; Psychiatrist in Chief, The New York Hospital; Training and Supervising Analyst, Columbia University Center for Psychoanalytic Training and Research, New York, New York

The
Psychiatric Interview
in clinical practice

W.B. SAUNDERS COMPANY
A Division of Harcourt Brace & Company
Philadelphia London Toronto Montreal Sydney Tokyo

W.B. SAUNDERS COMPANY
A Division of
Harcourt Brace & Company

The Curtis Center
Independence Square West
Philadelphia, PA 19106

Listed here is the latest translated edition of this book together with the language of the translation and the publisher.

Spanish (1st Edition)—NEISA, Mexico
                        D.F., Mexico

Portuguese (1st Edition) — Editora Artes Medicas Sul Ltda.,
                        Porto Alegra, Brazil

THE PSYCHIATRIC INTERVIEW in clinical practice   ISBN 0-7216-5973-X

Print No.: **36   35   34   33   32   31   30**

To our students and patients

FOREWORD

Those who have read and reviewed other psychiatrists' books, articles, or chapters on the interview will recognize my colleagues' work as a refreshing and illuminating presentation. So, too, is it thoroughly "au courant" with our times. The interview *is* the most important technical instrument of all those professions concerned with man and his social functioning.

Psychiatrists and psychoanalysts, with their particular goal of understanding and treating the more serious disturbances of personality functioning, have labored to improve the social relationship between interviewer and patient. By so doing, they strive to maximize their comprehension of the motivations, defenses, and patterns of psychological adaptation that determine human behavior. The wealth of clinical experience that these specialists have acquired over the years has provided them with the unique opportunity of careful examination, intensive analysis, and synthetic theorizing concerning the origin of symptoms and the psychodynamic bases of a wide variety of personality traits and behavioral patterns. This information is of value far beyond the range of interest of psychiatry or even of medicine, in which the understanding of the patient's report of his experience obtained through the medical interview lays the groundwork for the establishment of a medical diagnosis and eventual treatment.

Today the interview is used by members of all of the professions directly concerned with sustaining or improving mental health—psychologists, social workers, nurses. Others, including the clergy, lawyers, and those concerned with personnel assignments rely, too, on the interview. All are confronted with the abnormal from time to time. All elicit information concerning personality traits and symptoms that are distressing to the patient. All, too, must conduct themselves in such a way as to establish a compassionate understanding of the problems revealed to them by the person being interviewed.

What is refreshing about this book is the decision by the authors to describe the psychiatric interview in terms of the behavior, more or less specifically, for major forms of personality disturbance—various neurotic and psychotic syndromes. This is a new departure for such a work. Especially illuminating are their concrete descriptions of what these patients do in the course of the interview and, by means of their psychodynamic understanding, their explanations for these behaviors and the more effective and supportive responses used by experienced interviewers. Their discussions of the artifacts so often introduced into the conduct of interview through the circumstances of the situation or the mode of communication, particularly their discussion of that bit of modern technology, the telephone, reveal them as fully involved in our modern world.

Even the most knowledgeable and experienced will find much of interest here.

LAWRENCE C. KOLB, M.D.

PREFACE

After some years of experience in teaching interviewing to medical students, nurses, psychiatric social workers, psychologists and psychiatric residents, we felt there was a need for a book that provided a simple, dynamic, and practical guide to interviewing. Frequently it was necessary to interrupt our teaching with a beginning student in order to discuss basic principles that could have been better covered in a book. However, after attempting to describe the fundamental principles upon which interviewing is based, we finally appreciate the reasons behind our dissatisfaction with other books on the subject.

Although this volume is at times directed particularly to the psychiatric resident, it is our hope that much of the material will appeal to a wider audience, including medical students, nurses, social workers, psychologists, and others in the mental health professions. The book is intended to be read and re-read at different periods in the student's professional development. Unfortunately, it is difficult to avoid oversimplicity or overcomplexity in preparing a book for professionals of varying experience, and in attempting to reach such a wide audience, we have committed offenses in both directions.

The purpose of the book is to facilitate the acquisition of many of the basic skills that are required of a psychiatrist, as interviewing encompasses all of psychiatry. Obviously, clinical proficiency can only develop through actual work with patients. The interviewer must learn to observe the detailed and subtle aspects of the patient's behavior before he can hope to understand its meaning. There is no substitute for careful clinical teaching, and this book is designed only as an adjunct to the supervision of psychiatric interviews. However, for students in those programs who do not have experienced clinical teachers, the book may serve as a basis for self-criticism of interviewing technique.

We have made no attempt to review the vast literature on the subject, which has been done quite well elsewhere, an example being *The Initial Interviews in Clinical Practice,* by Gill, Newman, and Redlich (New York, International University Press, 1954).

As our many critics have uniformly advised us, the book is best in the clinical and management areas. We wished there were an easily understood, but comprehensive, textbook of psychodynamics that the student could read in preparation for a book on technique. Unfortunately, there is no single reference that could accomplish this purpose. Furthermore, psychodynamics is still a young science, with many areas of theoretical controversy and even more areas that are yet to be explored. Despite our frustration at the impossible task, we offer the reader a brief psychodynamic foundation upon which our practical discussion is based. Our theoretical framework is essentially psychoanalytic, although we have attempted to avoid more complex or controversial issues and have selected specific viewpoints that we find helpful in teaching. We considered omitting this theoretical material, but decided that the book would be too much of a "How-to-do-it" manual without a psychodynamic foundation for our practical recommendations.

There is some material in this book that, to the best of the authors' knowledge, cannot be found elsewhere. However, the justification for the book lies in its overall organization and the presentation of material that the reader would have to consult many sources in order to duplicate.

ACKNOWLEDGMENTS

The idea of teaching psychiatric interviewing in terms of the various clinical syndromes came from a series of seminars conducted by Nathan Ackerman at the Columbia University Psychoanalytic Clinic for Training and Research. His presentations of special problems in the treatment of obsessive, hysteric, and phobic characters were inspirational. This approach was broadened to include other syndromes and clinical situations and was applied to a course in interviewing for first year residents at the New York State Psychiatric Institute.

The presentation of this material in book form results from the encouragement and advice of numerous residents and medical students at Columbia Presbyterian Medical Center and at the St. Luke's Hospital Center. We particularly thank our resident groups of the past three years, who have read or listened to the various chapters and offered their extremely valuable criticisms. We have made no attempt to pay specific tribute to the hundreds of authors whose works have contributed to our material, as it is impossible to trace the source of each piece of knowledge. Obviously, we are indebted to Sigmund Freud for most of our current knowledge of psychodynamic theory.

At a more personal level, we owe a debt of gratitude to the teachers of the theoretical courses in psychodynamics and psychopathology and to our supervisors from the faculty of the Columbia Psychoanalytic Clinic for Training and Research. To the founder of the institute, Dr. Sandor Rado, we express great appreciation. Many of the modifications of Freud's ideas that we discuss are attributable to him, particularly in the areas of obsessive and hysterical characters.

We particularly wish to thank our patients and our students for the clinical vignettes that appear throughout the book. Some of them are used out of their original context in order to illustrate a particular point, but care has been taken to preserve their authenticity and to maintain their anonymity. We thank our families for the many hours of time given up as well as the encouragement offered when the work became burdensome. For countless hours of proof-reading, we thank Verena Michels, Carol MacKinnon, and Stuart MacKinnon.

For endless patience in the typing and preparation of the manuscript and bibliography, we thank Virginia Swift, Betty J. Lawrence, and Sally Goddard.

Our greatest debt is to the many colleagues who reviewed and criticized portions of the manuscript. Rather than acknowledge the specific areas to which they contributed, we shall list them:

Morton J. Aronson, M.D.

Michael Beldoch, Ph.D.

Arthur C. Carr, Ph.D.

Elizabeth Davis, M.D.

Bruce P. Dohrenwend, Ph.D.

Richard G. Druss, M.D.

B. Ruth Easser, M.D.

Eugene B. Feigelson, M.D.

Shervert H. Frazier, M.D.

Willard Gaylin, M.D.

Lothar Gidro-Frank, M.D.

Winslow Hunt, M.D.

David Kairys, M.D.

Lawrence C. Kolb, M.D.

Donald S. Kornfeld, M.D.

Louis Linn, M.D.

Irville H. MacKinnon, M.D.

Verena Michels, A.C.S.W.

Leonard Moss, M.D.

John F. O'Connor, M.D.

Paul Olsen, Ph.D.

George O. Papanek, M.D.

Arthur Peck, M.D.

David Peretz, M.D.

Ethel Person, M.D.

Stanley R. Platman, M.D.

James H. Ryan, M.D.

Jesse Schomer, M.D.

Leo Srole, Ph.D.

Editha Sterba, Ph.D.

Richard F. Sterba, M.D.

Alberta Szalita, M.D.

Milton Viederman, M.D.

Paul H. Wender, M.D.

We feel that our book is immeasurably improved by the suggestions they offered, which we endeavored to follow. Of this group, an extra vote of thanks is offered to Morton J. Aronson,

M.D., and Verena Michels, A.C.S.W., as they reviewed so many chapters.

We wish to thank Miss Carolyn Buckwalter for her careful editing of the manuscript and Miss Lorraine Battista for her work in designing the book.

Finally, we owe a special debt of gratitude to our publisher, for patience and encouragement in the face of our inexperience and slowness.

ROGER A. MACKINNON, M.D.

ROBERT MICHELS, M.D.

CONTENTS

Section Two: Special Clinical Situations

Section Three: Technical Factors Affecting the Interview

INTRODUCTION AND GENERAL PRINCIPLES

A clear understanding of psychopathology and psychodynamics is the foundation for the psychiatric interview. A brief historical perspective is followed by a consideration of the general principles of all interviewing and the specific aspects of the opening phase of the interview.

1
GENERAL PRINCIPLES OF THE INTERVIEW

INTRODUCTION

It has been said that interviewing is an art rather than a science, a skill that can be acquired but probably not taught. This may be true, but a great deal can be learned that will enhance the acquisition of interviewing skill.

The psychiatric interview is not a random or arbitrary meeting between doctor and patient. It evolves from the basic sciences of psychopathology and psychodynamics. The work of Sigmund Freud is the foundation of our current knowledge of psychodynamics, although others have broadened and extended his concepts. Freud delineated the psychological significance of specific psychiatric symptoms and formulated general principles for understanding the relation of psychopathology to emotional conflicts. The psychiatric interview is a systematic attempt to understand this relationship in a given individual.

The introductory section of this book is divided into two chapters. Chapter 1 considers the general principles of the psychiatric interview. Chapter 2 discusses the basic concepts of psychodynamic theory, psychopathology, and the structure and functioning of the personality. Since the symptoms and character style of the patient significantly influence the unfolding of the interview, Section One has been organized around major clinical syndromes. Each chapter in this section is divided into two parts.

3

The first offers a description of the psychopathology and clinical findings as well as a psychodynamic explanation. The second part discusses characteristic interview behavior and offers advice concerning the management of the interview with this specific type of patient.

Examples of interview situations and guidelines for the doctor are given throughout the book. This approach is not meant to imply that these are the "correct" techniques or that one can learn to interview by memorizing them. The authors' interviewing style will neither appeal to nor be equally suited to all readers. However, there are students who have little opportunity to observe the interviews of experienced psychiatrists or to be observed themselves. Although this book cannot substitute for good clinical teaching, it can provide some useful glimpses of how practicing psychiatrists conduct interviews.

A second reason for providing specific clinical responses stems from the common misinterpretations of abstract principles of interviewing. For example, one supervisor, who suggested that a resident "interpret the patient's resistance," later learned that the inexperienced therapist had told his patient, "You are being resistant." It was only after the patient reacted negatively and the resident shared this with his supervisor that the resident recognized his error. After the supervisor pointed out the patient's sensitivity to criticism and the need for tact, the resident rephrased his interpretation, and said instead, "You seem to feel that this is not a problem for a psychiatrist."

Section Two concerns interview situations that offer special problems of their own. These can involve patients with any syndrome or illness. Here, the emphasis shifts from the specific type of psychopathology to factors inherent in the clinical setting that may take precedence in determining the conduct of the interview. The consultation on the ward of a general hospital is an example.

The final section is reserved for special technical issues that influence the psychiatric interview, such as note taking and the role of the telephone.

This book is concerned with psychiatric interviews for the purpose of understanding and treating psychiatric illness and does not consider principles or techniques of interviews that are designed for research, court procedures, or assessment of suitability for employment. These often involve third parties or non-therapeutic motivation. Such interviews have little in common with those described here except that they may involve an interview conducted by a psychiatrist.

THE MEDICAL INTERVIEW

A professional interview differs from other types of interviews in that one individual is consulting another who has been defined as an expert. The "professional" is expected to provide some form of help, whether he is a lawyer, accountant, architect, or physician. In the medical interview, typically, one person is suffering and desires relief; the other is expected to provide this relief. The hope of obtaining help to alleviate his suffering motivates the patient to expose himself and to "tell all." This process is facilitated by the confidentiality of the doctor-patient relationship. As long as the patient views the doctor as a potential source of help, he will communicate more or less freely any material that he feels may be pertinent to his difficulty. Therefore, it is frequently possible to obtain a considerable amount of information about the patient and his suffering merely by listening.

THE PSYCHIATRIC INTERVIEW

The psychiatric interview differs from the general medical interview in a number of respects. As Sullivan pointed out, the psychiatrist is considered an expert in the field of interpersonal relations and, accordingly, the patient expects to find more than a sympathetic listener. Any person seeking psychiatric help justifiably expects expert handling in the interview. The psychiatrist demonstrates his expertise by the questions he both asks and does not ask and by certain other activities, which will be elaborated later. The usual medical interview is sought voluntarily and the patient's cooperation is generally assumed. Although this is also the case in many psychiatric interviews, there are occasions when the person being interviewed has not voluntarily consulted the psychiatrist. These interviews are discussed separately (see Chapters 8 and 12).

Interviews in non-psychiatric branches of medicine generally emphasize medical history taking, the purpose of which is to obtain facts that will facilitate the establishment of a correct diagnosis and the institution of appropriate treatment. The interview is organized around the present illness, the past history, the family history, and the review of systems. Data concerning the personal life of the patient are considered important if they have possible bearing on the present illness. For example, if a patient has gastrointestinal symptoms, the doctor will ask if he has visited the tropics in recent months. However, the patient's general subjective evaluation of himself will most likely be discouraged, and such information is certain to be omitted from the written history. The psychiatrist is also interested in the patient's symptoms, their dates of onset, and significant factors in the patient's life that may explain them. However psychiatric diagnosis and treatment are based as much on the total life history of the patient as on the present illness. This includes the patient's life style, self-appraisal, and traditional coping patterns.

The medical patient believes that his symptoms will help the doctor to understand his illness and to provide effective treatment. He is usually willing to tell the doctor anything that he thinks may be related to his illness. Psychiatric symptoms, on the other hand, involve the defensive functions of the ego, and represent unconscious psychological conflicts (see Chapter 2). To the extent that the patient defends himself from awareness of these conflicts he will also conceal them from the interviewer. Therefore, although the psychiatric patient is motivated to reveal himself in order to gain relief from his suffering, he is also motivated to conceal his innermost feelings and the fundamental causes of his psychological disturbance.

The patient's fear of looking beneath his defenses is not the only basis for concealment in the interview. Every person is concerned with the impression he makes on others. The doctor, as a figure of authority, often symbolically represents the patient's parents, and consequently his reactions are particularly important to the patient. Most often the patient wishes to obtain his love or respect, but other patterns occur. If the patient suspects that some of the less admirable aspects of his personality are involved in his illness, he may be unwilling to disclose such material until he is certain that he will not lose the doctor's respect as he exposes himself.

DIAGNOSTIC AND THERAPEUTIC INTERVIEWS

An artificial distinction between diagnostic and therapeutic interviews is frequently made. The interview that is oriented only toward establishing a diagnosis gives the patient the feeling that he is a specimen of pathology being examined, and therefore actually inhibits him from revealing his problems. If there is any single mark of a successful interview, it is the degree to which the patient and doctor develop a shared feeling of understanding. The beginner frequently misinterprets this statement as advice to provide reassurance or approval. As an example, statements that begin, "Don't worry," or "That's perfectly normal," are reassuring but not understanding. Remarks such as, "I can see how badly you feel about . . .," or those that pin-point the circumstances in which the patient became "upset," are understanding. An interview that is centered on understanding the patient provides more valuable diagnostic information than one that seeks to elicit psychopathology. Even though the interviewer may see a patient only once, a truly therapeutic interaction is possible.

Initial and Later Interviews

At first glance, the initial interview might logically be defined as the patient's first interview with a professional, but in one sense such a definition is inaccurate. Every adult has had prior contact with a physician and has a characteristic mode of relating in this setting. The first contact with a psychiatrist is only the most recent in a series of interviews with health professionals. The situation is further complicated by the patient who has had prior psychotherapy or has studied psychology, thereby arriving, before his initial psychiatric interview, at a point of self-understanding that would require several months of treatment for another person. There is also the question of time: How long is the initial interview? One hour, two hours, or five hours? Certainly there are issues that differentiate initial from later interviews; however, these often prevail for more than one session. Topics that may be discussed with one patient in the first or second interview might not be discussed with another patient until the second year of treatment. The authors are, at times, deliberately uninformative regarding those issues that should be discussed in the first few sessions and those that are more likely to emerge in later stages of treatment. Greater precision would require discussion of specific sessions with specific patients.

This book discusses the consultation and initial phase of therapy, which may last a few hours, a few months, or even longer.

The interviewer utilizes the same basic principles in the first few interviews as in more prolonged treatment.

DATA OF THE INTERVIEW

CONTENT AND PROCESS

The "content" of an interview refers both to the factual information provided by the patient and to the specific interventions of the interviewer. Much of the content can be transmitted verbally, although both parties also communicate through non-verbal behavior. Very often verbal content may be unrelated to the real message of the interview. Some common examples are the patient who tears an empty matchbook cover into small pieces or sits with a rigid posture and clenched fists, or the seductive woman who exposes her thighs and elicits a guilty non-verbal peek from the interviewer. Content involves more than the dictionary meanings of the patient's words. For example, it also concerns his language style—his use of the active or passive verb forms, technical jargon, colloquialisms, or frequent injunctives.

The "process" of the interview refers to the developing relationship between doctor and patient. It is particularly concerned with the implicit meaning of the communications. The patient has varying degrees of awareness of the process, experienced chiefly in the form of his fantasies about the doctor and a sense of confidence and trust in him. Some patients analyze the doctor, speculating on why he says particular things at particular times. The interviewer strives for a continuing awareness of the process aspects of the interview. He asks himself questions that illuminate this process, such as, "Why did I phrase my remark in those words?" or, "Why did the patient interrupt me at this time?"

Process includes the manner in which the patient relates to the interviewer. Is he isolated, seductive, ingratiating, charming, arrogant, or evasive? His mode of relating may be fixed or it may change frequently during the interview. The interviewer learns to become aware of his own emotional responses to the patient. If he examines these in the light of what the patient has just said or done, he may broaden his understanding of the interaction. For example, he may begin to have difficulty concentrating on the dissertation of an obsessive patient, thereby recognizing that the patient is utilizing words in order to avoid contact rather than to communicate. In another situation, the doctor's own emotional response may help him recognize a patient's underlying depression.

INTROSPECTIVE AND INSPECTIVE DATA

The data that are communicated in the psychiatric interview are both introspective and inspective. Introspective data include the patient's report of his feelings and experiences. This material is usually expressed verbally. The inspective data involve the non-verbal behavior of the patient and the interviewer. The patient is largely unaware of the significance of his non-verbal communications and their timing in relation to verbal content. Common non-verbal communications involve the patient's emotional responses, such as crying, laughing, blushing, restlessness, and so on. A very important way in which the patient communicates feelings is through the physical qualities of his voice. The interviewer also observes the patient's motor behavior in order to infer more specific thought processes that have not been verbalized. For example, the patient who plays with his wedding ring or looks at his watch has communicated more than diffuse anxiety.

AFFECT AND THOUGHT

Both the patient and the doctor experience anxiety in the initial interview, as in any other meeting between strangers. The patient is anxious about his illness, the doctor's reaction to him, and the practical problems of psychiatric treatment. Many people find the idea of consulting a psychiatrist extremely upsetting, which further complicates the situation. The doctor's anxiety usually centers on his new patient's reaction to him as well as on his ability to provide help. If the interviewer is also a student, the opinions of his teachers will be of great importance.

The patient may express other affects, such as sadness, anger, guilt, shame, pride, or joy. The interviewer should ask the patient what he feels and what he thinks elicited the feeling. If the emotion is obvious, the interviewer need not ask what the patient is feeling, but rather what has led to this emotion now. If the patient denies the emotion named by the interviewer, but utilizes a synonym, the physician accepts the correction and asks what stimulated that feeling, instead of arguing with the patient. Some patients are quite open about their emotional responses, whereas others attempt to conceal them. Although the patient's thoughts are important, his emotional responses are the key to understanding the interview. For instance, one patient who was describing details of her current life situation fought back her tears when she mentioned her mother-in-law.

The patient's thought processes can be observed in terms of quantity, rate of production, content, and organization. Is his thinking constricted? If so, to what topics does he limit himself? Are his ideas organized and coherently expressed? Gross disturbances in the pattern of associations, rate of production, and total quantity of thought are easily recognized.

THE PATIENT

PSYCHOPATHOLOGY.   Psychopathology refers to the phenomenology of emotional disorders. It includes neurotic or psychotic symptoms as well as behavioral or characterological disturbances. In the latter categories are defects in the patient's capacities for functioning in the areas of love, sex, work, play, socialization, family life, and physiological regulation. Psychopathology also deals with the effectiveness of defense mechanisms, the interrelationships between them, and their overall integration into the personality.

PSYCHODYNAMICS.   Psychodynamics is a science that attempts to explain the patient's total psychic development. Not only are his symptoms and character pathology explained, but also his strengths and personality assets. The patient's reactions to internal and external stimuli over the entire course of his lifetime provide the data for psychodynamic explanations. These topics are discussed in detail in Chapter 2.

PERSONALITY STRENGTHS.   Frequently, a patient comes to the psychiatrist with the expectation that the doctor is only interested in his symptoms and possible deficiencies of character. It can be reassuring for such a patient when the psychiatrist takes an interest in his assets, talents, and personality strengths. With some patients such information is volunteered, but with others the interviewer may have to inquire, "Can you tell me some things you like about yourself?" Often the patient's most important assets can be discovered through his reactions during the interview. Skillful interviewing is of great importance in helping the patient to reveal his healthier attributes. He may be tense, anxious, embarrassed, or guilty when revealing his shortcomings to the physician, who is, after all, a stranger. There is little likelihood that the patient will demonstrate his capacity for joy and pride if, just after he has tearfully revealed some painful material he is asked, "What do you do for fun?" It is often necessary to lead the patient away from upsetting topics gently, allowing him the opportunity for a transition period, before exploring more pleasant areas.

In this area, more than any other, the non-reactive interviewer will reach an inadequate impression. For example, if a patient asks, "Would you like to see a picture of my children?" and the interviewer appears neutral, the patient will experience this as indifference. If the doctor looks at the pictures and returns them without comment, it is unlikely that the patient will show his full capacity for warm feelings. Usually the pictures provide clues to appropriate remarks that will be responsive and will help to put the patient at ease. The doctor could comment on whom the children resemble or what feelings are apparent in the picture, indicating that he takes the patient's offering sincerely.

TRANSFERENCE.   Transference is a process whereby the patient unconsciously and inappropriately displaces onto individuals in his current life those patterns of behavior and emotional reactions that originated with significant figures from his childhood. The relative anonymity of the physician and his role of parent-surrogate facilitate this displacement to him. The patient's realistic and appropriate reactions to his doctor are not transference.

Transference is to be distinguished from the therapeutic alliance, which is the relationship between the doctor's analyzing ego and the healthy, observing, rational component of the patient's ego. The realistic cooperative therapeutic alliance also has its origin during infancy and is based on the bond of real trust between the child and his mother. Positive transference is often employed loosely to refer to all of the patient's positive emotional responses to the doctor. It should be confined to those responses that are truly transference—that is, attitudes or affects that are displaced from childhood relationships and are unrealistic in the therapeutic setting. An example is the delegated omnipotence with which the therapist is commonly endowed. It is desirable for treatment that the therapeutic alliance be strengthened so that the patient will place his trust and confidence in the doctor —a process that is mistakenly referred to as "maintaining a positive transference." The beginner may misconstrue such advice to mean that the patient should love him or should express only positive feelings. This leads to "courting" behavior on the part of the interviewer. Certain patients, such as paranoids, work better early in treatment if they are permitted to maintain a moderately negative transference. For other patients, such as many of those with psychosomatic or depressive disorders, negative transference must be interpreted and resolved promptly or the patient will flee treatment.

"Transference neurosis" refers to the development of a new form of the patient's neurosis during intensive psychotherapy. The physician becomes the central character in a dramatization of the emotional conflicts that began in the patient's childhood. Whereas transference involves fragmentary reproductions of attitudes from the past, the transference neurosis is a constant and pervasive theme of the patient's life. His fantasies and dreams center on the physician.

Realistic factors concerning the doctor can be starting points for the initial transference. Age, sex, personal manner, and social and ethnic background all influence the rapidity and direction of the patient's responses. The male physician is likely to elicit competitive reactions from male patients and erotic responses from female patients. If his youth and appearance indicate that he is a resident or a medical student, these factors also influence the initial transference.

Transference is not simply positive or negative, but is a re-creation of the various stages of the patient's emotional development or a reflection of his complex attitudes towards key figures of importance in his life. In terms of clinical phenomenology, some common patterns of transference can be recognized.

Desire for affection, respect, and the gratification of dependent needs is the most widespread form of transference. The patient seeks evidence that the interviewer can, does, or will love him. Requests for special time or financial considerations, pills, matches, cigarettes, or a glass of water can be common examples of such concrete evidence. The inexperienced interviewer has great difficulty in differentiating "legitimate" demands from "irrational" demands, and consequently many errors are made in the management of such episodes. The problem could be simplified if it is assumed that all requests have an unconscious transference component. The question then becomes when to gratify and when to interpret. The decision depends upon the timing of the request, its content, the type of patient, and the reality of the situation.

For example, at the first meeting a new patient might greet the interviewer saying, "Do you have a tissue, Doctor?" This patient begins his relationship with the doctor by making a demand. The physician will simply gratify this request, since immediate refusals or interpretations would be premature and quickly alienate the patient. However, once the initial relationship is established, the patient might ask for a tissue and add parenthetically, "I think I have one somewhere, but I'd have to look for it." If the physician wanted to interpret this behavior, he could simply raise his eyebrows and wait. Usually the patient will search for his own while commenting that the interviewer probably attributes some significance to the request. This provides an opportunity for further understanding of the patient's motives.

Another illustration is the patient who asks for a match. If the interviewer does not smoke, he can merely indicate that he has no matches. If he does have matches, his interpretation of the patient's behavior will encounter less resistance if he gratifies the request the first few times but later comments, "I notice that you often ask me for matches." The discussion will then indicate whether this request reflects a general practice or occurs only in the doctor's office. In either event, the doctor initiates a discussion of the patient's attitude toward self-reliance and dependency upon others.

On occasion, early transference feelings may appear in the form of a question, such as, "How can you stand to listen to people complain all day?" The patient is afraid he will not be accepted by the doctor. The comment reflects his own self-contempt as well. The interviewer might reply, "Perhaps you are concerned about my reaction to you?"

Omnipotent transference feelings are revealed by remarks such as, "I know you can help me!" "Why do I keep getting into these situations?" "You must know the answer" or, "What does my dream mean?" Hollywood has worn out the standard gambit of "What do you think?" Instead, the interviewer can reply, "You feel that I am holding something back?" "You feel that I know the answers?" or, "Do you feel that I am not being helpful enough?" A more difficult manifestation of this problem is seen in the younger patient who consistently refers to the doctor as "Sir" or "Doctor." The interviewer meets great resistance if he attempts to interpret this behavior prematurely.

Questions about the interviewer's personal life may involve several different types of transference. However, they most often reveal concern about his status or his ability to understand the patient. Such questions include, "Are you married?" "Do you have children?" "How old are you, Doctor?" "Are you Jewish?" "Do you live in the city?" The experienced interviewer usually knows the meaning of the question from prior experience and his knowledge of the patient. He also intuitively recognizes the few instances where it is preferable to answer the question directly. For the most part, the beginner is best advised to inquire of the patient, "What did you have in mind?" or, "What leads to your question?" The patient's reply may reveal his transference feelings. At that point, the interviewer could interpret the meaning of the patient's question by stating, "Perhaps you ask about my age because you're not sure if I'll be competent to help you?" or, "Your question about my having children sounds as if it really means, am I able to understand what it feels like to be a parent." On other occasions these questions signify the patient's desire to become a social friend rather than a patient, since he feels he can not be helped as a patient.

Later in therapy, the physician often becomes an ego-ideal for his patient. This type of positive transference is often not interpreted. The patient may imitate the mannerisms, speech, or dress of the therapist, usually without conscious awareness. Some patients openly admire the physician's clothing, furniture, or pictures. Questions such as, "Where did you buy that chair?" can be answered, "What makes you ask?" The patient usually replies that he admires the item and wants to obtain one for himself. If the doctor wishes to foster this transference he may provide the information; if he does not, he will explore the patient's desire to emulate him.

Competitive feelings stemming from earlier relations with parents or siblings are sometimes expressed in the transference.

An illustration occurred when a young man regularly arrived for morning appointments earlier than the physician. One day he arrived just after the interviewer and remarked, "Well, you beat me today." He experienced everything in his life as a competitive struggle. The therapist replied, "I didn't realize that we were having a race," thereby calling attention to the patient's comment and connecting it with those problems of which he had some awareness.

Other common manifestations of competitive transference include disparaging remarks about the physician's office, manners, and dress; dogmatic challenging pronouncements; or attempts to assess the doctor's memory, his vocabulary, or his fund of knowledge. Belittling attitudes may appear in other forms, such as referring to the physician as "Doc," or constantly interrupting him. In the case of obvious competitive remarks, the interviewer may ask, "Do you feel competitive with me?" If the doctor feels annoyed by the patient's remarks, he is advised to remain quiet. Patients behave in this way when they feel "one down." The physician can get directly at the underlying feeling by asking, "Do you feel there is something humiliating about talking to me?" However, competitive behavior usually is best ignored in the first interview.

Male patients show interest in the male physician's power, status, or economic success; with a female doctor they are more concerned with her motherliness, her seduceability, and whether she is dominating. Female patients generally react in the reverse. They are concerned about a male therapist's attitude concerning the role of women, whether he can be seduced, what sort of father he is, and what his wife is like. The female patient is interested in a female therapist's career and in her adequacy as a woman and mother.

The patient's competitive feelings may become manifest when he responds to the therapist's other patients as though they were his siblings. Psychiatrists often fall into the trap of interpreting all competitive material as related to the Oedipal conflict and pay only token attention to helping the patient resolve intense sibling rivalry.

Older patients may treat the physician as a child. Women patients may bring him food, knit socks for him, or caution him about his health, working too hard, and so on. Male patients may offer fatherly advice about investments, insurance, automobiles, and so on. These transference attitudes can also occur with younger patients. Such advice is well intentioned at the conscious level and is indicative of a positive transference. It is therefore often not interpreted, particularly in the first few interviews.

In general, transference is not discussed early in treatment except in the context of resistance. This does not mean that only negative transference is discussed; positive transference can also become a powerful resistance. For example, if the patient discusses only his affection for the doctor, the interviewer can remark, "You devote so much of our time to discussing your feelings about me that there isn't any opportunity to talk about yourself." Other patients avoid mentioning anything that is related to the interviewer. In this case, the physician waits until the patient seems to suppress or avoid a conscious thought and then inquires, "Did you have some feeling or thought concerning me?" When a patient who has spoken freely for the first few sessions suddenly becomes silent, it is usually because of feelings about the doctor. The patient may remark, "I have run out of things to talk about." If the silence persists, the interviewer could comment, "Perhaps you're uncomfortable because of some feeling concerning me?"

RESISTANCE.   Resistance is any attitude on the part of the patient that opposes the objectives of the treatment. Insight-oriented psychotherapy necessitates the exploration of symptoms and behavior patterns, and this leads to anxiety. Therefore, the patient is motivated to resist the therapy in order to maintain repression, ward off insight, and avoid anxiety. The concept of resistance is one of the cornerstones of all dynamic psychotherapy. Freud described five types of resistance from a theoretical viewpoint and classified them according to source.

Repression resistance results from the ego's attempts to ward off threatening impulses by holding them out of awareness. The same repression that is basic to all symptom formation continues to operate during the interview. This keeps the patient from developing awareness of the conflict which underlies his illness.

Transference resistance can develop from any of the transference attitudes previously described. Each of the major types of transference is at times utilized as a resistance. The patient attempts to elicit evidence of the doctor's love or expects a magical cure through his omnipotent power. Rather than resolving his basic conflicts, the patient may merely attempt an identification with the physician, or he may adopt an attitude of competition with the therapist instead of working together with him. These processes may assume subtle forms—for example, the patient may present material that is of particular interest to the physician simply in order to please him. Just as transference can be utilized as a resistance, so can it serve as a motivating factor for the patient to work together with the doctor.

Secondary-gain resistance is reflected by the patient's unwillingness to relinquish the secondary benefits that accompany his illness. Thus, the patient with a conversion symptom of back pain is legitimately unable to carry out her unwanted household tasks as long as she is sick, and at the same time she receives attention and sympathy.

Super-ego resistance is manifested by the patient's unconscious need for punishment. The patient's symptoms inflict suffering on himself that he is reluctant to relinquish. This is particularly prominent in the treatment of depressed patients.

The last, and most controversial from a metapsychological viewpoint, is what Freud called the *repetition-compulsion resistance*. He considered this resistance a manifestation of a biological aspect of the organism. Whether Freud's concept of adhesiveness of the libido or some other hypothesis is the best explanation is unsettled. The clinical phenomenon that Freud attempted to explain remains valid: Patients maintain fixed maladaptive patterns of behavior despite insight and the undoing of repression.

Clinical Manifestations of Resistance.   In the discussion of clinical examples of resistance, the above classifications will not be used, since most are overdetermined and represent mixtures of several psychodynamic mechanisms. Instead, they are classified in terms of their manifestations during the interview.

First are the resistances that are expressed by patterns of communication during the session. One that is most easily recognized and most uncomfortable for the interviewer is silence. The patient may explain, "Nothing comes to my mind," or, "I don't have anything to talk about." Once the initial phase of therapy is past, the doctor may sit quietly and wait for the patient. Except in psychoanalysis, such an approach is rarely helpful in the first few interviews.

The interviewer indicates his interest in understanding why

the patient is silent. Depending upon the emotional tone of the silence, as revealed by non-verbal communication, the doctor decides on a tentative meaning of the silence and then remarks accordingly. For example, he could say, "Perhaps there is something that is difficult for you to discuss," thereby addressing himself to the patient's discomfort in expressing himself. If the patient seems to feel helpless and is floundering for direction, the interviewer might interpret, "You seem to feel lost." If the silence is more a manifestation of the patient's defiance or retentive obstinacy, an appropriate remark would be, "You may resent having to expose your problems to me," or "You seem to feel like holding back."

Beginning interviewers often unwittingly provoke silences by assuming a disproportionate responsibility for keeping the interview going. Asking the patient questions that can be answered "yes" or "no" or providing the patient with multiple choice answers for a question discourage his sense of responsibility for the interview. Such questions limit the patient's spontaneity and constrict the flow of ideas. The patient retreats to passivity while the interviewer struggles for the right question that will "open the patient up."

The patient who speaks garrulously may use words as a means of avoiding engagement with the interviewer as well as warding off the patient's own emotions. If the physician is unable to get a word in edgewise, he can interrupt the patient and comment, "I find it difficult to say anything without interrupting you." The literal-minded patient may reply, "Oh, did you want to say something?" A suitable response would be, "I was wondering why you make it so difficult for us to talk together."

Censoring or editing thoughts is a universal resistance. Clues to this include interruptions in the free flow of speech, abrupt changes of subject, facial expressions, and other motor behavior. These are usually not interpreted directly, but the interviewer sometimes remarks, "You don't seem free to say everything that comes to your mind," or, "What was that thought?" or, "It seems that you're screening your thoughts." These comments emphasize the process of editing rather than the content. Another form of editing occurs when the patient comes to the appointment with a prepared agenda, thereby making certain that spontaneous behavior during the interview will be at a minimum. This resistance is not to be interpreted in the first few interviews, since the patient will be unable to accept that it is a resistance until later. Further discussion appears in Chapter 3.

Intellectualization is a form of resistance encouraged by the fact that psychotherapy is a "talking" therapy that utilizes intellectual constructs. Beginning interviewers have particular difficulty in recognizing the defensive use of the patient's intellect, except when it occurs in obsessive or schizophrenic patients, in whom the absence of affect is an obvious clue. However, in the case of the hysteric who speaks in a lively manner, often with more "emotion" than the interviewer, the process goes undetected. If the patient offers some insight into his behavior and then asks the interviewer, "Is that right?", resistance is operating regardless of how much affect was present. Although the insight may be valid, the editorial comment reveals the patient's concern with the interviewer's concurrence or approval. It is the use of intellectualization to win the doctor's emotional support that demonstrates the patient's resistance. At the same time, the patient is offering an opportunity to strengthen the therapeutic alliance as he attempts to collaborate with the psychiatrist in learning the doctor's "language" and concepts for the purpose of winning the therapist's approval. The interviewer can address himself to the transference resistance while supporting the therapeutic alliance. He might say to the patient, "Finding answers that are meaningful to you not only helps you understand yourself, but it also builds your self-confidence." The patient might not accept this answer and respond with, "But I need you to tell me whether I'm right or not." This is one of the most common problems in psychotherapy and one that will be analyzed repeatedly in a variety of different contexts. The doctor, by recognizing in an accepting way the patient's need for his reassurance and guidance, thereby offers some emotional support without infantilizing the patient.

There are several ways in which the interviewer can discourage intellectualization. First, he can avoid asking the patient questions that begin with "Why?" The patient usually does not know why he became sick at this time or in this particular way, or even why he feels as he does. The doctor wants to learn "Why?", but in order to do so he must find ways to encourage the patient to reveal more about himself. Whenever "why" comes to the doctor's mind, he could ask the patient to elaborate or provide more details. Asking, "Exactly what happened?" or "How did this come about?" is more likely to get the answer to a "Why?" question than is asking "Why." "Why" questions also tend to place the patient in a defensive position.

Any question that suggests the answer that the doctor is seeking will invite intellectualization. Furthermore, it will give the patient the idea that the doctor is not interested in his true feelings, but is attempting to fit him into a textbook category. The use of professional jargon or technical terms such as "Oedipus complex" or "sibling rivalry" also encourages intellectualized discussions.

Patients who use rhetorical questions for the effect that they produce on the interviewer become involved in intellectualization. For example, a patient says, "Why do you suppose I get so angry whenever Jane is home?" Any attempt to deal with the manifest question assures intellectualization. If the interviewer remains quiet, the patient usually continues to speak. The physician, on the other hand, may strategically utilize rhetorical questions on occasion when he wishes to stimulate the patient's curiosity or leave him with something to ponder. For instance, "I wonder if there is any pattern to these anxiety attacks?"

Reading about psychotherapy and psychodynamics is at times used as an intellectual resistance. It also may be a manifestation of a competitive or dependent transference. The patient is either attempting to keep "one up" on the doctor, or he is looking for the "magic answer." Some therapists give the patient injunctions against reading. Usually this avoids the issue. More fruitfully, the interviewer might explore the patient's motivation for reading, which almost always stems from transference feelings.

Generalization is a resistance in which the patient describes his life and reactions in general terms, but avoids the specific details of each situation. When this occurs, the interviewer can ask the patient to give additional details or to be more specific. Occasionally, it may be necessary to pin the patient down to a "yes" or "no" answer to a particular question. If the patient continues to generalize despite repeated requests to be specific, the therapist interprets the resistance aspect of the patient's behavior. That does not mean telling the patient, "This is a resistance," or, "You are being resistant." Such comments are experienced only as criticisms and will not be helpful. Instead, the doctor could say, "You speak in generalities when discussing your husband. Perhaps there are details concerning the relationship that you have trouble telling me." Such a comment, because it is specific, illustrates one of the most important principles in coping with generalization. The interviewer who makes vague interpretations such as, "Perhaps you generalize in order to avoid upsetting details," will encourage the very resistance he seeks to remove.

The patient's preoccupation with one phase of his life, such as symptoms, current events, or past history, is a common resistance. Focusing on symptoms is particularly common with psychosomatic and phobic patients. The doctor can interpret, "You seem to find it difficult to discuss matters other than your symptoms," or, "It is easier for you to talk about your symptoms than about other aspects of your life." The physician must find ways to demonstrate to the patient that constant reiteration of symptoms is not helpful and will not lead to the relief he seeks. The same principle applies to other preoccupations.

Concentrating on trivial details while avoiding the important topics is a frequent resistance with obsessives. If the interviewer comments on this behavior, the patient insists that the material is pertinent and that he must include such information for "background." One patient, for instance, reported, "I had a dream last night, but first I must tell you some background." Left to his own devices, the patient spoke most of the session before telling his dream. The interviewer can make the patient more aware of this resistance if he replies, "Tell me the dream first." In psychoanalysis, the patient might be permitted to discover for himself that he never allowed enough time to explore his dreams.

Affective display may serve as a resistance to meaningful communication. Hyperemotionality is common in hysterical patients; affects such as boredom are more likely in obsessives. The hysteric uses one emotion to ward off deeper painful affects; for example, constant anger may be used to defend against injured pride. Frequent "happy sessions" indicate resistance in that the patient obtains sufficient emotional gratification during the session to ward off depression or anxiety. This can only be dealt with by exploring the process with the patient and by no longer providing such gratification. In addition to resistances that involve patterns of communication, there is a second major group of types of resistance, called "acting in" and "acting out." These involve behavior that has meaning in relationship to the doctor and the treatment process. It does not necessarily occur during the session, but the doctor is directly involved in the phenomenon, although he may be unaware of its significance.

Frequent requests to change the time of the appointment are a resistance. One patient may look for an excuse to miss the appointment altogether, whereas another may become involved in a competitive power struggle with the doctor, the patient saying, in effect, "We will meet when it is convenient for me." A third patient may view the doctor's willingness to change the time as proof that he really wants to see the patient and therefore will be a loving, indulgent parent. Before interpreting such requests, the doctor needs to understand the deeper motivation. If the requests are excessive or are burdensome to meet, the doctor can indicate that he is *unwilling* to grant them. The physician who claims that he is *unable* to grant them is often afraid of displeasing his patient. The patient's emotional reaction to this frustration and his associations to it should make the underlying meaning clear.

The use of minor physical illness as an excuse to avoid the sessions is a common resistance in phobic, hysterical, and psychosomatic patients. Frequently, the patient telephones the doctor prior to the interview to report a minor illness and to ask if he should come. This behavior is discussed in Chapter 15. When the patient returns, the doctor explores how the patient felt about missing the interview before he interprets the resistance. Charging the patient for these sessions is usually an effective technique for bringing the patient's feelings into the treatment.

Arriving late or forgetting appointments altogether is an obvious manifestation of resistance. Early attempts at interpretation will be met with statements such as, "I'm sorry I missed the appointment, but it had nothing to do with you," "I'm late for everything; it has no bearing on how I feel about treatment," or, "I've always been absent-minded about appointments," or, "How can you expect me to be on time? Punctuality is one of my problems." If the interviewer does not extend the length of the appointment, the lateness will become a real problem that the patient must face. It will often become clear that the patient who arrives late expects to see the doctor the moment he arrives. It is not useful for the interviewer to deliberately retaliate, but it is not expected that he sit idly, waiting for the patient's arrival. If the physician has engaged in some activity and the patient has to wait for a few minutes when arriving late, additional information concerning the meaning of the lateness will emerge. In general, the motive for lateness involves either fear or anger.

Forgetting to pay the doctor's bill is another reflection of both resistance and transference. This topic will be considered in greater detail later in this chapter (see "Fees").

Second guessing or getting "one up" on the doctor is a manifestation of a competitive transference and resistance. The patient triumphantly announces, "I know what you are going to say about this," or, "You said the same thing last week." The interviewer can simply remain silent, thereby not encouraging the behavior, or he can ask, "What will I say?" If the patient has already verbalized his theory, the doctor might comment, "Why should I think that?" It is generally not a good idea to tell the patient if he was correct in second guessing the interviewer, but, like every rule, there are exceptions.

Seductive behavior is designed either to please and gratify the interviewer, thereby winning his love and magical protection, or to disarm him and obtain power over him. Illustrative are such questions as, "Would you like to hear a dream?" or, "Are you interested in a problem I have with sex?" The interviewer might reply, "I am interested in anything you would like to discuss." If these questions occur repeatedly, he could add, "You seem concerned with what I want to hear." Various "bribes" offered to the interviewer, such as gifts or advice, are common examples of seductive resistance.

Beginning interviewers are often made anxious by overt or covert sexual propositions. Most frequently these propositions involve a male physician and a female patient. The doctor knows better than to accept such an invitation and he recognizes it as a resistance. What, then, lies behind his discomfort? Most often, it is his guilt that he is pleased by the invitation and the fear that his feelings may interfere with proper management of the patient. Frequently, this is revealed by a statement such as, "That would not be appropriate in a doctor-patient relationship," or by a comment to the supervisor that "I don't want to hurt the patient's feelings by rejecting her." The doctor must explore in his own mind whether he subtly invited such behavior from the patient, as is often the case. If he did not elicit the invitation, he can ask the patient, "How would that help you?" If the patient indicates that she needs love and reassurance, the doctor can reply, "My job is to help you work out your problem, but your plan would make that impossible." When a doctor has acquired an adequate amount of professional self-confidence, he will no longer respond to overt seduction by feeling flattered and anxious, provided he also has adequate self-confidence as a man.

Asking the doctor for favors, such as borrowing small sums of money or requesting the name of his lawyer, dentist, accountant, or insurance broker, exemplifies resistance. It is not the purpose of insight psychotherapy to gratify the patient's dependent needs. One makes exceptions, at times, in the treatment of adolescent, depressed, borderline, or psychotic patients (see the appropriate chapters).

Other examples of the patient's "acting in" include behavior during the interview that is unconsciously motivated to ward off threatening feelings while allowing partial discharge of tension. Common illustrations are lighting a cigarette, leaving the interview to go to the bathroom, or walking around the office. For instance, the patient may be recounting a sad experience and is on the verge of tears when he interrupts himself to smoke. In the process he gains control of his emotions and continues the story, but without the same affect. The interviewer could comment, "Lighting your cigarette helps you to control your feelings." The patient often experiences these interpretations as critical or as being treated like a child. Rigidity of posture and other ritualized behavior during the session are other indications of resistance. For example, one patient always said, "Thank you" at the end of each session. Another went to the bathroom before each appointment. When asked about the "routine," she indicated that she did not wish to experience any sensations in that part of her body during a session.

"Acting out" is a form of resistance in which feelings or drives pertaining to treatment or to the doctor are unconsciously displaced to a person or situation outside the therapy. The patient's behavior is usually ego-syntonic and it involves the acting out of emotions instead of experiencing them as part of the therapeutic process. Genetically, these feelings involve the re-enactment of childhood experiences that are now re-created in the transference relationship and then displaced into the outside world. Two common examples involve patients who discuss their problems with persons other than the doctor and patients who displace negative transference feeling to other figures of authority and become angry with them rather than with the physician. This resistance usually is not apparent in the first few hours of treatment; but when the opportunity presents itself, the interviewer may explore the patient's motives for the behavior. In most cases the patient will change, but at times the doctor may have to point out the patient's unwillingness to give up the behavior despite his recognition that it is irrational.

A third group of resistances clearly show the patient's reluctance to participate in the treatment, but do not predominantly involve the transference. For example, transference seems not to develop with many psychopathic patients, with some who are forced into treatment by external pressures, or with some who have other motives for treatment, such as avoiding selective service. With certain combinations of therapist and patient, the true personality and background of the therapist is too far removed from that of the patient. In that case, a change in therapists is indicated, whereas in the former situation therapy is a waste of time unless the patient can be inspired to change his motivation.

Some patients do not change as a result of insight into their behavior. This is common in some character disorders and is to be differentiated from the patient who is psychologically obtuse and cannot accept insight. This resistance is related to the clinical phenomenon that led Freud to formulate the "repetition compulsion."

Super-ego resistance is common in depressed patients, as the patient only accepts insights and interpretations in order to further flagellate himself. He then says, "What's the use?" or, "I'm hopeless; nothing I do is right." This behavior is further discussed in Chapter 6.

The beginner may feel overwhelmed by such a detailed discussion of transference and resistance. Despite the complexity of these concepts, it is important to develop a framework for understanding the major aspects of the psychotherapeutic process.

THE INTERVIEWER

THE INEXPERIENCED INTERVIEWER.   The principal tool of the psychiatric interview is the physician himself. Each physician brings a different personal and professional background to the interview. His character structure, values, and sensitivity to the feelings of others influence his attitude toward fellow human beings—patients and non-patients alike. In spite of these variables, there are particular problems that beginning interviewers have in common.

The beginning interviewer is more anxious than his experienced colleague. The defense mechanisms that he employs to keep his anxiety under control diminish his sensitivity to subtle fluctuations in the emotional responses of the patient. Since the beginner is in a training institution, the major source of his anxiety is his fear that he will do something wrong and lose the approval of his teacher. There is also resentment, which results from not winning a supervisor's praise. His fear of being inadequate is often displaced onto the patient, who he imagines will become aware of his "student" status and lose confidence in him as a knowledgeable physician. The patient's references to such matters are best handled in an open and forthright manner, as patients are always aware that they have gone to a teaching hospital. The young doctor's calm acceptance of the patient's fears that he is inexperienced will strengthen the patient's trust and confidence.

The beginner commonly feels a desire to perform better than his peers in the eyes of the faculty. Not all of his competitive feelings are related to his sibling rivalry; he also wishes to perform more skillfully than his teacher. Defiant attitudes toward authority figures are another manifestation of competitiveness that prevent the novice interviewer from feeling at ease with his patient.

The inexperienced physician in any specialty feels guilty about "practicing" on the patient. This guilt is exaggerated in the medical student who fails three or four times while performing his first venipuncture, knowing that the intern could have succeeded at his first attempt. In every area of medicine, the young doctor has conscious or unconscious guilt feelings when he thinks that someone else could have provided better care.

In many medical specialties, a resident under supervision can provide approximately the same quality of treatment as a senior physician. However, the psychiatric interview can not be supervised in the same way, and it takes years to acquire skill in interviewing. Although his teacher may reassure him that he exaggerates the importance of this factor, the beginner continues to imagine how much faster the patient would recover if he were treated by the supervisor. The young physician projects the same feelings of omniscience onto his supervisor that the patient has projected onto the therapist.

The beginning psychiatrist's attitude toward diagnosis has been discussed. Not only does he become preoccupied with diagnosis, but often he feels that organic factors must be ruled out in each case, since he is more experienced and comfortable in the traditional medical role. He goes through the outline for psychiatric examination with obsessive completeness lest he overlook something important.

In other situations, the interviewer becomes so intrigued with psychodynamics that he neglects to elicit an adequate description of the psychopathology. One resident questioned a patient at length about her compulsive hair pulling. He asked questions pertaining to its origins, precipitating events in her daily life, how she felt about it, where she was when she did it, and so on. He failed to notice that she was wearing a wig and was surprised when she later told his supervisor that she was bald. Since the patient seemed to be quite "intact" and the resident had not encountered this syndrome previously, he would not have thought to ask the supervisor's next question: "Do you ever put the hair in your mouth?" The patient replied that she did and went on to disclose her fantasy that the hair roots were lice that she was compelled to eat. A comprehensive knowledge of both psychopathology and psychodynamics facilitates exploration of the patient's symptoms.

In some respects the inexperienced interviewer is similar to the histology student who first peers into the microscope and sees only myriad pretty colors. As his experience increases, he becomes aware of structures and relationships that had previously escaped his attention, and recognizes an ever-increasing number of subtleties.

The tendency of the novice is to interrupt the patient in order to hammer him with questions. With more experience, he learns whether a patient has completed his answer to a question or if he merely requires slight encouragement to continue his story. As his competence grows, it becomes possible to hear the content of what the patient is saying, and at the same time to consider how he feels and what he is telling about himself through inference or omission. For example, if the patient spontaneously reports several experiences in the past in which he felt that he was mistreated by the medical profession, the interviewer could remark, "No wonder you're uneasy with doctors."

The interview is most effectively organized around the clues provided by the patient and not around the outline for psychiatric examination. The new physician invariably feels more comfortable if he can follow a formal guide, but this gives the interview a jerky, disconnected quality and results in little feeling of rapport.

Although the neophyte may talk too much and not listen, he also tends toward passivity. His professional insecurity makes it difficult to know when to offer reassurance, advice, explanations, or interpretations. Wary of saying the wrong thing, the interviewer often finds it easier to overlook situations in which some active intervention is required.

A professional self-image is acquired through identification with teachers. The young psychiatrist often emulates the gestures, mannerisms, and intonations of an admired supervisor. These identifications are multiple and shifting, until after several years the interviewer integrates them into a style that is all his own. Then it is possible for him to relax while he is working and to be himself. In the meantime, he often resorts to gimmicks, which are sometimes used in a stereotyped manner; for example, repeating the patient's last word or phrase at frequent intervals or using clichés such as, "I don't understand, what do you think?", "Uh huh!" or, "And then what happened?" It is desirable for the interviewer to utilize a variety of comments of this type at appriate points during the interview.

COUNTERTRANSFERENCE.   Physicians have two classes of emotional responses to their patients. First are reactions to the patient as he actually is. The doctor may like the patient, feel sympathetic to him, or even be antagonized by him without countertransference implications, provided that these are reactions that the patient would elicit in most people. Countertransference responses are specific for an individual physician and are inappropriate. In this situation, the doctor responds to the patient as if he were an important figure from the doctor's past. The more intense the doctor's neurotic patterns, and the more the patient actually resembles such figures, the greater the likelihood of countertransference responses. In other words, the physician who had an intensely competitive relationship with his brother is more likely than other therapists to have irrational responses to male patients of his own age. If he reacts in this way to all patients, regardless of their age, sex, or personality type, the problem is more serious.

Countertransference responses could be classified into the same categories as are used in the discussion of transference. These responses are more frequent with beginning interviewers and with those who have major unresolved emotional conflicts.

The physician may become dependent upon his patient's affection and praise as sources of his own well-being, or, conversely, may feel frustrated and angry when the patient is hostile or critical. It takes an unbelievably secure therapist not to use the patient in this way occasionally when his personal life provides inadequate gratification. The doctor may unconsciously seek the patient's love by accepting gifts or favors. Beginning residents commonly find women patients writing love notes or poems, or proposing marriage. One resident commented that his only prior model for male-female relationships was that in dating. There are more subtle manifestations of this problem, such as offering excessive reassurance, helping the patient obtain housing, draft deferments, and so forth, when such assistance is not really necessary and serves as a bribe to earn the patient's love. Going out of one's way to rearrange time or fees, providing extra time, and being overly kind are all ways of courting the patient's favor. Not allowing the patient to get angry is the other side of the same coin.

The physician can utilize exhibitionism as a way of soliciting affection or admiration from his patients. Displaying one's knowledge or social or professional status to an inappropriate degree is a good illustration.

Experienced therapists have commented that it is difficult to have only one case in long-term therapy, as that patient becomes too important to them. Other factors can cause a psychiatrist to overemphasize the importance of a particular patient. The "V.I.P." creates so much difficulty for the doctor that a later section will be devoted to the discussion of this patient.

All persons in the healing arts react to the patient's need to endow them with magical power. The nature of the doctor-patient relationship reawakens the doctor's desire to be all-knowing and all-powerful. If the interviewer assumes such a role, the patient cannot overcome his basic feelings of helplessness and inferiority. Nevertheless, the wish to become omnipotent is universal and can often be recognized in the physician's behavior.

For instance, the interviewer may be unable to see inconsistencies or inaccuracies in certain interpretations, and he may refuse to examine his own comments. This insistence on his own infallibility may lead to his implying that previous psychotherapists did not conduct therapy properly, or did not accurately understand the patient.

This mechanism is demonstrated by the psychiatrist who tells his wife a clinical vignette that reveals how kind and understanding he was, or tells how desirable and attractive his women patients find him, or relates his brilliant interpretation. Discouraged with the slow progress of psychotherapy, he may subtly exaggerate and distort material from the sessions in order to impress his colleagues. He may exert pressure on the patient to improve for the purpose of enhancing his prestige and reputation. At times he may try to impress colleagues with the wealth, brilliance, or importance of his patients.

Countertransference is operating when the therapist is unable to recognize or refuses to acknowledge the real significance of his own attitudes and behavior. Such an admission might be phrased, "Yes, I was preoccupied last time" or, "My remark does sound belittling." If the patient tries to turn the tables by analyzing him further, the doctor might reply, "Finding out why I said that is my problem. It would be unfair to burden you with it. Instead, let's understand as much as we can about your reactions to me." The patient is concerned about whether the doctor lives by a double standard, analyzing his patient's behavior but not his own. Occasionally a patient may exploit his therapist's openness concerning a mistake. The doctor who allows the patient to treat him sadistically also has a countertransference problem. Similar issues are raised when the patient has information regarding his therapist that comes from outside the treatment situation. Common examples are the patient who lives in the same neighborhood, has children in the same school as the therapist's children, or works in the same institution as the therapist. The most usual example in the life of the psychiatric resident is the hospitalized patient who obtains information about his doctor from other patients, staff, bulletin boards, or his own direct observations.

In an attempt to maintain a professional role the doctor is defensively tempted to hide behind analytical clichés such as, "How do you feel about that?" or, "What meaning did that have "for you?" Often more subtle examples occur when the therapist's wording or the tone of his voice is crucial in revealing the implication of his remark. For example, "The idea of my flirting with the ward nurse seems to upset you," could be said so as to imply that the flirtation existed only in the patient's mind. However, if the interviewer remarks, "My flirting with the ward nurse upset you," the patient's perception is not challenged, and the interviewer can explore the impact of "reality" on the patient.

A common manifestation of countertransference is over-identification with the patient. In this situation, the physician attempts to make the patient over in his own image. Perhaps the universal pitfall for psychotherapists is to indulge their Pygmalion fantasies. Difficulty in paying attention or remembering what the patient has said may be the doctor's first clue to his countertransference. The doctor who overidentifies with his patient may have difficulty recognizing or understanding problems that are similar to his own. Or, he may have an immediate understanding of the problem, but be unable to deal with it. For example, an obsessive doctor, who is preoccupied with time, says after each hour, "I'll see you tomorrow at 3:30." It is unlikely that he will be able to help his patient work through a similar difficulty.

The beginning therapist tends to experience vicarious pleasure in the sexual or aggressive behavior of his patient. He may encourage the patient to stand up to his parents in a manner that he himself admires. He may cater to the patient's dependent needs because he would like to be treated in a similar fashion. Psychiatrists who are undergoing analytic treatment themselves find that their patients are often working on the same problem they are.

Power struggles, competition, and arguing with or badgering the patient are familiar examples of countertransference. The interviewer's task is to understand how the patient views the world and to help the patient better understand himself. It is not useful to force the interviewer's concepts on the patient. More subtle manifestations of this problem include the use of words or concepts that are slightly over the patient's head and thereby demonstrate the doctor's "one up" position. Other illustrations include the tendency to say, "I told you so," when the patient discovers that the doctor has been correct, or laughing at the patient's discomfort.

The countertransference response of wishing to be the patient's child or younger sibling most often occurs with older patients. Once again, the more the patient actually resembles the therapist's parent or sibling, the greater the likelihood of such responses. With female patients the therapist might accept gifts of food or clothing; with a male patient he might accept business advice or other such assistance.

There are a variety of non-specific manifestations of countertransference. Sometimes an interviewer will experience anxiety, excitement, or depression, either while he is with a certain patient or after the patient leaves the office. His reaction might involve a countertransference problem or it might reflect anxiety or neurotic triumph about the way in which he dealt with the patient.

Boredom or inability to concentrate on what the patient is saying most often reflects unconscious anger or anxiety on the part of the interviewer. It can be caused by several different countertransference responses. Although certain patients tend to be boring, to a large extent boredom is due to the fact that they easily elicit countertransference responses. If the doctor regularly is late or forgets the session, this behavior usually indicates avoidance of hostile or sexual feelings toward the patient.

Another common countertransference problem stems from the therapist's failing to see occasions when the apparent "observing ego of the patient" is actually a transference masquerade. The result is an overly intellectualized therapy that is relatively devoid of emotion.

The direct expression of emotion in the transference will frequently provide an opportunity for countertransference responses. For example the doctor tells the patient, "It isn't really me you love (or hate); it's your father." Transference does not mean that the patient's feelings toward the therapist are not real. Telling the patient that his feelings are displaced is disrespectful and belittling. Similarly, beginning therapists sometimes respond to the patient's expression of anger by a comment such as, "It is a real sign of progress that you are able to get angry at me." Remarks of this type are contemptuous of the patient's feelings. Although the transference neurosis involves the repetition of past attitudes, the emotional response is real; in fact, it is often stronger than it was in the original setting because less defense is necessary. The therapist's discomfort with the patient's intense emotional reactions may lead to a subtle defensiveness. An example is provided by the doctor who asks, "Isn't this the same way you felt toward your sister?" or, "We know that you have had similar feelings in the past." These comments divert the patient away from the transference rather than encouraging exploration of it. Both the doctor and the patient will understand the patient's feelings better if the interviewer asks, "How am I a son-of-a-bitch?" or, "What is it that you love about me?" Such an approach takes the patient's feeling seriously. When the patient elaborates his feeling, he will usually discover the transference aspect of his response by himself. As he fully delineates the details of his reaction, he often volunteers, "You don't react the way my father did when I felt like this," or, "This makes me think of something that happened years ago with my brother." Then the interviewer can demonstrate the transference component of the patient's feeling.

In the pursuit of the details of the patient's emotional reactions, distorted perceptions of the therapist frequently emerge. For instance, when describing why she felt that she loved her doctor, a patient said, "For some strange reason I pictured you with a mustache." Exploration of such clues identified the original object of the transference feeling from the patient's past.

Discussions of countertransference typically leave the beginner feeling that this reaction is bad and must be eliminated. It would be more accurate to say that the doctor tries to minimize the extent to which his neurotic responses interfere with the treatment. Neurotic conflicts that have not been resolved should be recognized by the interviewer. The physician who is aware of his countertransference can use it as another source of information about the patient. In interviews with schizophrenic patients, the mutual recognition of the doctor's countertransference can be particularly useful in the process of therapy (see Chapter 7).

THE SPECIAL PATIENT.   The special patient is discussed at this point because the chief distinguishing features of this interview center on the interviewer's reactions to the status of his patient. The problem continues to occur throughout a physician's career, although the criteria that define the patient as "special" may change. In the early years of a doctor's training, this patient may be a medical student, a fellow house staff officer, the relative of a staff member, or a patient who is known by a prestigious teacher.

As the physician's experience and status increase, so does the status of his special patients. No matter how experienced the physician, or how secure, there always exists a person of such renown that the doctor will feel uneasy with him. There is as much variety in the attitude of special patients about their status as there is in any other group of people. Those whose special status depends upon their significance to the interviewer usually expect to be treated like any other patient.

Some patients do expect and warrant special consideration. The interviewer may be uncertain where reality ends and neurotic expectations begin. Resolution of the quandary involves a consideration of the rights of the ordinary patient. The status of the special patient may deprive him of these basic rights. The doctor's making extraordinary arrangements that, in effect, place this patient on a par with other patients is not likely to harm his treatment. For example, consider the nationally prominent political figure, whose position could be jeopardized if the public discovered that he had consulted a psychiatrist. The psychiatrist, by conducting a consultation in the patient's home, offers the same privacy that another patient can maintain while seeing the doctor in his office. In this case the application of the principle is clear, but in other instances the doctor must decide whether to side with the reality situation of the patient's life or with the principle that neurotic demands should not be gratified. If the consequences are high, it is preferable to risk gratifying the patient's neurosis.

Problems arise in the treatment of this patient not only because his situation is special, but also because he becomes special to the doctor. The success of his treatment assumes an urgent importance, and the physician is overly concerned with maintaining the good will of the patient, his relatives, and his associates. One protection for both the patient and doctor is to make special arrangements in the selection of a doctor. The senior physician who is hospitalized for a major depression or the psychotic son of a prominent person should not be assigned to a first year resident. By choosing a psychiatrist who is less likely to be made insecure, many problems are minimized.

The physician-patient presents particular problems. The treating doctor offers more detailed explanations on some occasions, but no explanation at all on others, assuming that the patient already has sufficient knowledge. The physician patient sometimes expects to be treated as a colleague and to have a "medical" discussion about his own case. He may fear asking questions that would make him appear ignorant or frightened. If he is receiving professional courtesy, he feels that he should not complain, express anger, or take too much of his physician's time. The young doctor is prone to use jargon or to give intellectualized formulations to physician-patients. One physician-patient described a terrifying experience during which a urologist gave a continuous monologue of his maneuvers while passing a cystoscope, and then described the clinical findings in the doctor's bladder which, unbeknownst to the patient, had little pathological significance. The urologist apparently felt that a physician-patient might be reassured by this extra information.

THE ROLE OF THE INTERVIEWER. The most important function of the interviewer is to listen and to understand the patient in order that he may help. An occasional nod or "un-huh" is sufficient to let the patient know that the interviewer is paying attention. Furthermore, a sympathetic comment, when appropriate, aids in the establishment of rapport. The physician can use remarks such as, "Of course," "I see," or, "Naturally" to support attitudes that have been communicated by the patient. When the patient's feeling is quite clear, the doctor can indicate his understanding with statements such as, "You must have felt terribly alone," or "That must have been very upsetting." In general, the interviewer is non-judgmental, interested, concerned, and kind.

The interviewer frequently asks questions. These may serve to obtain information or to clarify his own or the patient's understanding. Questions can be a subtle form of suggestion, or, by the tone of voice in which they are asked, they may give the patient permission to do something. For example, the interviewer might ask, "Did you ever tell your boss that you felt you deserved a raise?" Regardless of the answer, the interviewer has indicated that such an act would be conceivable, permissible, and, perhaps, even expected.

The interviewer frequently makes suggestions to the patient either implicitly or explicitly. The recommendation of a specific form of treatment carries the physician's implied suggestion that he expects it to be helpful. The questions that the doctor asks often give the patient the feeling that he is expected to discuss certain topics, such as dreams or sex. In psychotherapy, the doctor suggests that the patient discuss any major decisions before acting on them, and he may suggest that the patient should or should not discuss certain feelings with important persons in his life.

He may help the patient with practical matters. For instance, a young married couple requested psychiatric help because of difficulty getting along with each other. At the end of the consultation they asked if it would be helpful if they tried to have a baby. A well-intentioned family doctor had suggested that a child might bring them closer together. The psychiatrist advised that it would not be a good idea to have a child at that time and recommended that they wait until their relationship had improved.

The doctor provides the patient with certain gratifications and frustrations in the process of treatment. He helps the patient by his interest, understanding, encouragement, and support. He is the patient's ally, and in that sense offers him opportunities to experience closeness. When the patient becomes unsure of himself, he may provide reassurance with a comment such as, "Go ahead, you're doing fine." Generalized reassurance such as, "Don't worry, it will all work out," is of limited value for most patients. It is preferable to offer support in the form of understanding that is founded on specific formulations of the patient's problem. At the same time, the doctor seeks to remove the patient's symptoms and the gratification that they provide. He makes the patient aware of conflicts—an awareness that can be painful and frustrating.

The most important activity in psychoanalytically oriented psychotherapy is interpretation. The aim of an interpretation is to undo the process of repression and allow unconscious thoughts and feelings to become conscious, thereby enabling the patient to develop new methods of coping with his conflicts without the formation of symptoms (see Chapter 2 on the formation of symptoms). The preliminary steps of an interpretation are confrontation, which is pointing out that the patient is avoiding something, and clarification, which is formulating the area to be explored.

A "complete" interpretation delineates a pattern of behavior in the patient's current life, showing the basic conflict between wish and fear, the defenses that are involved, and any resulting symptom formation. This pattern is traced to its origin in his early life, its manifestation in the transference is pointed out and, in addition, the secondary gain is formulated. It is never possible to encompass all of these aspects at the same time.

Interpretations can be directed at resistances and defenses or at content. In general, the interpretation is aimed at the material closest to consciousness, which means that defenses are interpreted earlier than the unconscious impulse that they help to ward off. In practice, any single interpretation involves both resistance and content, and is usually repeated many times, although with varying emphasis, the therapist shifting back and forth as he works on a given problem. The earliest interpretations are aimed at the area in which the conscious anxiety is greatest, which usually is the patient's presenting symptoms, his resistance or transference. Unconscious material is not interpreted until it has become preconscious.

To illustrate these issues, consider a young man with a phobic anxiety neurosis. The therapist's first confrontation was aimed at the patient's resistance, with the remark, "You spend a good portion of our time talking about your symptoms." The patient answered, "What would you like me to talk about?", and the interviewer indicated that he would like to know more about what had been happening just before the last attack began. The patient's reply led to a clarification by the interviewer, "This is the third time this week that you had an attack after becoming angry with your wife." The patient accepted this remark, but it was not until a subsequent session that he added that he became angry whenever he felt that his wife was closer to her mother than to him. Still later it was learned that the patient felt intensely competitive with his sister and feared that their mother preferred her to him. At this time it was possible to interpret the patient's wish to kill his sister, and his fear that he would be killed in return. The same feelings were re-created in his current relationship with his wife. The physician not only interpreted the patient's jealousy of his wife's attention to her mother, but also his jealousy of the love that his mother-in-law bestowed on her daughter. At a different time, the secondary gain of the patient's symptom was interpreted as the fact that his attack invariably brought forth sympathetic indulgence from his wife. The entire process was repeated in the transference, in which the patient became enraged that the therapist did not demonstrate more sympathy for his symptoms, and then described a dream in which he was the doctor's favorite patient.

Interpretations are more effective if they are specific. In the above example, a specific interpretation is, "You become angry when you feel that your wife cares more about her mother than about you." A general statement would be, "Your anger seems to be directed at women." An initial interpretation is, of necessity, incomplete. As shown in the example, many steps are required before one can formulate a complete interpretation. When the interviewer is uncertain, interpretations are better offered as possibilities for the patient's consideration than as dogmatic pronouncements. He might introduce an interpretation with "Perhaps," or, "It seems to me."

Timing is a critical aspect of interpretation. A premature interpretation is threatening; it increases the patient's anxiety and intensifies his resistance. A delayed interpretation slows treatment and the physician is of little help to the patient. The optimal time to interpret is when the patient is not yet aware of the material, but is able to recognize and accept it. In other words, the patient will not find it too threatening.

Whenever there is a strong resistance operating in the transference, it is essential that the interviewer direct his first interpretations to this area. One patient began each session with a discussion of her most recent dates. She felt that the therapist, like her father, was concerned about her sexual activity. A more obvious example is the patient who only wishes to discuss her erotic interest in the physician. The doctor might comment, "It seems that your feelings for me are disturbing you more than your symptoms." Other dramatic examples occur with those patients who are unwilling to speak with the psychiatrist.

The impact of an interpretation upon a patient may be viewed in three main ways: first, the significance of the content of the interpretation upon the patient's conflicts and defenses; second, the effect of the interpretation upon the transference relationship; and third, the effect on the therapeutic alliance, which is the relationship between the doctor and the healthy, observing portion of the patient's ego. Each interpretation simultaneously operates in all three areas, although sometimes more in one than another.

The clinical manifestations of the patient's responses are quite varied. The patient may display emotional responses such as laughter, tears, blushing, or anger, indicating that the interpretation was effective. New material might emerge, such as additional historical data or a dream. The patient sometimes reports that his behavior in the outside world has changed. He may or may not have awareness of the confirmatory significance of such material. In fact, the patient may vigorously deny that the interpretation is correct, only to change his mind later, or he may agree immediately, but only as a gesture to please the doctor. If the patient negates or rejects an interpretation, the interviewer should not pursue the matter. Argument is ineffective and therapeutic impact is not necessarily correlated with the patient's conscious acceptance.

Interpretations are deprivations in so far as they are aimed at removing a patient's defense or blocking a symbolic or substitute route for obtaining gratification of a forbidden wish. Certain patients are able to defend themselves against this aspect of an interpretation by accepting it as another form of gratificaiton, i.e., the doctor is talking to them, wants to help them, and therefore must love them. This is easily recognized when the doctor makes an interpretation and the patient replies, "You're so smart; you really understand my problems." A change may take place in the quality of the therapeutic alliance following a correct interpretation, as an increased feeling of trust in the doctor. One patient was less preoccupied with fantasies about the doctor as the result of a transference interpretation.

The interviewer is expected to set limits on the patient's behavior in the office anytime the patient seems unable to control himself or uses inappropriate judgment. For example, if an enraged patient gets out of his seat and walks menacingly toward the interviewer, this is not the time to interpret, "You seem angry." Instead, the interviewer would raise his own voice and say, "Sit down!" or, "I can't help you if I'm scared of you, so why don't you sit down." Likewise, the patient who refuses to leave at the end of the session, uses the shower in the doctor's bathroom, reads his mail, or listens at his office door should be told that such behavior is not permitted before the doctor attempts to analyze its meaning.

THE PSYCHIATRIC EXAMINATION

The outline for organizing the data of the interview is referred to as the psychiatric examination. It is emphasized in a number of psychiatric textbooks and will, therefore, be discussed here in terms of its influences on the interview. It is usually divided into the history (or anamnesis) and the mental status. Although this organization is modeled after the medical history and physical examination, it is actually much more arbitrary. The medical history includes subjective findings such as pain, shortness of breath, or digestive problems; the physical examination is limited to objective findings such as heart sounds, reflexes, skin discoloration, and so forth. Many of the findings pertaining to the mental status are subjectively revealed and the interviewer may not be able to observe them directly. Hallucinations, phobias, obsessions, feelings of depersonalization, previous delusions, and affective states are examples. Furthermore, the general description of the patient is technically part of the mental status. However, it is more useful if it is placed at the start of the written record.

THE HISTORY

The history is usually much more important than the physical examination or laboratory studies in the diagnosis and treatment of the patient. The written history is better understood if it is organized into present illness, past history, and family history. The past history is further subdivided into infancy, childhood, adolescence, and adulthood. The interviewer must be familiar with characteristic landmarks and milestones of each period and inquire about them if they are omitted by the patient. The vast majority of patients do not offer this material chronologically. Since the beginning interviewer is usually required to prepare a written history, he is tempted to gather the data in a manner that simplifies the preparation of this record, Thus, a written history is too often a conglomeration of data that tells no story about the patient. Instead, the psychiatric history should convey a picture of a person and his individual characteristics, including his strengths and weaknesses. In addition, it should provide insight into his relationships with other human beings, particularly those closest to him. The history is never complete, and the interviewer must direct the patient to the information that is most pertinent for the treatment. The interviewer usually begins with the patient's reasons for seeking help and the immediate precipitating factors that led him to do so at this time. The consultation usually is sought because the patient is suffering, but in some instances the request for help is at someone else's behest, thereby creating special problems that are discussed in Chapters 8, 9, 11, 12, and 14.

The doctor encounters difficulty in attempting to discover emotional conflicts that may have led to the patient's symptomatology. If asked directly, the patient can rarely delineate cause and effect relationships between his conflicts and his symptoms, and finds the subject uncomfortable. Direct inquiry invites attempts at intellectualization and feelings of inadequacy. Therefore, questions about the onset and the ways in which symptoms developed are more effective. Either actual or impending shifts or changes in significant interpersonal relationships, as well as changes of residence or job, will frequently offer relevant clues.

These clues are important, even though the patient is unaware of the significance of what he is saying. For instance, a woman reported that her anxiety attacks "began two years ago, right after we moved to our present neighborhood." Later in the interview she revealed that a man with whom she had previously had an affair lived in the same neighborhood and she feared that they would meet on the street. More often, these factors are not so easily correlated, particularly with more sophisticated patients.

Often the patient's symptom represents his identification with an important figure. Hence, it is useful to ask if he has ever know anyone else with similar symptoms.

When the physician inquires about the developmental history, valuable information is obtained by allowing the patient to describe the events of his past life in the order of his choice. He may begin with a topic about which he feels most comfortable, an area in which he feels the interviewer is interested, or one that is dynamically related to his problem. It is particularly illuminating to note the subjects that the patient avoids as well as those to which he consistently returns. Sometimes the patient defensively offers a story of traumatic events in order to establish an external cause for symptoms.

The interviewer can direct the patient's thoughts to his earlier life by such general statements as, "Tell me about your family." In this way he can see whom the patient mentions first, his father, mother, siblings, or other relatives. Another useful question is, "Can you tell me about your background?" or, "Could you describe your earlier life?" In some instances this is sufficient to get the patient started on the story of his development. Others may reply, "Can't you ask me questions?" "It would be easier if you gave me some leads," or, "I don't know where to begin." Experience will teach the interviewer that if he remains silent for a few moments the patient will continue. At other times the physician might reply, "Begin anywhere." This places some of the responsibility for the interview upon the patient.

As the patient covers the major periods of his life, the interviewer asks for elaboration or for material that has obviously been omitted. For example, if the patient is discussing grammar school, but omits mention of friends, the interviewer might inquire, "And what about your playmates?" The minimal directiveness that characterizes this approach is not adequate for certain patients, and more structured questions are required. The principle involved is that the less organized the patient's current ego functioning is, the more structure must be provided by the interviewer. It is desirable to offer the least amount of structure that will enable the patient to communicate. If the question is, "Tell me about your schooling," the patient can discuss his emotional responses, academic performance, or relationships with peers and teachers. The patient's choice is illuminating, but it would be lost if the question had been, "How did you do in school?" The experienced interviewer obtains further details by gently prodding the patient when necessary with questions such as, "And then what happened?" or, "What did you do after that?"

The interviewer is interested in a description of the home in which the patient was reared and the important people with whom he lived. A comprehensive picture of the family involves areas of conflict as well as areas of cooperative and affectionate interaction. Other topics include the patient's thoughts regarding the personality of his parents and the manner in which they reared him, parents' or relatives' preferences among the children, illnesses or deaths, the patient's age at the time of these events or perceptions, and his reactions to them.

Early memories reveal the patient's most lasting emotional impressions of his childhood, and they are often dynamically related to dominant aspects of character structure. Dreams, particularly repetitive dreams, and fantasies remembered from the past elucidate the inner emotional life of every developmental period. Of significance is the age of the patient and existing circumstances at the time of his first separation from his parents, as well as his reaction of homesickness or other related disturbances.

The development of the patient's attitudes toward authority, methods of parental discipline, and the consistency in their attitudes is important. Also vital is an understanding of any feelings of inferiority and their sources during each period. Another critical area is the patient's expression and control of hostility, anger, and aggression, including their chief targets. The history includes the details of the patient's sexual development in childhood, adolescence, and adult life. Any disturbances, including the absence of normal experience, are of importance.

THE MENTAL STATUS

The mental status is the systematic organization and evaluation of information about the patient's current psychological functioning. The developmental picture of the person revealed by the history is thus supplemented by a description of the patient's current behavior, including aspects of his intrapsychic life. Although the mental status is separated in the written record, such a separation is artificial in the interview and will be resented by the patient. The interviewer is increasingly professional as he develops skill in evaluating the patient's mental status while simultaneously eliciting the history.

At some point in the interview, the neophyte may say, "Now I'm going to ask you some questions that may sound silly." This apology usually precedes mental status questions that the physician consciously or unconsciously realizes are most likely inappropriate. There is no excuse for asking a patient "silly questions." Instead, the interviewer might pursue a more detailed discussion of problems in the patient's daily living that reflect potential difficulties in his mental processes. A senile woman became distressed during an interview by a noise from a steam pipe. She asked, "Do you hear that?" The physician replied, "Yes, do noises bother you?" She nodded, and the doctor inquired further, "Do you sometimes hear things when other people don't?" In this way the inquiry followed a natural course in the interview. Another patient seemed unaware that she was in a hospital and thought that she was in a hotel. Now the interviewer's questions about orientation seemed quite appropriate. An elderly man revealed some memory difficulties. The physician asked if he had any problem counting change when shopping. The patient answered, "Well, most people are honest, you know." At this point a question about change from a dollar after a 53-cent purchase would not seem silly.

One would no more ask an obviously non-psychotic patient if he hears voices than ask an obviously comfortable medical patient if he is in great pain. The interviewer will inhibit the development of rapport by asking a patient who has no suggestion of impaired orientation or cognition to subtract serial 7's or to identify today's date.

Detailed instruction on this subject can only be provided by the demonstration and supervision of interviews. The greatest difficulties are encountered in interviews with borderline patients, during which it may be necessary to ask formal questions designed to test the patient's psychological capacity. For further consideration of specific examples, the reader is referred to the appropriate chapters.

THERAPEUTIC FORMULATION

Although the techniques of case formulation exceed the scope of this book, it has been demonstrated that those physicians who have carefully formulated their understanding of the patient make more successful therapists. Statements about the patient's clinical condition (psychopathology) should be kept separate from speculative hypotheses that attempt to explain the intrapsychic forces at work (psychodynamics) and from constructs that suggest how the patient became the person he is (genetic theories).

As the interviewer attempts a psychodynamic formulation, he will quickly become aware of the areas of the patient's life about which he has obtained the least knowledge from the patient. He can then decide whether these omissions are caused by his lack of experience, or possibly by countertransference, or are manifestations of the patient's defenses. In any case, he will be well rewarded for his efforts.

PRACTICAL ISSUES

TIME FACTORS

DURATION OF THE SESSION. Psychiatric interviews last for varying lengths of time. The average therapeutic interview is about 45 or 50 minutes. Often interviews with psychotic or medically ill patients are briefer, whereas in the emergency room longer interviews may be required. This is discussed in the appropriate chapters.

Frequently new patients will ask about the length of the appointment. Such questions usually represent more than simple curiosity, and the physician might follow his answer with, "What makes you ask?" For example, the patient may be making a comparison between the interviewer and previous psychiatrists.

Another common experience is for patients to wait until near the end of an interview and then ask, "How much time is left?" When the interviewer inquires, "What did you have in mind?" the patient usually explains that there is something he does not wish to talk about if there are only a few minutes remaining. At this point the physician comments that his putting it off to the last few minutes has significance. He might suggest that the patient bring the topic up at the beginning of the next appointment, or, if there is enough time, that they begin now and then continue in the following interview.

THE PATIENT. The patient's management of time reveals an important facet of his personality. Most patients arrive a few minutes early for their appointments. Very anxious patients may arrive as much as a half hour early. This behavior usually causes little problem for the interviewer, and it is often not noted unless the patient mentions it. Likewise, the patient who comes precisely on time or even a few minutes late does not often provide an opportunity to explore the meaning of his behavior in the early weeks of treatment.

A difficult problem is created by the patient who arrives very late. The first time this occurs the interviewer might listen to the patient's explanation, if one is volunteered, but avoid making comments such as, "Oh, it's quite all right," or, "That's o.k.," or, "No problem." Instead, he calls the patient's attention to the realities of his own schedule with a remark such as, "Well, we'll cover as much as we can in the time remaining." On occasion, the patient's reason for being late is a blatant resistance. For instance, he might explain, "I forgot all about the appointment until it was time to leave." In this situation the interviewer can ask, "Did you feel some reluctance about coming?" If the answer is "Yes," the physician might continue his exploration of the patient's feeling. If the answer is "No," he should allow the matter to rest for the time being. It is important that the interview be terminated promptly in order to impart the message that lateness is against the patient's own best interests.

An even more difficult situation exists when the patient

arrives quite late for several interviews, each time showing no awareness that his actions might be caused by factors within himself. After the second or third time, the doctor might remark, "Your explanations for being late emphasize factors outside yourself. Do you think that the lateness may have something to do with your feelings about coming here?" Another method is to explore the patient's reaction to the lateness. The physician could ask, "How did you feel when you realized you would be late today?" or, "Did it bother you that you were late?" Such questions may uncover the meaning of the lateness. The main concern is that the doctor does not become angry with the patient.

THE PHYSICIAN. The physician's handling of time is also an important factor in the interview. Chronic carelessness regarding time indicates a countertransference problem. However, on occasion the physician is unavoidably detained. If it is the first interview, it is appropriate for the doctor to express his regret that the patient was kept waiting. After the first few interviews, other factors must be considered before the physician offers any apology for his lateness. For certain patients, any apologetic comment from the doctor only creates more difficulty in expressing their annoyance. Usually they seem to accept the physician's lateness most graciously. With such patients, the doctor could call attention to his lateness by glancing at his watch and remarking on the number of minutes. The patient may say, "Oh, that's all right," or some similar comment. The doctor could reply, "You don't appear to be annoyed at my lateness." Depending on the effectiveness of his repression and reaction formation, the patient will either acknowledge some mild irritation or say that he did not mind waiting. The interviewer can then look for indications that the patient had some unconscious response which should be explored.

When the doctor is late he should extend the length of the interview to make up the time. He will show respect for the patient's other time commitments if he inquires, "Will you be able to remain 10 minutes longer today?"

THE TRANSITION BETWEEN INTERVIEWS. It is a good idea for the interviewer to have a few minutes to himself between interviews. This provides an opportunity to "shift gears" and to be ready to start fresh with the next interview rather than continue to think about the patient who has just left. A telephone call or glancing at the mail or at a magazine will facilitate this transition.

SPACE CONSIDERATIONS

PRIVACY. Most patients will not speak freely if they feel that their conversation might be overheard. Quiet surroundings also offer fewer distractions that might interfere with the interview, and psychiatrists try to avoid interruptions, except perhaps to receive a brief telephone call (see Chapter 15). These conditions are more often available for the private practitioner than for the psychiatric resident. Nevertheless, privacy and some degree of physical comfort are minimal requirements.

SEATING ARRANGEMENTS. Many psychiatrists feel more "secure" if they conduct interviews while seated at a desk, but even then it is preferable not to place the chairs so that there is furniture between the doctor and patient. Both chairs should be of approximately equal height, so that neither party is looking down on the other. If the room contains several chairs, the doctor can indicate which chair is for himself and then allow the patient to select the location in which he will feel most comfortable. The main factors that influence the patient's choice involve the physical distance and location in relation to the doctor's chair. Overtly dependent patients, for example, prefer to sit as close to the doctor as possible. Oppositional or competitive patients will sit farther away and often directly across from the doctor.

FEES

Money is the common unit of value for goods and services in our culture, and the fee that the patient pays symbolizes the value of treatment. The payment of a fee can reflect the patient's desire to be helped. The fee signifies that the relationship is mutually advantageous, but it is not true that a patient must undergo some financial hardship or sacrifice in order to benefit from psychotherapy. Although the examples are extreme, consider the millionaire and the welfare patient, neither of whom directly feels the financial burden of treatment.

The average physician has little opportunity to determine and collect fees before he has completed his training. It is easy for the beginning resident to remain aloof from the fee-setting arrangements of the hospital registrar. Under this system, patients are able to have their fees changed without the need for discussion with the doctor, with the unfortunate result that the entire subject is ignored in the therapy.

Residents become involved in financial arrangements with clinic patients that they would never permit with a private patient. The doctor may ignore the fact that the patient pays little or nothing. The doctor may feel that because he is so inexperienced, his services are not worth money, or that he owes the patient something because he is learning at the patient's expense, or even that he is underpaid by the hospital and can retaliate by allowing the patient to cheat the "establishment." In one case, a patient had concealed financial assets from the registrar only to confess to the resident, who then passively became a collaborator in "stealing from the hospital." It was some months before he realized that, in the patient's unconscious, he was the "establishment." Supervisors, too, often pay no attention to the handling of fees, thereby losing valuable opportunities to explore transference and countertransference.

The fee assumes various meanings in the therapeutic relationship. The patient may use the fee as a bribe, offering to pay a larger fee than the doctor would customarily charge. One woman came for a consultation regarding a possible therapeutic abortion. She stated, "I hope you realize that I would be willing to pay you any fee you ask." Another patient utilized the fee as a means of control. He had already determined the doctor's fee per session; he multiplied it by the number of visits and presented the doctor with a check before receiving his bill. He was symbolically in control; the doctor was not charging him, he was giving the doctor money.

Masochism or submissiveness may be expressed by payment of inordinately high fees without protest. The patient may express anger or defiance to the therapist by not paying, or by paying late. He may test the therapist's honesty by offering to collaborate in a deal, such as paying cash, with the inference that the doctor will not report it on his income tax. These maneuvers are discussed in greater detail in Chapter 9.

With private patients, the subject of fees usually does not arise until the end of the interview. The doctor can wait until the patient raises the issue, which may not happen for two or three visits. If the interviewer suspects that the patient cannot afford a private fee, he can mention the subject at the time when the patient is on the topic of his finances. If the patient describes difficult financial problems, but plans to continue therapy, the doctor might ask, "How do you expect to manage the cost of private treatment?" If the patient has no realistic plan, the interviewer could explore the meaning of this behavior.

Occasionally, a patient will ask about the doctor's fee at the beginning of the interview, or on the telephone. Rather than answer directly, the physician might inquire if the patient is worried about the cost of treatment. If such is the case, the doctor could suggest that the subject of cost be deferred until the end of the consultation, since the major factors of frequency of visits and possible duration of treatment must also be taken into account and those questions must wait until the doctor has learned about the problems. Affluent patients may never ask about the fee, but if the patient should be concerned about the cost of therapy and does not inquire after several sessions, the doctor might say, "We have not discussed the fee." In this way the physician may learn something about the patient's attitude toward money.

CHANCE MEETING OF THE PATIENT OUTSIDE THE INTERVIEW

Occasionally the physician may meet his new patient outside of the consulting room either before or after the interview, in a lobby, hospital dining room, elevator, or subway. This situation may be uncomfortable for the young psychiatrist, who is not sure whether to speak or what to say. The simplest procedure is to take one's cue from the patient. The doctor is not obligated to make small talk, and he is well advised to wait until he is inside the office before entering any discussion of the patient's problems. In the majority of situations, the patient will feel uncomfortable in the presence of his doctor outside the office. If the patient makes small talk, the interviewer can reply in a brief but friendly manner, without extending the conversation. When the patient does ask a question which the physician feels should not be answered, he can suggest that they wait to discuss that until they have more time or are in more private surroundings. When the therapist meets the patient outside the office and the patient becomes intrusive, the physician can use small talk to control the situation and keep the conversation on neutral ground. Occasionally the doctor's admission of his own uneasiness after meeting a patient outside the office can be useful for the therapy.

PRE-INTERVIEW CONSIDERATIONS

THE PATIENT'S EXPECTATIONS

The patient's prior knowledge and expectations of the doctor play a role in the unfolding of the transference. During the physician's early years of training, these factors are less often significant, since the patient did not select the doctor personally. On the other hand, the "institutional transference" is of considerable importance, and the doctor can explore the reasons for the patient's selection of a particular hospital or clinic. In addition, the patient usually has a mental image of a psychiatrist. This pre-interview transference may be disclosed if the patient seems surprised by the doctor's appearance, or remarks, "You don't look like a psychiatrist." The doctor could ask, "What did you expect a psychiatrist to be like?" If the patient replies, "Well, someone much older," The doctor might answer, "Would it be easier to speak to an older person?" The patient may indicate that he is actually relieved and that he had imagined the psychiatrist to be a more frightening figure. At times a patient enters the physician's office and jokes, "Well, where are the guys with the white coats?", thereby revealing his fear of being considered crazy. He sees the doctor as a dangerous and authoritarian person.

In private practice, patients are usually referred to a specific doctor. The interviewer is interested to learn what the patient was told about the doctor at the time of the referral. Was he given one name or a list of names? In the latter case, how did he decide which doctor to call first, and was the interviewer the first one he contacted? One patient may indicate that he was influenced by the location of the doctor's office, to another the doctor's name may have suggested an ethnic background similar to his own.

THE DOCTOR'S EXPECTATIONS

The interviewer usually has some knowledge of the patient prior to their first meeting. This may have been provided by the person who referred the patient. Some clues about the patient have often been obtained directly by the physician during the initial telephone call that led to the appointment (see Chapter 15).

Experienced psychiatrists have personal preferences concerning the amount of information they want from the referring source. Some prefer to learn as much as possible; others desire only the bare minimum, on the grounds that it allows them to interview with a fully open mind.

Any time the interviewer experiences a feeling of surprise when he meets his new patient, he must question himself. Was he misled about the patient by the person who referred him, or was his surprise due to some unrealistic anticipation of his own?

THE OPENING PHASE

Meeting the Patient

The doctor obtains much information when he first meets a new patient. He can observe who, if anyone, has accompanied the patient, and how the patient was passing the time while waiting for the interview to begin.

One interviewer begins by introducing himself; another prefers to address the patient by his name and then introduce himself. The latter technique will indicate that the doctor is expecting the patient, and most people like to be greeted by name. As a rule, social pleasantries, such as "It is nice to meet you," are not warranted in the professional situation. However, if the patient is unduly anxious, the doctor might introduce a brief social comment, perhaps inquiring if he had any trouble finding the office. It is inappropriate to use the patient's first name except in the case of children or young teenagers. Such familiarity would put the patient in the "one down" position, since the patient is not expected to use the doctor's first name.

Important clues to the conduct of the interview can often be obtained during these few moments of introduction. The patient's spontaneity and warmth may be revealed in his handshake or greeting. Dependent patients question where to sit and what to do with their coats. Hostile, competitive patients may sit in the chair that quite obviously is reserved for the interviewer. Suspicious patients might carefully glance around the

office searching for "clues" about the physician. The specific behavior of different patients is elaborated in the chapters in Section One.

THE DEVELOPMENT OF RAPPORT

The experienced interviewer learns enough about the patient during the initial greeting that he may appropriately vary
the opening minutes of the interview according to the needs of
the patient. The beginner usually develops a routine way of
starting the interview and then attempts variations later in his
training.

A suitable beginning is to ask the patient to be seated and
then inquire, "What problem brings you here?" or, "Could you
tell me about your difficulty?" A less directive approach would
be to ask the patient, "Where shall we start?" or, "Where would
you prefer to begin?" Sometimes a very anxious patient will
speak first, inquiring, "Where shall I begin?" As indicated, the
beginner will do better to reply, "Let's start with a discussion
of your problem." After some years of experience, the physician
knows when the patient will continue easily without a reply
and when to say, "Begin anywhere you like."

Sullivan discussed the value of a summary statement about
the referring person's communications concerning the patient,
or a restatement of what the physician learned during the initial
telephone conversation. It is comforting for the patient who is
not self-referred to feel that the physician already knows something about his problem. A presentation of all the details is
likely to be harmful, as they will rarely seem completely accurate
to the patient, and the interview gets underway with the patient
defending himself from misunderstanding. General statements
are preferable. For example, the physician might say, "Dr. Jones
has told me that you and your husband have had some difficulties," or, "I understand that you have been depressed." Most
patients will continue the story at this point. Occasionally, the
patient may ask, "Didn't he tell you the whole story?" The interviewer could reply, "He went into some of the details, but I
would like to hear more about it directly from you." If the patient has difficulty continuing, the physician might remark sympathetically, "I know it is difficult to talk about some things."
This gives the patient a feeling that the doctor understands him,

but, depending on how he chooses to interpret the remark, he might take it as permission to begin by discussing some less painful material.

In the event that the patient brings something with him to the interview, it will help the development of rapport to examine what the patient has brought. For example, one patient was referred for treatment by a psychologist who had tested him for career aptitude. The psychiatrist refused to read the psychologist's report and the patient was offended. Another doctor never asked about some art work that a young woman had brought to show him. She failed to return for a second visit.

At some point during the initial interview, the physician will want to write down the patient's name, address, telephone number, and referral source. This can be done either at the beginning or end of the interview or at the first transition period, when the physician leaves the topic of the present illness to learn more about his patient as a total human being and what sort of place the patient has made for himself in the world.

To establish rapport, the interviewer must communicate a feeling of understanding the patient. This is accomplished both by the doctor's attitude and by the expertise of his remarks. He does not wish to create the impression that he can read the patient's mind, but he does want the patient to realize that he has treated other people with emotional difficulties and that he understands them. This includes not only neurotic and psychotic symptoms, but ordinary problems in living. For example, if a harried housewife reveals that she has six children under the age of 10 and no household help, the interviewer might remark, "How do you manage?" The young physician who has had little experience in life and has no imagination might ask, "Do you ever find your children a strain?" The successful interviewer will broaden his knowledge of life and human existence through the empathic experience associated with gaining an intimate understanding of the lives of so many others.

The doctor's interest helps the patient to talk. However, the more the doctor speaks, the more the patient is concerned with what the doctor wants to hear, instead of what is on his own mind. On the other hand, if the doctor is unresponsive, the patient will be inhibited from revealing his feelings.

Some patients are reluctant to speak freely because they fear that the doctor might betray their confidence. The patient might say, "I don't want you to tell this to my wife," or, "I hope you won't mention my homosexuality to my internist." The interviewer might reply, "Everything you tell me is in confidence." When this behavior occurs in later sessions, the patient's mistrust and fear of betrayal can be explored.

Sometimes a patient will ask, "Are you Freudian?" Usually this means, "Do I have to talk about sex?" In any event, the patient is not really interested in the doctor's theoretical orientation, and such questions require exploration of their meaning to the patient instead of a literal reply.

THE MIDDLE PHASE

An abrupt transition is sometimes required after the patient has discussed the present illness. For example, the physician can say, "Now I would like to learn more about you as a person," or, "Can you tell me something about yourself other than the problems that brought you here?" The interviewer now devotes his attention to the history. Just where to start depends upon what aspects of the patient's life have been revealed while discussing his present illness. Most patients talk about their current life before revealing their past. If the patient has not already mentioned his age, marital status, length of marriage, ages and names of spouse, children, and parents, occupational history, description of current living circumstances, and so on, the interviewer can ask for these details. It is preferable to obtain as much of this information during the description of the present illness as possible. Rather than following the outline used for the organization of the written record, it is much easier for the physician to draw conclusions about the significance and interrelationship of this data if the patient offers them in his own way. For instance, if the interviewer asks, "How do your symptoms interfere with your life?", the patient may provide information pertaining to any or all of the topics mentioned above.

It is a mistake to permit the first interview to end without knowing the patient's marital status, occupation, and so forth. These basic identifying data are the skeleton of the patient's life, upon which all the other information is placed. When this material does not emerge spontaneously during the discussion of the present illness, it is often possible to obtain much of it with one or two questions. The interviewer could inquire, "Tell me about your present life." The patient may then interpret the question as he sees fit, or he may ask, "Do you mean, am I married and what sort of work do I do, and things like that?" The interviewer merely has to nod and then see if the patient omits anything, and then point out that the patient has not mentioned thus and such. Most patients will provide more useful information if they are given a topic to discuss rather than a list of questions that can be answered briefly. Specific exceptions are discussed in the section on the disorganized patient and Chapter 10.

The number of possibilities in the middle portion of the interview are infinite, and consequently it is impossible to provide precise instructions about which choices to make. For example, the patient might indicate that she is married, has three children, that her father is dead, and that her mother lives with her. Experience, skill, and personal style all influence what the interviewer will do now. He could be quiet and permit the patient to continue, or he could ask about the marriage, the children, the mother, or the father's death, or ask the patient, "Could you elaborate?" without indicating a specific choice. The feeling tone of the patient's description is another important aspect that could be focused upon. If she seems anxious and pressured, the interviewer might remark, "It sounds as if you have your hands full."

In the above example, some psychiatrists would argue in favor of one approach over another. However, the authors feel that there is no single right answer and that they would probably make different choices with different patients and even with the same patient on different occasions.

Most leads provided by the patient should be followed up at the time of presentation. This gives smooth continuity to the interview even though there may be numerous topical digressions. To continue with the last vignette, let us suppose that the patient goes on to reveal that her mother has only been living with her family for a year. It would be logical to assume that the patient's father had died at that time, and therefore the interviewer might ask, "Is that when your father died?" If the patient replies, "Yes," the doctor might assume that the patient's parents had lived together until that time, but rather than jump to false conclusions, it is better to ask, "How did it happen that your mother came to live with you after your father's death?"

The patient might surprise the doctor by saying, "You see, Mother and Dad were divorced 10 years ago, and she moved in with my brother's family, but now that Dad is gone, my brother moved to Chicago to take over his business. Mother's friends are all in this area and she didn't want to move to Chicago, so she moved in with us." The interviewer might ask, "What was the effect on your family?" or, "How did your husband feel about this arrangement?" At the same time, the interviewer notices that the patient did not provide any information about the circumstances of the father's death. When the patient "runs down" on the present topic, the physician could reopen that area.

Now that the interviewer has some ideas concerning the present illness and the patient's current life situation, he might turn his attention to what sort of person the patient is. A question such as "What sort of person are you?" will come as a surprise to most people, as they are not accustomed to thinking of themselves in that fashion. Some patients will respond easily and others may become uncomfortable or offer concrete details that reiterate facts of their current life situation, such as, "Well, I'm an accountant," or "I'm just a housewife." Nevertheless, such replies provide both phenomenological and dynamic information. The first reply was made by an obsessive-compulsive man who was preoccupied with numbers and facts, not merely in his job, but in his human relationships as well. What he was telling the interviewer was, "I am first and always an accountant, and, in fact, I can never cease being an accountant." The second reply was offered by a phobic woman who had secret ambitions for a career. She was letting the physician know that she had a deprecatory view of women and, in particular, of women who are housewives. Like the first patient, she was never able to forget herself.

Often the patient's self-perception will vary, depending upon the situation in which he finds himself. Consider the businessman who is a forceful leader in his job, but is timid and passive at home, or the laboratory scientist who is active and creative in his work but feels shy and reserved in social situations. Then there is the man who is a sexual athlete with numerous affairs who perceives himself as inadequate and ineffectual at work. The interviewer does not elicit all of the material pertinent to the patient's self-perception in one portion of the interview. However, it is an important question to keep in mind at all times, so that gradually a more complete picture emerges.

Other questions that pertain to the patient's view of himself are, "Tell me the things you like about yourself," or, "What would you consider your greatest assets?" or, "What things bring you the most pleasure?" The interviewer might ask the patient to describe himself as he appears to others, and to himself, in the major areas of his life, including family, work, social situations, sex, and situations of stress. It is often revealing to ask the patient to describe a typical 24-hour day. The patient may even experience some increase in his self-awareness while reflecting on this question. Topics and questions that have a direct bearing on the present illness and current life situation are most meaningful to the patient.

Depending on the amount of time available and whether there will be more than one interview, the physician will plan his inquiry into the patient's past. The question of which past issues are most significant varies with the problems of the patient and the nature of the consultation.

At various times during the interview, the patient may become uncomfortable with the material he is discussing. This is not only due to his wish to be accepted by the interviewer but also, and often more importantly, because of his fear concerning partial insights into himself. For example, he may pause and remark, "I know lots of people who do the same thing," or "Isn't that normal, doctor?" or, "Do you think I'm a bad father?" Certain patients may require reassurance in order to become engaged in the interview, whereas others will profit by the doctor's asking, "What did you have in mind?" or, "Just what are you concerned about?"

Stimulating the patient's curiosity is a fundamental technique in all interviews aimed at uncovering deeper feelings. Basically, the doctor uses his own genuine curiosity to awaken the patient's interest in himself. The question of where the physician can best direct his curiosity is related to the principles of interpretation discussed earlier in the chapter. In summary, the curiosity is not directed at the most deeply repressed or most highly defended issues, but rather at the most superficial layer of the patient's conflict. For instance, a young man describes how he first experienced his anxiety attack after he saw a man collapse in a railroad station. Later he reveals that he often experiences attacks in situations in which he feels that he is winning an argument with someone he considers an inferior. The interviewer would not express curiosity about an unconscious wish to destroy his father, whom he considered passive and helpless, but would direct his curiosity to situations which seem to be exceptions to the patient. Thus, he might ask, "You mentioned that on some occasions winning an argument doesn't seem to bother you; I wonder what could be different about those situations?"

The doctor's expressed curiosity about motives of both the patient and his loved ones is seldom therapeutic in the first few interviews, as it is too threatening to the patient's defenses. For example, the physician might say, "I wonder why your husband spends more time at his office than is necessary?" Although the interviewer has the right to be curious about this phenomenon, a direct question could be construed by the patient as an accusation or innuendo.

THE CLOSING PHASE

The closing phase of the initial interview varies in length, but 10 minutes is generally sufficient. The interviewer might indicate that time is drawing to a close by saying, "We have to stop soon; are there some questions that you would like to ask?" If the patient has no questions, the interviewer could comment, "Perhaps you could suggest something for us to talk about during the remaining time," or, "Is there something we should discuss further?" Most often the patient will raise questions pertaining to his illness and treatment.

Each person who consults an expert expects and is entitled to an expert opinion about his situation as well as recommendations for therapy or some other helpful advice. It has long been a medical tradition to tell the patient as little as possible about his diagnosis and the therapeutic rationale of the treatment plan. In recent years, the publication of medical information through the lay press, as well as changes in the training of doctors, has led to a better informed and more questioning public. Psychiatry particularly has been the recipient of such attention, and many patients have questions about psychotherapy, hypnosis, psychoanalysis, behavioral therapy, shock therapy, and various drug therapies. Although the patient has a right to receive direct answers about such issues at the completion of the consultation, the interviewer can assume that these questions will reveal important transference attitudes as well.

Although it is artificial to distinguish between diagnostic and therapeutic interviews, it is nevertheless valuable to present the patient with a clinical formulation and a treatment or other plan when the consultation is completed. Usually this presentation occurs at the end of the second or third interview, but in some cases it may require months of exploratory meetings. Beginning therapists often neglect this phase, and, much to their surprise, a patient they have been seeing for six months will suddenly ask, "Why am I still coming?" or say, "I don't think I need to see you anymore!" Such neglect is disrespectful of the patient's right to question the doctor's treatment plan and of his right to seek a different therapist. The patient is entitled to state his own goals for treatment. He may only desire symptomatic improvement, and this may be good judgment; there are patients whose basic character structure is best left alone. An example is the patient with a very limited life expectancy.

This phase of the interview provides a useful opportunity for the physician to uncover resistance and to alter his treatment plan accordingly. Although the doctor is the expert, his recommendations cannot be handed down like royal decrees. Often the physician must modify his treatment plan as he learns more about the patient. By presenting a treatment plan in a stepwise fashion, the interviewer can discover in what areas the patient has questions, confusion, or disagreement. This cannot happen if the doctor makes a speech.

If the consultation is limited to one interview, more of that interview must be devoted to such matters than if a second or third meeting can be arranged. The physician should avoid giving the patient a formal diagnostic label. Such terms have little use for the patient, and may be quite harmful, since the interviewer may be unaware of the meaning that the patient or his family attaches to them. The patient often provides clues to the proper terms to use in giving the formulation. One patient acknowledges a "psychological problem"; another says, "I realize it's something emotional," or, "I know I haven't completely grown up," or, "I realize it isn't right for me to have these fears." Although the patient's statement may have been made earlier in the session, the doctor can utilize it as a springboard for his own formulation, provided the patient truly believes what he is saying. This is not the case with the psychosomatic patient who says, "I know it is all in my mind, doctor." (See Chapter 11.)

The doctor might begin, "As you have already said, you do have a psychological problem." He might refer to what he considers the chief symptoms and indicate that they are all related and part of the same condition. He might separate acute problems from those that are chronic and concentrate first on treatment for the acute ones. Since it is not a good idea to overwhelm the patient with a comprehensive statement of all his pathology, the formulation should be confined to the major disturbance. For example, in the case of a young man who has difficulty getting along with authority figures, including his father, the interviewer would state, "It appears that you do have a problem getting along with your father, which has influenced your attitude toward all figures of authority."

Now that the physician and patient are each clear on what they believe constitutes the problem, it is time to consider the subject of treatment. The doctor may be confident of his opinion without making a dogmatic pronouncement. For example, he might state, "In my experience, the most effective approach is . . . . ," or, "A variety of therapies are used for this condition, but I would suggest . . . ." This pays proper respect to the fact that, whatever the doctor's therapeutic orientation, the patient probably knows that there are other treatments available. Often the patient will bring up a question he has kept back pertaining to the effectiveness of one of the other therapies.

It is rarely useful in analytically oriented psychotherapy to give the patient prepared speeches about the method of treatment, how psychiatry works, or free association. However, less sophisticated patients do require some preparation. This may involve an explanation that the doctor is interested in all of their thoughts and feelings, whether or not they seem important. It takes a long time and a great deal of trust before a patient can associate freely. Some patients may ask, "Shall I just talk?" or, "Shall I just say anything that comes to mind?" The interviewer can answer such questions affirmatively.

Frequently the patient will inquire, "How long will treatment take?" or, "It isn't serious, is it?" It is difficult to predict the duration of treatment except in general terms. Once again, the best indication is found in the patient's own productions. It is usually helpful, when acute symptoms can be differentiated from chronic ones, to point out that more recent symptoms are usually the first to improve and that problems of long duration often require long treatment. Sometimes the patient will ask about a more specific period of time. It is unfair to make misleading statements concerning the duration of therapy in order to reassure the patient. Few patients respond favorably to learning in the first interview that they require years of treatment. The patient's concern with the duration of treatment is not entirely a manifestation of resistance or the desire for a magical cure. Therapy is costly in terms of both expense and time involved that interferes with other activities in the patient's life. If there is a time limit on the duration of therapy, as is often the case in clinics, or if the doctor is not going to be available as long as the patient expects treatment to last, the patient should be told at once. Also, the patient deserves to know from the outset if the consultant will not be the treating physician. This is the time in the interview to consider the financial aspects of treatment, which have been discussed earlier in the chapter.

If the patient was upset during the interview, the closing phase also serves as an opportunity for him to pull himself together again prior to leaving the doctor's office and returning to the outside world.

Some patients ask about prognosis, either seriously or in a pseudo-jest. Common examples are, "Well, Doctor, is there any hope?" or, "Have you ever treated any cases like mine?" or, "Is there anything I can do to speed things up?" The doctor is advised to be careful in dealing with these questions. Prognosis is difficult to determine with accuracy in the first few visits. The patient may not have revealed all of his problem. In cases in which statements about prognosis are indicated, such as with the depressed patient, the doctor's encouraging reassurance is of great importance.

Before the interview is terminated, the physician can set the time and date of the next appointment. The end of the session is indicated by the doctor's saying, "Let's stop now," or, "We can go on from here next time," or, "Our time is up for now." Although it is not a universal practice, the authors feel that it is common courtesy to arise and escort the patient to the door.

Occasionally, an interview must be terminated prematurely because the doctor receives an emergency call. This is a more common experience for resident psychiatrists. The doctor can explain the situation to the patient and arrange to make up the time on another occasion. A related but more infrequent occurrence is that the patient gets angry and leaves before the session is over. The doctor can attempt to stop the patient verbally by saying firmly, "Just a minute!" If the patient waits, he can continue, "If you are angry with me, it is better that we discuss it now." The doctor neither rises from his chair nor indicates that he condones the patient's action.

LATER INTERVIEWS

Often the consultation is completed in two interviews, but it may take longer. The second interview is best scheduled from two days to a week later. A single meeting with the patient permits only a cross-sectional study. If several days are allowed to intervene before the next session, the doctor will be able to learn about the patient's reactions to the first visit. In this way he can determine how the patient will handle treatment. There is also an opportunity for the patient to correct any misinformation that he provided in the first meeting. One way to begin the second interview is for the doctor to comment, "I suspect that you have thought about some of the things we discussed last time," or, "Frequently, people think of things they wanted to discuss after the first meeting; what thoughts did you have?" When the patient answers, "Yes" to the former, the doctor might say, "I would like to hear about that," or, "Let's start there, today." If the patient says, "No," the doctor might raise his eyebrows questioningly and wait for the patient to continue.

There are several common patterns of response. The patient might have pursued the self-inquiry that began in the previous meeting, often providing additional pertinent history related to a previously raised point. He might have reflected further on a question or on suggestions of the doctor and come to some greater understanding. Such activity is subtly rewarded by interviewers who in one way or another let the patient know that they are on the right track. This response has more important prognostic significance for analytically oriented psychotherapy than whether the patient felt better or worse after the session.

Another group of responses have more negative implications.

The patient might have thought about what he reported the first time and decided that it was wrong, or that he didn't understand why the doctor had asked about a certain topic, or felt that the doctor didn't understand him. He might state that he had ruminated about something the doctor had said and felt depressed.

Frequently these responses occur when the patient feels guilty after talking "too freely" in the first interview. He then either withdraws or becomes angry with the doctor. In this patient's mind, criticizing his loved ones or expressing strong emotions in the psychiatrist's presence is personally humiliating.

While on the topic of the patient's reactions to the first interview, the doctor might inquire whether the patient discussed the session with anyone else. If he did, the interviewer will be enlightened by learning with whom the patient spoke and the content of the conversation. After this topic has been explored, the physician will continue the interview. There are no set rules concerning the questions that are better put off until the second meeting. But, in general, whatever inquiries the doctor senses to be most embarassing for this patient are postponed unless the patient has already approached this material himself or is consciously preoccupied with it. If the doctor asks about dreams in the first interview, the patient will frequently have dreams prior to the second meeting. It is useful to inquire directly about such dreams, as they reveal the patient's unconscious reactions to the physician as well as showing key emotional problems and dominant transference attitudes.

SUMMARY

This chapter has considered the broader aspects and general techniques of the psychiatric interview. Subsequent chapters will discuss specific variations that are determined either by the type of patient or by the clinical setting of the interview. It must be emphasized that real people do not fit into the discrete diagnostic categories outlined in this book. Every person is unique, integrating a variety of pathological mechanisms in a characteristic way. In discussing different clinical syndromes, the authors are not merely considering patients who fall into the associated diagnostic categories. For example, obsessive defenses will be encountered in phobic, hysterical, depressive, hypochondriacal, paranoid, organic, schizophrenic, and sociopathic patients and may be integrated into neurotic or psychotic patterns. The techniques of working with a patient who has a given cluster of defenses will be similar regardless of his diagnosis. The reader is left with the task of resynthesizing the material that has been separated for pedagogic purposes. In any given interview the patient will utilize defensive patterns that are described in several different chapters, and he may shift his defenses during the course of treatment or even within a single interview.

The interviewer can function effectively without having a conceptualized understanding of resistance, transference, counter-transference, and so forth. Furthermore, intellectual mastery of these concepts does not itself produce clinical proficiency. However, an organized framework is necessary for the systematic study and conceptualization of the factors that contribute to the success or failure of an interview. A theoretical understanding of psychodynamics is vital if the student plans to study his own intuitive functioning and thereby improve his clinical skill. It will allow each interview to contribute to the progressional growth of the psychiatrist.

References

Adler, M. H.: Psychoanalysis and psychotherapy. Int. J. Psycho-Anal., *51*:219, 1970.

Colby, K. M.: A Primer for Psychotherapists. New York, Roland Press Co., 1951.

Freedman, A., and Kaplan, H.: Comprehensive Textbook of Psychiatry. Baltimore, Williams & Wilkins Co., 1967.

Gill, M., Newman, R., and Redlich, F.: The Initial Interview in Psychiatric Practice. New York, International Universities Press, 1954.

Greenson, R. R.: The Technique and Practice of Psychoanalysis. New York, International Universities Press, 1967.

Greenson, R. R., and Wexler, M.: The non-transference relationship in the psychoanalytic situation. Int. J. Psycho-Anal., *51*:143, 1970.

Group for the Advancement of Psychiatry. Report #49: Reports in Psychotherapy: Initial Interviews. June, 1961.

Saul, L. J.: The psychoanalytic diagnostic interview. Psychoanal. Quart., *26*:76, 1957.

Saul, L. J.: The Technique and Practice of Psychoanalysis. Philadelphia, J. B. Lippincott Co., 1958

Stevenson, I.: The psychiatric interview. In Arieti, S. (ed.): American Handbook of Psychiatry, Vol. 1. New York, Basic Books, Inc., 1959, Chap. 9, pp. 197–214.

Stevenson, I.: Medical History Taking. New York, Hoeber, 1960.

Stevenson, I., and Sheppe, W., Jr.: The psychiatric examination. In Arieti, S. (ed.): American Handbook of Psychiatry, Vol. 1. New York, Basic Books, Inc., 1959, Chap. 10, pp. 215–234.

Sullivan, H. S.: The Psychiatric Interview. New York, Norton Press, 1954.

Tarachow, S.: An Introduction to Psychotherapy. New York, International Universities Press, 1963.

Whitehorn, J. C.: Guide to interviewing and clinical personality study. Arch. Neurol. Psychiat., *52*:197, 1944.

2 GENERAL PRINCIPLES OF PSYCHODYNAMICS

INTRODUCTION

Psychiatry is the medical specialty that studies disorders of human behavior and experience. Like other branches of medicine, it considers (1) the phenomenology of the normal and abnormal; (2) systems of classification and epidemiological information; (3) etiology; (4) diagnosis; and (5) prevention and treatment. Since human behavior is complex, psychiatry employs many fields of knowledge, ranging from biochemistry, genetics, embryology, and physiology to psychology, anthropology, sociology, and general systems theory, in order to understand its subject matter.

The interview is the basic technique of psychiatry and most other clinical specialties. Other methods may also be employed, such as biological or psychological diagnostic tests or pharmacological and physical treatments, but even these usually occur within the setting of a clinical interview. In fact, the psychiatric interview is by far the most important diagnostic and therapeutic tool of today's psychiatrist. With our current knowledge, physiological and biochemical studies of behavior offer little assistance in understanding interviews, whereas psychodynamic concepts have proved most valuable.

In the psychodynamic frame of reference, behavior is viewed as the product of hypothetical mental forces, motives or impulses, and the psychological processes that regulate, inhibit, and channel them. Thoughts and feelings are of central importance, and overt behavior is understood in terms of inner psychological processes that are inferred from the patient's words and acts.

A psychodynamic formulation offers a means of describing abnormal mental states, understanding their origins, and developing a rational basis for their treatment. Although it may be possible to develop a theory of behavior, including the causes and cures of mental illnesses, that ignores psychodynamics, no one has yet been able to do so. Furthermore, as long as the interview is the central tool of psychiatry, psychodynamics will remain the essential basic science. At present, it also provides the most comprehensive understanding of pathology, pathogenesis, and treatment.

This chapter presents the basic assumptions of psychodynamics and psychoanalysis, the school of psychodynamics started by Freud that has been the source of most of our knowledge and has almost become synonymous with psychodynamics. It will then discuss the basic psychodynamic model of psychopathology, various types of pathological formations, and those psychoanalytic concepts that are most crucial in understanding the interview. Space does not permit a complete consideration of psychoanalysis, which includes a theory of personality development, a technique of treatment, a specific method for obtaining information about the psychodynamic determinants of behavior, and a metapsychology, or series of abstract hypotheses about the nature of mental functioning and the source of human motives. These aspects of psychoanalysis go beyond the scope of a book on interviewing and are discussed in the books on psychoanalytic theory listed in the References.

BASIC ASSUMPTIONS OF PSYCHODYNAMICS AND PSYCHOANALYSIS

MOTIVATION

Behavior is seen as purposeful or goal-directed, and as being a product of hypothetical forces—drives, urges, impulses, or motives. Motives are represented subjectively by thoughts and feelings and objectively by a tendency toward certain patterns of action. Hunger, sex, and aggression are examples of important motives.

The early years of psychoanalysis were extensively concerned with the origin of basic human motives and, specifically, with developing a model that would relate them to their biological roots. Freud used the German term "trieb," which has usually been translated as "instinct," to refer to these basic drives, which were assumed to involve a form of "psychic energy." This drive theory was helpful in focusing on the complex shifts or "vicissitudes" in motivations that are found in the course of development and it was essential in understanding the psychodynamic basis of neurotic behavior. For example, the idea of a sexual drive with many and varied manifestations makes it easy to conceptualize the link between hysterical seizures and sexual inhibitions. However, in recent years, some aspects of psychoanalytic drive theory have been strongly criticized as tautological and unscientific. At the same time, attention has shifted from the origins of basic human motives to the various means by which they are expressed. To many, the biological basis of motivations is a physiological problem that cannot be explored by psychoanalysis, a psychological science. In any event, it is an issue that has little direct bearing on the interview. By the time a child is able to talk, he has strong drives that will be present for the rest of his life, and that form the foundation of our understanding of his behavior in psychodynamic terms. The extent to which they are constitutional or acquired is of great theoretical, but little clinical, importance.

DYNAMIC UNCONSCIOUS

Many of the important determinants of behavior occur outside the individual's subjective awareness, and are not normally recognized by him. The existence of unconscious mental activity was apparent long before Freud—events that are forgotten but later remembered are obviously stored in some form during the interim. However, this would be of little clinical importance were it not for the dynamic significance of these unconscious mental processes. That is, they exert great influence on behavior, and are particularly important determinants of abnormal behavior.

The early history of psychoanalysis is a record of the discovery of the role of unconscious mental processes in determining almost every area of human behavior—neurotic symptoms, dreams, jokes, parapraxes, artistic creations, myths, religion, character structure, and so forth.

REGULATORY PRINCIPLES

Behavior is regulated in accordance with certain basic principles. These organize the expression of specific motives and select among them when they come into conflict with each other or with external reality. For example, someone may be impelled to act in an angry or violent fashion, but his awareness of the painful consequences of doing so leads to a modification of his behavior. This illustrates the pleasure-pain principle (or simply, "pleasure principle"), which states that behavior is designed to pursue pleasure and to avoid pain. Although this seems obvious, much of the behavior that psychiatry studies appears to violate this principle. Pathological or maladaptive behavior frequently seems designed to seek pain, and often even a casual observer will tell the patient that he is acting foolishly and that he would be much happier if he simply changed his ways. Every paranoid person has been told that his suspiciousness is self-defeating, every obsessive that his rituals are a waste of time, and every phobic that there is no reason to be frightened. Perhaps one of the major contributions of dynamic psychiatry has been the demonstration that these apparent paradoxes are really confirmations of the pleasure principle once the underlying emotional logic is revealed, and that even the individual with an apparently inexplicable desire to be beaten or tortured is following this basic principle.

With maturity, the capacity for abstract symbolic thought provides the basis for mental representations of the distant future. The elementary pain-pleasure principle rooted in the immediate present is modified, as the rational determination of behavior includes the willingness to tolerate current discomfort in order to achieve future pleasure. This is called the reality principle. However, at an unconscious level, much behavior continues to be regulated by the more primitive pleasure principle.

FIXATION AND REGRESSION

Childhood experiences are critical in determining later adult behavior. Neurotic psychopathology can often be seen as the re-emergence of fragments or patterns of behavior that were prevalent, and often appropriate, during childhood, but that are mal-adaptive in the adult. Regression refers to this return to an earlier adaptive mode, while fixation describes the failure to mature beyond a developmental stage that is usually associated with an earlier age. Both of these are selective processes, and affect only certain aspects of mental functioning. The result is that the neurotic individual has a mixture of age-appropriate and regressive behavior patterns. For example, his cognitive functioning might be unimpaired but his sexual fantasy life immature. The most normal adult has some behavior that is characteristic of earlier developmental stages, and even the sickest patient retains some aspects of mature functioning.

Fixation and regression can affect motives, ego functions, and conscience mechanisms, or any combination of these. Often the most important indication of pathology, especially in children, is not the extent of the regression, but the unevenness with which it has affected some psychological processes while sparing others. Regression is universal during illness, stress, sleep, intense pleasure, love, strong religious feeling, artistic creativity, and many other unusual states, and is not pathological in these situations. In fact, the capacity to regress and to make adaptive use of regressive experiences is an essential prerequisite for creative thinking, for empathetic understanding, and even for conducting a psychiatric interview. To be able to feel what the patient feels while at the same time observing and studying that feeling is the essence of the psychiatrist's skills, and is an excellent example of regression in the service of the most mature aspects of the personality.

EMOTION

Emotions are states of the organism that involve both the mind and the body. They include characteristic physiological responses, subjective affects, thoughts and fantasies, modes of interpersonal relations, and styles of overt action. Anxiety, a key emotion in the development of psychopathology, serves as an example. The anxious individual is aware of inner feelings of diffuse, unpleasant, anticipatory fear or dread. His cognitive functioning is impaired, and he is likely to be preoccupied with fantasies of magical protection or escape. His overt behavior is dominated by his own characteristic response to threat—fight, flight, or helpless surrender. There are alterations in pulse, blood pressure, respiratory rate, gastrointestinal functioning, bladder control, endocrine function, muscle tone, the electrical activity of the brain, and other physiological functions. No one of these phenomena is itself an emotion, but the syndrome as a whole constitutes the organismic state which we call anxiety.

Emotions occupy an intermediate position between the more elementary regulatory principles of pleasure and pain and the more refined and abstract rational thought. They play a critical role in the development of the personality as a whole, and especially of symptoms, which will be explored in greater detail below.

PSYCHODYNAMICS OF PSYCHOPATHOLOGICAL CONDITIONS

NORMALITY AND PATHOLOGY—
THE NATURE OF NEUROTIC BEHAVIOR

There are no generally accepted definitions of the terms "normal" and "pathological" or "health" and "disease," and yet the daily practice of medicine requires frequent decisions based on these concepts. Psychopathology refers to behavior that is less than optimally adaptive for a given individual at a given stage of his life and in a given setting. The psychodynamic study of psychopathology investigates the mental processes that lead to maladaptive behavior. There is, of course, psychopathology that cannot be understood in psychodynamic terms alone—the automatic behavior of a psychomotor seizure and the hallucinations that result from taking a psychedelic drug are examples. Conversely, normal as well as pathological behavior has psychodynamic origins. The description of a given piece of behavior as resulting from the resolution of an inner conflict, or as the product of mental mechanisms of defense, does not yet distinguish whether it is normal or pathological. The critical question is whether the individual in resolving his conflict has significantly impaired his capacity to adapt to his environment while maintaining his capacity for pleasure. Everyone has inner psychological conflicts and everyone responds to the anxiety that they evoke by the use of mental mechanisms. In a general sense, a discussion of the psychodynamics of a piece of behavior is independent of whether it is normal or pathological. This is somewhat more complex in practice; some psychodynamic constellations are almost always associated with pathological behavior, and, in general, any defense that threatens the individual's contact with reality, the maintenance of his interpersonal relationships, or the possibility of pleasurable affects is likely to be pathological. However, there is no single defense mechanism that is not found in normal individuals.

In clinical practice, the physician is not primarily concerned with assessing whether the patient's interview behavior is healthy or sick. He is more interested in what it means and what it tells him about the patient. This is particularly true of interviews with patients who do not have major emotional problems. Knowledge of psychodynamics is vital for the skillful conduct and thorough understanding of interviews with these psychiatrically normal individuals. However, it is important for every clinical interviewer to study psychopathology as well as psychodynamics, not only in order to understand interviews with patients who are not psychiatrically normal but also because psychodynamic principles are learned most easily from individuals with emotional difficulties.

THE STRUCTURE OF NEUROTIC PATHOLOGY

Basic motives, such as sex, aggression, or dependency, impel the individual toward behavior that should lead to their gratification. However, due to internal psychological conflict, the expression of this behavior may be partially or completely blocked, with a resulting increase of intra-psychic tension. The opposing forces in this conflict result from an anticipation of unpleasant or dangerous consequences of acting on the motive involved. In the simplest situation, this is manifested by an emotional state, fear, related to the perception of an immediate real danger. For example, a man may feel angry and want to attack a policeman who treats him unfairly; however, his fear of retaliation will lead him to control and suppress his rage. In this example, the outcome is highly adaptive, and it makes little difference whether the perception of danger and the resulting inhibition of the impulse occurred consciously or unconsciously.

The situation becomes more complex when the dangerous consequences that are feared are neither real nor immediate, but rather fantasies, imaginary fears that result from formative experiences in childhood, i.e., when the shadow of the past falls on the present. Such fears are almost always unconscious, and since they result from dynamically significant unconscious memories rather than conscious current perception, they are not easily corrected even by repeated exposure to a contradictory reality. It is difficult to unlearn attitudes that are rooted in unconscious mental processes. The fear of an unconsciously imagined danger, called anxiety, leads to an inhibition of the relevant motive. In this case, the inhibition is not a response to the real world in which the individual is currently living, and therefore is more likely to be maladaptive or pathological. However, there are some exceptions. Inhibitions of basic motives that stem from unconscious fantasies of imagined dangers may be highly adaptive if the original unconscious fantasies themselves developed in a situation that is closely analogous to the individual's current reality.

An example will illustrate this. A man who has warm and loving feelings toward his wife has unconscious fears of being castrated should he participate in adult sexual activity. A potency disturbance and inhibition of sexual impulses result, an obviously maladaptive solution in his current life, however appropriate it might have been in the childhood setting in which it originally developed. Another man who is momentarily sexually attracted to a woman at a cocktail party loses interest when he learns that she is his boss's wife. This may also be the result of an inhibition of sexual impulses based on the unconscious fear of castration, but the result is now highly adaptive, since the setting closely parallels that of early childhood, when the expression of such impulses was clearly limited.

The anxiety that results from a conflict between a wish and an unconscious fear is one of the most common symptoms of psychological distress. It is the dominant feature of the classic anxiety reaction and is also found in many of the symptomatic neuroses. However, some people with symptomatic neurotic psychopathology, and many individuals with personality or character disorders, experience little or no anxiety. Their problems are manifested by phobias, obsessions, compulsions, conversion phenomena, or various character traits, and anxiety may be a less important part of the clinical picture, or may even be absent altogether.

The psychoanalyst understands these more complex conditions as the result of defense mechanisms. These automatic unconscious patterns of behavior are elicited by psychological conflicts that threaten the individual's emotional equilibrium. The resulting threat or anticipation of anxiety, called "signal anxiety," never becomes conscious because of the mental mechanisms that defend the individual from it. In other words, the individual responds to the unconscious threat of anxiety resulting from a psychological conflict by utilizing mechanisms that lead to a symptom or behavior pattern in order to ward off that anxiety.

A clinical example will illustrate the theory. A young woman who had had a somewhat restrictive and Puritanical upbringing developed a phobia, a fear of going outdoors alone. She recalled a brief period of anxiety at the time that her phobia began. However, she experienced no anxiety at present as long as she remained indoors. When asked why she was afraid of going outdoors, she described episodes of palpitations and dizziness, and her concern about what would happen if these occurred while she was on the street. Later she told of women in her neighborhood who had been accosted by strange men, and of her fear of being attacked. She had repressed sexual impulses toward attractive men whom she saw on the street, and she feared that her family would strongly disapprove and punish her for these, although both the wish and the fear were unconscious. Here we see a number of defenses: repression of sexual wishes, the displacement of a fear of sex to a fear of the outdoors, avoidance of the outdoors, and the projection of sexual impulses onto strange men. These mechanisms were effective in controlling her anxiety, but at the price of sexual inhibitions, frigidity, and the restriction of her freedom to travel. This inhibition of healthy behavior is a constant feature of symptom formation.

Symptoms not only defend against forbidden wishes, they also serve, symbolically and partially, to gratify them. This is necessary if symptoms are to be effective in protecting the individual from discomfort, since the ungratified wish would continue to press for satisfaction until the psychological equilibrium was disturbed and the fear and anxiety returned. An example of the gratification provided by symptoms is seen in the case of the woman described above, who was only able to venture outdoors in the company of her older brother, who had always been a romantic partner in her unconscious fantasies. Symptoms may also provide symbolic punishment, which is related to the original unconscious fear. As a small child, the same young lady had been punished for naughtiness by being locked in her room, and her phobic symptom recreated that long-repressed experience.

SYMPTOM AND CHARACTER

All neurotic psychopathology represents a compromise between a repressed unacceptable wish and an unconscious fear. Whereas all behavior represents a compromise between the demands of inner drives and external reality, neurotic behavior is a second-best solution, reflecting the individual's effort to accommodate not only to the real world but also to the restrictions imposed by his unconscious fear. The two basic ways in which these neurotic patterns can be integrated into the general personality structure are described by the terms "symptom" and "character."

Neurotic symptoms are relatively sharply delineated behavior patterns that are experienced by the individual involved as undesirable "ego-alien" phenomena, not truly part of his self or personality. He consciously desires to be free from them, and they not infrequently lead him to seek help. Anxiety, depression, phobias, obsessions, compulsions, and conversion phenomena are typical examples. In time the patient may adjust to his symptoms and learn to live with them, but they always remain a foreign body that is fundamentally experienced as "not me."

Character traits are more generalized behavior patterns that merge imperceptibly into the individual's total personality. They are ego-syntonic in that he sees them as part of himself, and either fails to recognize them as pathological or, realizing that they are undesirable, simply feels that they reflect what he is "really" like. These traits rarely lead the individual to seek assistance, although their indirect secondary social consequences are frequent precipitants of psychiatric consultations. Mistrust, stinginess, irresponsibility, impulsiveness, aggressiveness, and timidity are illustrations of character traits.

Although the underlying psychodynamic structures of symptoms and character traits are closely related, they present quite different technical problems in psychiatric interviews and in treatment. In general, when treating patients who seek relief from symptoms, the doctor considers the underlying character structure along with such factors as motivation and life setting in planning the therapy, since it is only by viewing the symptoms in terms of the individual's overall functioning that a rational program for treatment can be developed. For instance, two men may experience depressive symptoms of the same severity. One is young, articulate, and intelligent, has an obsessive personality structure, and has considerable motivation for treatment, great flexibility, and few irreversible life commitments. Intensive exploratory, analytically oriented psychotherapy is recommended for this person. The other is older and has married a woman whose personality problems complement his. She responded quite negatively to an earlier attempt at treatment on his part. He is now suspicious and mistrustful of psychiatry and tends to think concretely, with little sensitivity to psychological issues. For this person a briefer, more supportive treatment is preferable, perhaps using drugs, with the aim of removing symptoms.

Conversely, with individuals who present predominantly characterological pathology, the interviewer must uncover symptoms that the patient has not acknowledged, since it is only by doing so that he can develop the patient's motivation for change. In a sense, the interviewer tries to intensify the awareness of symptoms in individuals with character disorders, attempting to make the patient dissatisfied with his pathological traits and to expose hidden concerns and doubts about himself. This has led to the often misunderstood maxim that treatment is not really working until the patient becomes symptomatic. It would be more accurate to say that the patient with a character disorder becomes either anxious or depressed as he begins to gain some insight into his pathology. For example, an extremely obsessive man prided himself on his punctuality and his general perfectionism. One day he arrived at his session exactly on the hour, proudly explaining to the therapist that he had timed it perfectly, just glancing at his watch in time to make the train. Later he revealed that he had been lunching with his daughter, an unusual event, and that she had been somewhat surprised and hurt when he had left so abruptly. The therapist agreed that he had made the appointment on time, but suggested that he had traded an experience of intimacy and warmth for a "perfect record." The patient became quite gloomy—a necessary step before his treasured virtue could be seen as a psychological problem.

In the interview, symptoms are most clearly reflected in what the patient talks about; character traits are revealed in the way he talks and the way he relates to significant other people, particularly to the interviewer. From another point of view, the patient describes his symptoms, whereas his character traits are observed by the doctor. The beginning interviewer tends to focus on symptoms, since they are easiest to recognize and to understand. The more experienced interviewer may also talk about the patient's symptoms, but more of his attention is directed to the patient's character structure as it emerges during this discussion. One of the major contributions of psychoanalysis is the recognition of the importance of dealing with the patient's characterological pathology if treatment is to be effective.

NEUROTIC AND PSYCHOTIC

There is no single criterion that differentiates psychotic from neurotic patients. In general, psychotics are sicker; that is, they have more pervasive and widespread difficulties in adaptation. More specifically, areas of functioning that are considered to be essential for a minimal level of adaptation and that are usually intact in neurotics may be impaired in psychotics. These would include the perception and testing of reality, the capacity for sustained interpersonal relations, and the maintenance of autonomous ego functions such as memory, communication, and motor control. The distinction between psychotic and non-psychotic organic brain syndromes is based on related criteria, and is discussed in Chapter 10.

Studies of the psychological processes involved in neuroses and psychoses have repeatedly raised the question of whether these are fundamentally and qualitatively different disorders or merely quantitative variations of the same basic mechanisms. Those who hold the former view usually suggest that one or another basic defect is primary in the psychotic process, and that the other phenomena of the illness can then be explained as the result of defensive and reparative responses similar to those seen in neuroses. The central defect has variously been described as a diminished capacity for affectivity, a disturbance in the perception or testing of reality, abnormal cognitive processes, poor interpersonal relations, or a primary deficit in the synthetic function of the ego, which integrates other mental functions into an harmonious whole.

Specific mechanisms of defense are not psychotic rather than neurotic, or, for that matter, pathological rather than healthy.

However, some mental mechanisms, including projection and denial, are commonly associated with psychotic processes. These interfere with autonomous ego functions and the perception of reality, and are therefore closely related to psychosis.

Hallucinations and illusions are gross disorders in the perception of reality, delusions represent severe disturbances in reality testing, and all three of these symptoms are usually associated with psychosis. However, subtler disturbances in the subjective sense of the "real" world, such as derealization or depersonalization, are common in neuroses as well as psychoses. Furthermore, all neurotic symptoms, insofar as they are maladaptive, are in some sense "unrealistic." However, the defective contact with reality found in neurosis is more sharply circumscribed and most areas of the patient's life are unaffected.

The disturbance in interpersonal relations is, in a sense, more fundamental than the other differentiating characteristics, and probably stems from an earlier stage of the patient's development, as the beginnings of the child's capacity for perception and testing of reality, thought, language, and affectivity all grow out of his early relationship with his mother. The neurotic patient tends to force his current relationships into the mold created by his childhood experiences, and the result can be a serious disturbance in his friendships and his love life. However, he does have the capacity to develop and maintain relationships with others, and if his neurotic problems are resolved, these are major sources of gratification. The psychotic individual, particularly the schizophrenic, has a more basic defect in his capacity for relating to others. This is seen clinically in his tendency to isolation and withdrawal, with few lasting friendships and a shallowness and superficiality in those that do develop. He may be less troublesome to get along with than the neurotic, but his friends and acquaintances will often find him a less stable and less important part of their lives.

The doctor may experience this defect in the nature of the patient's relationships during the interview. The psychotic patient "feels" different; it is harder to make contact with him and to empathize with his emotional responses. For example, if the doctor is unable to remember the patient several hours after the first visit, it may reveal in retrospect that little real contact was established. The patient's shifting sense of personal identity may leave the doctor feeling that there is not a specific other person there with him. Experienced psychiatrists are more likely to detect psychosis by this kind of feeling than by the pathological criteria that are used to justify the diagnosis. Every relationship that the psychotic establishes need not be shallow or superficial. There are striking exceptions, and often there is one person with whom he has an intense symbiotic relationship that is far more all-encompassing than any that the neurotic develops. This may become the psychotherapist, and therefore has special relevance to the interview.

When sufficient information about the patient's life is available, most neurotic psychopathology can be understood in great detail within the psychodynamic frame of reference. Even with this information, however, much psychotic psychopathology is difficult to understand. This has led to the view that psychoses have a major organic determinant, although neuroses do not. In any case, the psychodynamic explanation of any type of pathology is more helpful in understanding its meaning than in clarifying its etiology. Indeed, it should be recalled that Freud felt that there was an organic basis to neuroses as well as to psychoses.

Psychotic patients can, and usually do, have neurotic problems in the form of both symptoms and character traits in addition to their more serious pathology. The interviewer must take into account both the psychotic and the neurotic pathology of the psychotic patient. This may be quite difficult, since the psychotic disturbance can interfere with the ability of the patient to participate in the interview itself. The patient's tendency to be mistrustful of others makes it difficult for him to feel comfortable with the interviewer, and his diminished capacity for interpersonal relations together with his disturbed thought processes leads to major problems in communication. Psychosis is not a constant phenomenon, and many psychotic patients move in and out of psychotic states over a span of days or weeks, or even within a single interview. Often the dilemma in treatment is to work on the patient's conflicts and problems while providing enough emotional support that the stress of the therapy does not push him toward psychosis.

Two clinical examples may help to illustrate these issues. A young man arrived at a hospital emergency room in a state of extreme anxiety. He felt that he had had a heart attack and was dying, and complained of chest pains and a choking sensation. Although cooperative, he was sweating and trembling with fear.

He denied any psychological or emotional difficulties. There had been several similar episodes in the past, each ending quickly and without incident. The remainder of the brief initial history was unremarkable, and as the doctor spoke with the patient, his symptoms subsided and he began to feel better. A normal electro-cardiogram offered further reassurance, and after the intern told him that he seemed to be in good physical health, the patient began to relax and to speak more comfortably. He spoke of his family and early life experiences, and revealed that he had led a sheltered and protected childhood. He was still closely tied to his family, and particularly to his mother, who strongly disap-proved of the girl he had been seeing recently. It was while on his way to see her that the attack occurred.

A second young man also arrived at the hospital in a panicky state. He complained of strange feelings in his back and "electric shocks" in his legs, which he thought might be related to physical exhaustion. He had not slept for several days, staying up in order to protect his apartment and possessions from attack. He was vague about who might want to hurt him, but felt certain that he had been followed on the street in recent days. As he discussed these thoughts, he lowered his voice and leaned forward to tell the interviewer that several men had made homosexual advances toward him earlier that day. The doctor, inexperienced in psychiatry, asked if the patient had ever had homosexual ex-periences. The patient became wildly excited, screaming that the doctor was trying to frame him, and tried to run from the examining room. Later, after he had received some tranquilizing medication, he readily agreed to hospitalization in order to pro-tect himself from his enemies. The first patient had a classic neurotic anxiety attack with hyperventilation and the second an early psychotic paranoid schizophrenic break, although they both had virtually the same initial complaints.

PSYCHOANALYTIC MODEL
OF MENTAL FUNCTIONING

As psychoanalytic theory was applied to the study of psy-chopathology, personality development, dreams, art, culture, and other areas of human activity, a series of models were developed in order to conceptualize the role of psychodynamic factors in behavior. The first of these, the so-called "topographic" model, described mental activity as conscious or unconscious. Although this scheme was easy to apply, it soon became apparent that it was not helpful in discussing the central psychodynamic issue in psychopathology, that of intra-psychic conflict. In clinical practice, most conflicts were entirely unconscious, with the patient unaware of both the basic drive or motive and the fantasied danger.

As a result, the "structural" theory was developed by Freud, and it has largely supplanted his earlier topographic one. In it the mind is viewed as consisting of more or less autonomous structures that are most sharply defined at times of conflict. Each structure consists of a complex array of psychological functions that act in concert during conflict. Therefore most, if not all, conflict is seen as occurring between two structures. Three basic structures are generally recognized: the id, which consists of the basic drives, impulses, and needs, the ego, which includes the psychological functions that control and regulate these drives, the defenses, and all other psychological coping devices, and the superego, a specialized aspect of the ego that develops in the early relationship with the parents and embodies the ethical, moral, and cultural standards acquired during socialization. The ego ideal, usually considered a component of the superego, refers to the goals and aspirations that the individual develops through identification with parents and that are elaborated and modified through his later contact with peers and the larger culture.

EGO

The term "ego" describes those psychological functions that help the individual to adapt to the environment, respond to stimuli, and alter basic biological functions, while insuring survival and the satisfaction of needs. Historically, the concept originated from studies of psychological conflict, in which the ego represented those forces that opposed, controlled, and regulated basic biological drives. Later it was extended to include functions that were not involved with conflict, and that could even operate in concert with basic drives to serve the organism's adaptive needs. The ego is the executive organ of the mind, mediating between the internal demands of the biologically determined motives (the id), the socially determined goals and values (the superego), and the external demands of reality. It is the final common pathway that integrates all of these determinants and then controls the organism's response. The ego develops through interaction of the maturing infantile psyche with external reality, particularly that portion of external reality that consists of significant other humans. There is on the one hand an unfolding biological potential for memory, learning, perception, cognition, communication, and other vital adaptive functions, and on the other a highly specialized environment composed of need-gratifying and stimulus-controlling devices encompassed within a human object, the attentive and responsive mother.

The ego includes both conscious and automatic unconscious psychological processes. The conscious portion is roughly equivalent to the common concepts of "self" or "personality," which before Freud were considered to be the subject matter of psychology. The ego also includes the unconscious defense mechanisms and the forces of repression that Freud discovered in his early work. Although they operate outside the patient's awareness, they are directed against the expression of basic needs and drives and are, therefore, considered part of the ego.

Id

The term "id" describes the biologically based drives and motives that are at the source of much behavior. Sex, aggression, and the craving for security are examples of such motives. Other needs develop as the result of exposure to society and are determined by the demands of that society. Status, prestige, and power are examples of the goals related to such needs. Classic psychoanalytic theory would consider them part of the id, since they can ultimately be related to biologically determined factors. As these biological or socially determined motives press for satisfaction, they become one of the major factors impinging on the ego and, therefore, determining the individual's behavior. Freud's early explorations of the unconscious determinants of neurotic symptoms uncovered the phenomena encompassed by the term id.

In more recent years, psychoanalytic investigation has been directed toward the psychology of conscious mental processes and patterns of behavioral integration, as well as toward the influence of unconscious drives. In other words, there has been a shift from an exclusively id psychology to a more balanced view that includes ego psychology. This shift became possible after the unconscious determinants of behavior were better understood, and it was paralleled by a growing interest in psychiatric problems that involve ego pathology, such as character disorders and psychoses.

Freud described the primitive mental activity of the id and the unconscious ego by the phrase "primary process," in contrast to the "secondary process" thinking of the conscious adult ego. Primary process thinking is childlike, prelogical, and self-centered. It is controlled by the pleasure principle, tolerates contradictions and inconsistencies, and employs such mental mechanisms as symbolization, condensation, and displacement. Secondary process thinking, in contrast, is logical, rational, reality-centered, goal-directed, and relatively free of emotional control. Most thought processes combine elements of both.

SUPER-EGO

This term refers to psychological functions that involve standards of right and wrong together with the evaluation and judgment of the self in terms of these standards. In general usage, it also includes the ego ideal, the psychological representation of what a person wishes to be like, his ideal self. The super-ego was originally considered to be a portion of the ego, but it has been found to operate independently of, and often at odds with, other ego functions, particularly in conflict situations and pathological conditions. It develops out of the young child's relationship with his parents, who initially provide him with external judgments, criticism, and praise for his behavior. As he grows away from his parents, he nevertheless maintains a perpetual relationship with them by internalizing a psychological representation of them. This process, termed introjection, creates a dynamically significant psychic agency that carries on those functions that formerly belonged to the parents.

The super-ego is also influenced by parental surrogates, such as teachers, by peers, and by society at large. This is even more true of the ego ideal, which at the age of latency is often concretely symbolized by popular cultural heroes.

REALITY

At first it might seem superfluous to include a section on reality in a discussion of psychological functioning, but a distinction must be made between psychological reality and the more familiar concept of physical reality. The real world influences psychological functions only as it is registered and perceived by the individual. This can be illustrated by considering the most important aspect of external reality, the social reality of important other people. An individual reacts not to his real mother or father, but to internal object representations, which inevitably involve some distortion. There has been repeated misunderstanding of this critical distinction, even by Freud himself. During their childhoods, neurotic patients frequently experienced adults as highly seductive or callously indifferent. It took Freud some time to recognize that this was not necessarily an accurate portrayal of real experiences. However, it is even more inaccurate to discard this psychic reality, for without it the child's fears and adult's neuroses are meaningless. The conclusion is that reality must be considered as another psychic structure that is responsive to the external environment, but that involves a creative personal interpretation for any given individual. When we tell someone, "Don't be silly" (i.e., "You're crazy"), it usually means that we do not perceive their psychological reality, but only our own. Their behavior probably makes sense in the context of their own psychic reality.

SUMMARY

In summary, then, we see that any piece of behavior results from the interaction of innate and socially determined motives, the goals and standards acquired during early socialization, the perception of external reality, and the individual's own unique personality, talents, defensive style, and integrative capacity. It is the product of id, ego, super-ego, and psychic reality.

This psychodynamic framework provides a means of thinking about clinical data in general, and about psychiatric interviews in particular. The physician can consider the patient's predominant wishes or motives, his unconscious fears, and his characteristic defenses. How are these integrated; what symptoms or character traits are present? How do these interfere wih his adaptation, and what secondary adjustments have been necessary? Each individual is unique, but there are certain typical patterns of drive, fear, and defense; symptom and character style, that have led to the description of the well-known clinical syndromes in psychiatry. The discussion of more specific problems in the psychiatric interview will begin with one of the most sharply defined and easily recognizable syndromes—the obsessive character.

REFERENCES

Arieti, S. (ed.): American Handbook of Psychiatry (3 vols.). New York, Basic Books, Inc., 1959.

Arlow, J., and Brenner, C.: Psychoanalytic Concepts and the Structural Theory. New York, International Universities Press, 1964.

Brenner, C.: An Elementary Textbook of Psychoanalysis. New York, International Universities Press, 1955.

Cameron, N.: Personality Development and Psychopathology. Boston, Houghton-Mifflin, 1963.

Engel, G.: Psychological Development in Health and Disease. Philadelphia, W. B. Saunders, 1962.

Erikson, E.: Childhood and Society. New York, W. W. Norton, 1950.

Fenichel, O.: The Psychoanalytic Theory of Neurosis. New York, W. W. Norton, 1945.

Frazier, S. H., and Carr, A. C.: Introduction to Psychopathology. New York, Macmillan, 1964.

Freud, A.: The Ego and the Mechanisms of Defense. New York, International Universities Press, 1946.

Freud, S.: Introductory lectures on psychoanalysis. Standard Edition of Complete Psychological Works of Sigmund Freud, Vols. XV and XVI. London, Hogarth Press, 1963.

Freud, S.: The ego and the id. Standard Edition of Complete Psychological Works of Sigmund Freud, Vol. XIX. London, Hogarth Press, 1961, pp. 3–66.

Freud, S.: Neurosis and psychosis. Standard Edition of Complete Psychological Works of Sigmund Freud, Vol. XIX. London, Hogarth Press, 1961, pp. 149–153.

Freud, S.: The loss of reality in neurosis and psychosis. Standard Edition of Complete Psychological Works of Sigmund Freud, Vol. XIX. London, Hogarth Press, 1961, pp. 183–187.

Freud, S.: Inhibitions, symptoms and anxiety. Standard Edition of Complete Psychological Works of Sigmund Freud, Vol. XX. London, Hogarth Press, 1959, pp. 77–174.

Freud, S.: The question of lay analysis. Standard Edition of Complete Psychological Works of Sigmund Freud, Vol. XX. London, Hogarth Press, 1959, pp. 197–258.

Freud, S.: An outline of psychoanalysis. Standard Edition of Complete Psychological Works of Sigmund Freud, Vol. XXIII. London, Hogarth Press, 1964, pp. 141–207.

Kardiner, A., Karush, A., and Ovesey, L.: Methodological study of Freudian theory. I. Basic concepts. J. Nerv. Mental Dis., 129:11, 1959.

Kardiner, A., Karush, A., and Ovesey, L.: A methodological study of Freudian theory. II. The libido theory. J. Nerv. Mental Dis., 129:133, 1959.

Kardiner, A., Karush, A., and Ovesey, L.: A methodological study of Freudian theory. III. Narcissism, bisexuality and the dual instinct theory. J. Nerv. Mental Dis., 129:207, 1959.

Kardiner, A., Karush, A., and Ovesey, L.: A methodological study of Freudian theory. IV. The structural hypothesis, the problem of anxiety, and post-Freudian ego psychology. J. Nerv. Mental Dis., *129*:341, 1959.

Kolb, L. C.: Noyes' Modern Clinical Psychiatry, 7th ed. Philadelphia, W. B. Saunders Co., 1968.

Lidz, T.: The Person. New York, Basic Books, Inc., 1968.

Mayer-Gross, W., et al.: Clinical Psychiatry, 3rd ed. Baltimore, Williams & Wilkins Co., 1969.

Rado, S.: Adaptational Psychodynamics. New York, Science House, 1969.

Redlich, F., and Freedman, D.: Theory and Practice of Psychiatry. New York, Basic Books, Inc., 1966.

Sandler, J., Holder, A., and Dare, C.: Basic psychoanalytic concepts. I. The extension of clinical concepts outside the psychoanalytic situation. Brit. J. Psychiat., *116*:551, 1970.

Sandler, J., Holder, A., and Dare, C.: Basic psychoanalytic concepts. II. The treatment alliance. Brit. J. Psychiat., *116*:555, 1970.

Sandler, J., Holder, A., and Dare, C.: basic psychoanalytic concepts. III. Transference. Brit. J. Psychiat. *116*:667, 1970.

Sandler, J., Holder, A., and Dare, C.: Basic psychoanalytic concepts. IV. Countertransference. Brit. J. Psychiat., *117*:83, 1970.

Sandler, J., Holder, A., and Dare, C.: Basic psychoanalytic concepts. V. Resistance. Brit. J. Psychiat., *117*:215, 1970.

Sandler, J., Holder, A., and Dare, C.: Basic psychoanalytic concepts. VI. Acting out. Brit. J. Psychiat., *117*:329, 1970.

Sandler, J., Holder, A., and Dare, C.: Basic psychoanalytic concepts. VII. The negative therapeutic reaction. Brit. J. Psychiat., *117*:431, 1970.

Sandler, J., Holder, A., and Dare, C.: Basic psychoanalytic concepts. VIII. Special forms of transference. Brit. J. Psychiat., *117*:561, 1970.

Sandler, J., Holder, A., and Dare, C.: Basic psychoanalytic concepts. IX. Working through. Brit. J. Psychiat., *117*:617, 1970.

Sandler, J., Holder, A., and Dare, C.: Basic psychoanalytic concepts. X. Interpretations and other interventions. Brit. J. Psychiat., *118*:53, 1971.

Section one:

MAJOR CLINICAL SYNDROMES

This section deals with the major clinical syndromes. Each type of patient is described as he will appear during the interview. A brief psychodynamic explanation of the conflicts and psychopathology is offered. Within this framework, specific instructions are presented on alterations and modifications of the interview for each syndrome.

3 THE OBSESSIVE PATIENT

Psychopathology and Psychodynamics

THE CENTRAL CONFLICT

The obsessive individual is involved in a conflict between obedience and defiance. It is as though he constantly asks himself. "Shall I be good, or may I be naughty?" This leads to a continuing alternation between the emotions of fear and rage—fear that he will be caught at his naughtiness and punished for it, rage at relinquishing his desires and submitting to authority. The fear, stemming from defiance, leads to obedience, while the rage, derived from obedience, leads back again to defiance.

This conflict has its orgins in childhood experience, and therefore is couched in childish terms. Obedience and defiance are equated with humiliating subjugation and murder. Issues lose their proportion, and the problem of whether one finishes a sentence or permits an interruption is a problem of whether one annihilates the other or is annihilated by him. Vital issues require extreme defenses, and the rigidity and totality of obsessive defenses are extreme. The obsessive is the easiest patient to recognize and the most stereotyped of the major clinical syndromes.

Most of the character traits that classically define the obsessive personality can be traced to this central conflict. Thus his punctuality, conscientiousness, tidiness, orderliness, and reliability are derived from his fear of authority. These can be highly adaptive traits of great social value. It is important to realize that, for the obsessive individual, such behavior is not motivated by mature, healthy, constructive forces, but stems from unrealistic fear. This understanding will bring much behavior that appears at first to be uninvolved in psychopathology, into dynamic significance. If the patient is early for the appointment, it is not simply an accident or a sign of enthusiasm, but a symbolic placation to avoid punishment for transgressions of which he is quite aware, even if the doctor is not. If the interviewer is hesitant or asks the patient his preference in arranging the time of the next appointment, the patient does not respond to the doctor's consideration or interest, but as if he had obtained a special privilege.

Another set of obsessive traits is derived from the rage portion of the conflict. Untidiness, negligence, obstinacy, parsimony, and sadism can be traced to defiant anger. It is apparent by now that this list of traits includes many opposites—conscientiousness and negligence, orderliness and untidiness, and so on. These contradictory traits are not only essential features of the obsessive individual, but they even appear in the same person at the same time! He may meticulously clean his overshoes before entering the office, but later drop ashes on the rug. Contradictory motives can be seen within a single act. The patient, in his eagerness to pay the bill as soon as he receives it, will delay the therapist for several minutes while he carefully fills out his check. The apparent contradictions vanish when one remembers that the origin of these traits is embedded in the conflict of defiance and obedience, rage and fear. The essence of the obsessive is not either side of this conflict, but the conflict itself.

Issues Involved in the Conflict

Three key issues are inevitably involved and frequently appear in the interview situation. They are dirt, time, and money. Although the earliest power struggles between parent and child center about feeding and sleeping, the battle soon includes toilet training. Parental concern with the child's bowel habits extends into other areas that involve dirt and cleanliness. These include the struggles that develop over the child's washing behind his ears, cleaning his room, and even drying dishes and raking leaves. Dirt and time provide the most common issues for the formal structure of the child's struggle with parental authority. The child develops magical concepts that associate dirt with aggression and defiance. The defiance then leads to guilty fear and expectation of punishment through illness or even death. These concepts are based on parental and cultural edicts concerning the dangers of dirt, germs, and the defiance of authority. The obsessive patient will be fearful to reveal his secret dirty habits, whether picking his nose or wearing yesterday's socks. He will be particularly concerned about the dirt he brings into the interview—the mud on his shoes or the ashes on his cigarette. Both sides of the conflict may be seen as he expresses regret over soiling the therapist's attractive ashtray and then permits the ashes to fall on the carpet. Exposure of this behavior leads to intense shame and humiliation. It can only be discussed after many sessions, and even then the therapist must utilize tact.

Time is another key area in the child's battle with his parents. Dawdling and procrastination are prominent in the battles at bedtime, mealtime, playtime, and homework time. It is also related to current power struggles, as it deals so directly with control and mastery. The amount of time that is spent in the interview has a special significance to the obsessive patient. He will want to know how long the interviews are going to be, as though there were a direct proportion between quantity and quality. At the close of the session, the obsessive patient will consult his watch to be sure he "got his money's worth," as though his watch would measure the value of the experience. An additional two minutes could cause him to leave feeling expanded and important, as if he were the recipient of a gift. It could also lead to a sense of having gotten away with something, and to a fear that the interviewer is unable to maintain proper control over his time. The obsessive looks at his watch rather than looking at his feelings to see what he will do next. In this way, the motivation of behavior is externalized. He may look at his watch shortly before the end of a session to see if there is enough time to bring up a matter he has been avoiding.

The obsessive tends to use money and status, rather than love, as his foundation for emotional security. Finances are one of the most threatening topics for discussion, and the physician's motivation for prying into such matters is immediately suspect. Money comes to represent the innermost source of self-esteem, and is treated with the secrecy and privilege that others reserve for the intimate details of love relationships. This is all the more striking when love relationships can be discussed with an apparent lack of anxiety or emotion. Social prohibitions against the discussion of money may lead the interviewer to collaborate with the obsessive in avoiding this important area.

Indeed, in many ways the obsessive is a caricature of social tact. Customs of etiquette are designed to avoid hurting or offending others. The exaggerated etiquette of the obsessive is designed to control his inordinately hostile impulses. The skillful interviewer is working for emotional rapport and honesty rather than a sham of social form. This requires maneuvers that may seem tactless or rude to the beginner. This apparent tactlessness strives for an understanding relationship, sympathetic with the patient's difficulty with both anger and friendship.

In his preoccupation with time, money, status, and power struggles, the obsessive is an intensely competitive individual. Although he fears the consequences of open competition with anyone of equal or greater status, he imagines himself to be in competition with everyone. All behavior is viewed in terms of its competitive implications. This is related to a later phase of his conflict with parental authority. He struggles over sleeping, feeding, toilet training, and the other issues of the first two years of life with his mother. Toward the end of this period the father becomes included in the battle. His authority is dominant, so that the child's fear of authority now represents a fear of competition with a more powerful male figure. The emerging dynamics of the Oedipal stage are superimposed on this struggle. The boy symbolically experiences fear of retaliation for his Oedipal desires as a fear of castration. It is therefore easy to understand how the anxiety manifested in the clinical interview often relates to fears of castration rather than to fears of loss of dependency. The initial power struggle is similar with the female obsessive patient, but the battle with the father may not occur until a later age.

DEFENSES DERIVED FROM THE CONFLICT

The obsessive patient must keep his conflicting emotions and indeed all emotion, as secret as possible—secret not only from the therapist, but also from himself. This leads to one of his most characteristic defense mechanisms: emotional isolation. He prefers to operate as though emotion did not exist and tries to "feel with his mind."

The obsessive uses his intellect to avoid his emotions; he thinks rather than feels. Conflicts involving emotion are reflected by his rational doubting. He struggles to engage other people on the level of theories and concepts, leading to an endless discussion of details and situations in order to avoid true engagement on the level of feelings and emotions. Thoughts should be related to motives, emotions, and actions in the real world. For the obsessive, thought serves to avoid awareness of motives and emotions and to delay adaptive action.

Words and language, the tools of thought, are also utilized in a special way by the obsessive. They are used in order not to communicate. The obsessive will provide a flood of speech, but the interviewer is left with useless residue. Details are used to obscure rather than enlighten, producing a great deal of data but no real information. Boredom is the common response to the patient's preoccupation with minutia, his struggle to find just the right word, and his emphasis on irrelevant detail. The physician's boredom is a signal that the patient is successfully avoiding emotion and that the interviewer has not been able to effectively challenge this defensive behavior.

The avoidance of such painful affects as fear and rage is easily understood, but the obsessive is even more anxious to avoid affection, warmth, and love. His sense of strength and pride is tied to his ever-present, defiant rage, causing him to mistrust any feelings of warmth or tenderness. In his earlier life, the emotions that normally accompany closeness have occurred in the context of dependency relations. Therefore, he reacts to his warm emotions with dependent and helpless feelings that stimulate fears of possible ridicule and rejection. Pleasurable experiences are postponed, for pleasure is also dangerous. The obsessive is intensely efficient in planning for future happiness, but cannot relax enough to enjoy it when that time arrives. His avoidance of pleasure is based upon unconscious guilt. He atones for his transgressions, appeases his conscience, and rigidly controls his forbidden impulses.

In the initial interviews, the obsessive patient usually denies problems in his sexual relations. His inhibition will emerge only when he perceives his general constriction of pleasurable functioning. The partner of the obsessive patient knows that sexual relations are always the same. There is either little variety or compulsive variety, as true spontaneity is viewed as dangerous. The obsessive has a particular fixation and conflict in the area of

masturbation, which has become projected into heterosexual experience. The partner becomes a new and more exciting instrument for accomplishing masturbation. The partner is expected to
be under the control of the obsessive patient during the sexual
relationship, and neither is allowed to do anything different.
This kind of control is a direct extension of the masturbatory
fantasy, where the fantasy partner is exclusively controlled by the
individual creating the fantasy. It comes as a startling revelation
to the obsessive that no two people make love exactly the same
way. The concept of the sexual relation as an opportunity for two
persons to discover and explore one another while expressing
feelings of love and tenderness is quite foreign. Instead, obsessive
individuals experience the bed as a proving ground where they
must demonstrate their prowess and work to conceal their feelings
of inadequacy. The obsessive man is preoccupied with his performance; the obsessive woman is more likely planning the next
day's grocery list. Either may be preoccupied with getting into
just the right position, and if both are obsessive a power struggle
will ensue over that issue. Performance for the obsessive can be
measured. It is measured by duration, frequency, or the number
of orgasms. Often the number of orgasms given to the partner is
more important than the pleasurable aspects of the experience.

The need to avoid feelings leads to evasiveness and suspiciousness. Emotions are frequently hidden behind token representa-
tives of their opposites. Angry at the therapist's lateness, the
patient will thank the physician for managing to find time for
him in a busy schedule. Moved by the doctor's warm spontaneity
in response to a tragedy in his life, the obsessive may complain
that the interviewer is only pretending to be concerned as a paid
listener. These token emotions are coupled with a kind of
deviousness. An apparent gift usually contains a hidden dagger.
The patient who compliments a drab piece of furniture may be
indirectly telling the interviewer that he has no taste. The patient
is even more likely to disguise warm feelings, and consequently
suffers from loneliness, social isolation, and diminished capacity
for pleasure. He pays a heavy price for avoiding his fear and
rage by minimizing emotional contact with others.

Analogous to the use of token emotions is the experience of
emotions after the fact. Unresponsive during the interview, the
patient will experience feelings of rage after leaving the office.
Once he has left the interview, the need for repression is no

longer so great. Depending on the severity of the isolation, only the ideas may come to consciousness. An illustration is the patient who says, "After the last session, the thought of punching you in the nose came to mind." If the doctor inquires whether this was accompanied by anger, the patient might reply, "No, the thought just passed through my head." The less severe obsessive might work himself into a rage and declare, "If only he were here, I would really tell him." It will be ancient history by the next appointment, back in the box with the lid nailed down. The obsessive lives a vivid secret inner life that he fears sharing with anyone. The interviewer must convince the patient that he can accept and understand these feelings without disapproval. The patient's shame and mistrust make this difficult, and he often provokes the angry or disapproving behavior that he fears. Every obsessive is somewhat paranoid.

Unable to experience love and affection, the obsessive substitutes respect and security. This leads to a desire for dependent attachments to others, but such dependency is experienced as a form of inadequacy and submission. The obsessive usually responds by avoiding the dependency gratification that he craves; therefore, he is frequently depressed. This is aggravated by the diminished self-confidence and self-esteem that follow his inhibition of assertion and aggression. The depression may not be apparent to the patient, as he handles depression, along with other emotions, by isolation. The interviewer should anticipate its appearance as soon as the isolation is broken through. From this renunciation of dependency gratification, together with his need for respect from others, the obsessive forges a subjective sense of moral superiority. This compensates for his refusal to accept dependency gratification from others by providing a fantasy of constant approval from internalized objects. Moral superiority colors the obsessive's every act. This can be a particularly difficult resistance to interpret, as it converts many symptoms and character traits, however painful or maladaptive, into ethical virtues.

It has already been mentioned that the obsessive suffers from exaggerated feelings of dependence and helplessness. Dynamically, such feelings occur whenever his omnipotent status is threatened. Omnipotence is a function of two people who are joined together in symbiotic partnership. The original omnipotent partnership was that of the infant and his mother, who seemed to be all-knowing, all-powerful, and all-providing. He continually seeks to re-establish such a partnership, in which he can again substitute grandiose omnipotence for effective coping mechanisms. This alliance does not have to be with an individual, but can be with a system of thought, a religion, a scientific doctrine, and so forth. When you separate the obsessive from his omnipotent partner, he becomes overwhelmed with feelings of helplessness, inadequacy, and dependence. The scientist who feels insecure when away from his science is a clear example. Not infrequently, the obsessive will attempt to re-establish his grandiosity by appearing to be an expert in matters about which he actually knows very little. In each new situation, he will quickly rush about amassing facts, upon which he then proceeds to expertize. Typical of the obsessive in his compensatory grandiosity is his refusal to delegate. He feels he can do everything better for himself than anyone else can do it for him, and he hates to admit to himself that he needs another person. Possessiveness and the need to save everything relate to his fear of separation from any loved object as well as to the defiant aspects of the power struggle.

Management of the Interview

THE PATTERN OF THE INTERVIEW

An interview with most patients develops like a play, or a game of chess, with a beginning, a middle, and an end. Problems and events characteristic of each phase appear in the expected order, and a brief vignette taken out of context can frequently be identified as coming from one or the other portion of the interview. The characteristic sequence is a product of the developing emotional interplay between two people, just as a play or a game of chess reflects the developing interaction between protagonists.

With the obsessive, however, the picture is somewhat different. There is often a particular flavor to the initial or final moments, but the bulk of the interview, at least in initial interviews, is marked by almost monotonous homogeneity. While the interviewer is attempting to encourage the development of emotional contact, the patient is struggling to avoid such contact by controlling the interview. When the interviewer penetrates his defenses, the patient controls his angry or frightened response by renewed isolation. Thus there is a constant alternation between isolation and engagement with anger and fear. The problems will be illustrated by presenting them in a sequence that will recur many times within the interview: the emotional isolation of the patient, the manuevers of the therapist to establish contact, the resulting emergence of the patient's fear and rage, and finally, the utilization of the sequence itself to establish both insight and a firmer therapeutic alliance.

DEFENSES AGAINST ENGAGEMENT WITH THE INTERVIEWER

The obsessive may approach the interviewer by attempting to reverse the roles. He may begin by asking, "How are you today?" and then continue with other questions, seizing the aggressive role. Another pattern is to wait for the doctor to initiate the interview and then turn the tables by saying, "Could you explain what you mean by that?" It is not unusual for the neophyte to respond with annoyance to the patient's manuevers. It is more useful to respond sympathetically with a casual comment such as, "Your interest in interviewing me suggests that it must be difficult for you to be the patient." Later in the interview, the therapist responds to these maneuvers by telling the patient that there are no right or wrong answers and that he should reply to the questions with whatever comes into his mind.

The chief problem in the interview is to establish genuine emotional contact. The emotional responses of the interviewer are an excellent guide to success. If the interviewer is interested, involved, "tuned in," contact has been established. If he is anxious or angry, contact has been established, but the secondary defenses of the patient are at work. If the interviewer is bored or indifferent, there is little contact.

The obsessive will misuse every mode of communication in the service of isolation. To reach someone, it is necessary to look at the person, talk to him, listen to him, and attend to what he says; it is also necessary to be spontaneous and expressive, and to avoid silence.

The obsessive will come into the interview and will not look at the interviewer, or possibly will only peek at him. He will look at the floor, the wall, the ceiling, or anyplace except at the interviewer. The eyes are important mediators of emotional contact with people. To avoid looking helps to avoid emotional contact. On occasion the patient may appear to be looking at the interviewer, but he is only pretending, and is really looking beyond the interviewer. It is the same avoidance, but with token appeasement added.

He can also avoid engagement with his voice. He can whisper, mumble, or speak in such a way that the interviewer will have difficulty hearing what is said. The patient will not listen. He will not hear the interviewer's comments and will ask to have them repeated. When the interviewer repeats, the patient will interrupt to complete the sentence and ask for verification. The patient may hear, but not comprehend the meaning of the words. The obsessive is a master at concealing his inattentiveness. While appearing to pay complete attention, in reality he is thinking about something totally different. Some individuals are highly skilled at this and are able to repeat the interviewer's words upon request. On such occasions, one may notice that although the words were registered in the patient's mind, the significance of the thought content was not comprehended until the patient repeated the statement.

Repeating the interviewer's phrases and questions allows the obsessive to avoid contact; he is really talking to himself. He is not answering questions or following rules, but, in his fantasy, is controlling the entire interchange without the interviewer's participation. Another common way of accomplishing this is by lecturing to the interviewer. It is important that one not hurt the patient unnecessarily when interrupting this tendency. Rather than utilize the patient's device of phony tact, it is more to the point to comment in an accepting tone, "You feel in a lecturing mood today?"

The patient will utilize a variety of defenses for the same purpose. The interviewer should avoid interpreting every defense, or the patient will feel attacked and the interview will have the quality of constantly putting the patient down, increasing his self-consciousness. Instead, the interviewer observes what is happening and directs his comments to a key or central defense. It is far better to err by choosing a less important defense than to bombard the patient with the table of contents of a psychodynamics textbook. This error is more likely to occur when one has had enough training to recognize the many defensive maneuvers but has not yet had the experience to use this knowledge at the proper time.

While the interviewer is inquiring about the chief complaint and basic identifying data, he may notice that the patient is facing the window, quietly repeating the interviewer's questions verbatim, and answering them with little feeling. The interviewer should discontinue the questioning without further comment. The ensuing silence will attract the patient's attention—he didn't expect it. At this point, the interviewer might say, "I see that you are looking out of the window; what is going on?" The patient will say his mind was on what the doctor was saying and he was thinking of the questions. The interviewer will not argue, but instead will say, "Perhaps you were thinking of something else at the same time?" Another time the patient may reply, "What I was thinking about has nothing to do with the subject." The interviewer will answer, "Let's hear about it anyway." This may allow the patient to reveal some of his inner thoughts.

The pursuit of these inner thoughts frequently leads to a process similar to the unraveling of a sweater. As the initial clue is followed, the entire neurosis will gradually emerge. At certain points it may appear that the end has been reached, only to discover later that this was merely a point of great resistance. It is valuable for future work to label such points by making a comment that will cause this issue to stand out, or to suggest an idea that will germinate in the patient's mind after the interview is over. These goals may be achieved through comments such as: "I guess we have pursued this topic as far as we can at present," or, "We seem to have encountered something here that you don't understand," or, "There seems to be something about this matter that is upsetting to you." Then the interviewer will let the subject drop, but he must remember, in listening to the patient's subsequent comments, that there is an unconscious connection between all ideas that evolve through free association.

Another approach with the same patient would focus on his block of communication rather than on his secret inner thoughts. The interviewer might say, "Your quiet tone of voice makes it difficult for us to really talk." The patient will protest, saying that he is talking as loudly as possible. Again the interviewer will not argue, but will focus on the patient's feeling: "What is it like when people have trouble understanding you?"

A third possibility would be for the interviewer to comment, "I've noticed that you repeat everything I say after I've said it." The patient will reply, "I want to make sure I have it right." The interviewer may inquire, "What makes you so concerned that you might get it wrong?" The patient will then reveal that he is anxious and that he feels the doctor's comments are very important. He is then questioned about the anxiety, and the interviewer will reassure him that it is preferable for him to reply to whatever he hears the question to be. Later in the interview, it might even be suggested that it seems as though the patient is talking to himself rather than to the interviewer.

Another common means of avoiding involvement is the use of notes or lists, consisting of topics to be discussed or questions to be asked. These may be utilized before or during the interview. Notes represent a central defense, and the interviewer must show immediate interest, firmly but gently suggesting that the patient attempt to manage without them. This will lead to anxiety and immediate engagement. The interviewer will focus upon the difficulty that requires the use of notes. What is their function? These individuals do not trust their spontaneity. They are not sure what is going to come forth. They may forget all the important things that they really want to discuss and their anger might sneak out instead. The notes provide a secure, comfortable structure to follow. When it is apparent that the patient is following an outline, inquiry should be made as to mental notes if no written ones are visible. Did the patient feel it was important to plan the interview before it occurred and decide his initial words in advance, scrutinizing them carefully for objectionable revelations of feeling? The patient may not be aware of his motivation, and with certain patients it may be necessary to compromise in an attempt to gradually wean them from their dependency on the notes.

The obsessive interviewer may use notes in a similar way. They protect him from genuine involvement with the patient. Instead of the primary relationship being between two individuals, it is between an individual and a piece of paper.

The obsessive patient will waste time on irrelevant detail. He is so convinced that the interviewer will not understand him that he must provide volumes of background information before he can come to the point of his story. This becomes so complex that, when he finally arrives at what he wanted to say, either the interviewer has lost interest or the time is up. Eventually, this defense must be interpreted; it is an error to let him finish, although he will plead that it will only take another minute. He is inordinately sensitive to criticism, which makes interruptions or admonitions to get to the point particularly difficult. The interviewer can say, "I don't understand how this is related to the question that I asked you," to which the patient may respond, "Oh, it's related. You've got to know about this and this and this." The physician's reply might be, "Do you feel that I won't be able to understand you if I don't have all this detailed background?" "Indeed," the patient will answer, to which the interviewer comments, "Well, let's try going directly to whatever the specific matter is, and if I don't understand I'll ask you for some more background information." The patient may hesitate while deciding whether to appease the interviewer or to proceed as before. If he persists with irrelevant details, the interviewer may point out, "You seem very determined to do it your way rather than follow my suggestion." The patient will probably become angry, and this anger should be used constructively. The manner in which this is done will be considered later in the chapter.

Silence is the ultimate technique in avoiding emotional rapport. The obsessive can endure prolonged silence to a greater extent than most patients can, with the exception of those who are grossly psychotic or deeply depressed. The interviewer must learn to tolerate longer silences than the patient. If the patient breaks the silence, a piece of spontaneous behavior emerges from an individual who avoids spontaneity. If the patient remains silent, the interviewer may inquire, "You feel quiet now?" or, "What have you been involved in during the silence?" The patient may reply, "I was just waiting for your next question." If this is indeed what the patient was doing, and it is very unlikely, the reply might be, "Yes, I can see that you were waiting for me to do something next, but how were you occupying yourself in the meantime?" His evasion should not be accepted, but instead an exploration of his spontaneous emotional processes would be attempted. If the therapist interrupts the silence, it is not to introduce a new topic, but rather to focus on the meaning of the silence itself.

The obsessive patient's attempts to do the interviewing do not all occur at the beginning of the session. He may refer to a comment the interviewer made earlier, with a request that some confusing aspect be explained. If the interviewer complies, more questions ensue, and soon the patient will have the interview well in hand—his hand. This both assures him that he will not be caught off guard, saying the wrong thing, and allows him to control and direct the interview.

Toward the middle or later portion of the interview, one could explore the patient's financial status. This is useful in exposing the patient's fear and mistrust of the doctor. It is equally productive with private patients and clinic patients, with whom the doctor may not have direct responsibility for setting the fee. Fees and the hours of the appointments are two issues that the physician should not allow the patient to control through bargaining. The obsessive is a "wheedler." If the fee is reduced, the patient feels either that the physician was overcharging him in the first place or that he, the patient, has succeeded in gaining an advantage, which increases his guilt feelings. It is equally destructive to allow the patient to bully and inconvenience the physician with frequent requests to change the time of his appointments.

DEFENSES AGAINST
EXPOSURE OF THE CONFLICT

When the patient's defensive attempts at emotional isolation are penetrated, he is immediately confronted with a problem. He fears that his anger may emerge, and therefore he must conceal it. One of his favorite techniques involves his peculiar use of intellect and language. He is preoccupied with finding just the right word to describe the quantitative aspect of emotion. Words have become more than symbols and have an importance of their own. He was not "angry," he was "annoyed," or he was not "angry" or "annoyed," he was "perturbed," and so on. A related way of avoiding emotion is through the use of scientific terms and technical jargon. The psychiatrist must avoid such terms in his own comments and should translate the patient's technical terms into every-day language. The obsessive will often utilize euphemisms to describe a basically unpleasant or embarrassing situation. These misleading terms should also be rephrased by the doctor in basic, direct words. For example, if the patient states that he and his wife had a "slight tiff," the doctor might reply, "You mean a fight?" In another instance, a patient might refer to a recent sexual experience by saying, "We were close last night." The interviewer can reply, "Do you mean you had sexual relations?"

The patient's tendency toward intellectualization can also be minimized if the doctor avoids asking questions that contain the word "think." "What did you think about this?" is a typical obsessive question, and leads to intellectualization. Instead, the interviewer asks, "How did you feel?" When the obsessive is asked how he feels, he will relate what he thinks. The doctor can interpret this, saying, "I didn't mean, 'what did you think?' I meant, 'how did you feel?'" It requires persistence to reach feelings if the person has no awareness of them himself. The doctor should also avoid asking questions that require the patient to make a decision, thereby triggering the doubting mechanism in the intellectual defenses. If the patient is asked, "Who are you closer to, your mother or your father?", his answer may offend someone, and therefore his doubting serves as a defense. It is better to say, "Tell me about your parents," and notice which parent is mentioned first and what information is volunteered.

Another technique for concealing feelings is the use of denial. The obsessive patient will frequently tell more about himself in the negative than in the positive. "It isn't that I feel thus and such," or, "It isn't that this happened to be troubling me at such and such a time." In the unconscious there are no negatives; he is revealing the underlying problem in his own way. Do not directly challenge this denial, but encourage him to elaborate. The more this is done, the more he begins to reverse himself. When the reversal is complete, the interviewer is in a position to return to the original statement and expose the conflict. He may point out that the patient is describing the feelings that he denied only a few minutes before, and that this is puzzling.

For example, a patient described her eagerness to visit her sister as motivated by fondness for her and not by any feeling of competition between them. Inquiry about the relationship led to a discussion of the sister's dependence on their parents, and finally to the patient's irritation that the sister received more than her share of presents from the parents. The visit emerged as an attempt to ascertain what recent gifts her sister might have received. At this point the interviewer said, "I'm not sure I understand. You said that there is no competition, but it seems that you are envious of the things she receives from your parents."

The patient struggled to explain that there was no contradiction, but finally admitted that the visit would help to suppress her competitive feelings, since the sister's gifts were always more attractive in the patient's fantasies than in reality.

A specific type of denial commonly found is the introductory or parenthetical statement, such as "To tell the truth," "My real feelings are . . . ," or "Let me be frank with you." These apparently innocuous assurances are purposeful. The patient has something to hide, and is denying it. Again, direct contradiction will only lead to more indignant denial, but these are invaluable clues to distortions and hidden feelings that the patient feels are reprehensible.

The patient has other techniques that are designed to control and conceal anger. He may shake the interviewer's hand at the end of every appointment, thereby gaining assurance that parting is on friendly terms and that his aggression did no harm during the interview. After this has occurred repeatedly, the interviewer could remark casually, "I've noticed that you want to shake hands with me after every interview. What is that about?" The patient will insist that this is routine social behavior and suggest that the interviewer may be deficient in this area. An appropriate reply would be, "I have the impression that you would be upset if we didn't shake hands, which suggests that it means more to you than routine social behavior."

More seriously ill patients may utilize the handshake as a means of establishing contact with the doctor. It is important that one accept whatever form of contact a schizophrenic patient offers initially in treatment. Early interpretive comments would alienate such patients. The doctor should wait until the patient says, "The only time I can really feel you is when we shake hands." Another frequent pattern is exemplified by the patient who remarks at the end of the session, "Thank you, Doctor." After this has become a ritual, the patient could be told, "I'm not sure I understand exactly what you are thanking me for." In being direct with the obsessive, it must be realized that the patient feels more underneath than he will show on the surface. If the interviewer bases his behavior on the patient's outward show of feeling, he will grossly misjudge the patient. For example, when the obsessive patient grins, he is probably angry, and it is important for the interviewer to ask, "Why are you smiling?" or, "What is the joke?"

Any spontaneity is disturbing to an obsessive individual. The rigidity of his defenses and controls is threatened by surprise or by the unpredictable. His emotions may be revealed; his friendly or angry feelings may be exposed. The interviewer should strive for spontaneity and pursue it whenever it is shown by the patient. What the patient volunteers is of much greater significance than specific answers to specific questions. Often his choice of words or a parenthetical expression that is supposed to be off the record is a major clue. The doctor should temporarily abandon the "official" subject and ask him to elaborate on these comments.

When discussing an uncle whom he has mentioned many times, the patient might add, "He is my uncle." The interviewer can stop him and inquire, "Did you think I didn't remember who he was?", to which the patient may reply that he was only making certain that the therapist was able to follow his story. The doctor could then ask, "Do you feel that the things you tell me are of such little concern to us that I don't remember people who are important to you?"

Even the most carefully guarded obsessive has two episodes of spontaneous behavior in each interview: the beginning and the end. Most patients exclude these episodes from their mental picture of an interview, but they provide a wealth of information to the attentive interviewer who excludes nothing. The patient reveals feelings in the corridor or the waiting room that he carefully conceals in the office. Rather than start a new conversation after the patient and interviewer are seated, the doctor might continue the original conversation. The patient's activity in the waiting room should be observed, for example, the magazine he reads, the chair he selects, and the objects in which he becomes interested. He will compliment or criticize the office furniture as a means of communicating his feelings about the interviewer. When the session is finished, he will relax, and with this relaxation, his feelings will emerge. He may allude to the secret he has been guarding, "I wonder why you didn't ask about such-and-such," or reveal his disappointment in the interview by saying, "I thought you were going to tell me what to do."

MAINTAINING THE THERAPEUTIC ALLIANCE

There are a number of problems in the interview that relate to the patient's feelings of dependency and helplessness and their humiliating implications for him. He may indicate that he has several topics and does not know which would be most important to discuss first. He may ask, "What do you think thus-and-such means?" or, "What do you think my problems are, Doctor?" The interviewer soon recognizes that the patient seems to feel that the doctor should have all the answers or that he is all-powerful. It is the physician's task to teach the patient to formulate his own answers and to develop confidence in his own reactions. On the other hand, when the patient has his own answer, he finds it very upsetting if the doctor does not agree with him. At times he may seem to flounder during the interview and may say to the doctor, "Help me," or, "Can't you ask me something else?" Instead of suggesting a topic, the doctor can either inquire into the patient's feeling of helplessness and fear of being abandoned or return the responsibility to the patient with a question such as, "Is there anything in particular that you would like me to ask about?" or, "What problem would you like me to help with?" At such times it is common for male patients to mention their fears of homosexuality. This fear may also be activated by their awareness of some warm or tender emotional response. Such emotions are typically accompanied by embarrassment. The therapist might comment at such times, "You are blushing," or, "You seem embarrassed," or, "You felt friendly toward me just then."

No matter how correct and insightful an interpretation is, if it is expected by an obsessive patient he will remain emotionally unaffected. He has prepared himself and is able to listen from a distance or to disagree completely without being involved in the interchange. The interviewer should say and do the unexpected, trying not to use gimmicks that have a stereotyped quality—such as constantly saying, "I don't understand," or repeating the patient's last word in order to draw him out further. Beginners often search for rules or standard formulas. It is a rule to avoid standard formulas with an obsessive patient.

Emotional engagement is such a difficult and trying experience that once the patient achieves it he does not want to lose it; at the end of the interview he often does not want to leave the office. There is one more question to ask, and one more thing to discuss. The interviewer may say, "We will talk about that next time." However, the patient may not be deterred by this, and may continue speaking. An appropriate reply would be, "It seems to be difficult for you to stop now. Next time we can look into why you have so much trouble with this." If the patient tries to flee after revealing his feelings, the opposite approach may be effective—he should be called back into the office for a brief discussion of what he just said. At this time his guard is down and important feelings can emerge. If the patient is anxious to escape from the office, a few extra minutes could be spent, but if he is clinging to the interviewer, it is better to suggest that the matter be discussed the next time.

INTERPRETATION OF
THE DEFENSIVE PATTERN

We have enumerated a number of methods that the obsessive uses to control and conceal his feelings. He can negate and deny them, try to reverse the relationship with the interviewer, use magical symbolic devices, avoid spontaneity, and try to confine his feelings to a portion of the interview where he believes that they will not be detected. The various means of dealing with these problems frequently lead to the patient's becoming overtly angry or upset. This must be dealt with constructively, but what does that mean?

The obsessive is usually secretly angry; when he becomes overtly angry he can show intense feeling, particularly if he feels entitled to his emotion. This should not be evaded or minimized. It is defensive for the interviewer to say, "Now there's really nothing to get mad about," or, "You must have misunderstood me." He should not hasten to explain or modify, to patch things up, or to reassure. The patient will benefit from experiencing the feeling that he so rarely allows himself.

The interviewer should not argue with the patient or collaborate in recreating a power struggle. The patient's love of logic tempts one to influence him by reason. When this approach fails, there is a tendency to redouble the effort to convince him. Such efforts are doomed; furthermore, it is not the purpose of the interviewer to impose his opinions on the patient.

The patient should experience his feelings openly, without fear of punishment or retaliation. By doing so, he finds them less violent and overwhelming than he had feared. The physician can relate in an easy manner, feeling neither fear nor anger toward the patient. He should not placate the patient's emotional reactions or retaliate because of them. This accepting attitude will help the patient to identify and to live with a part of himself that he finds reprehensible. No matter how bright the patient is in other areas, he is slow to recognize his emotions. Simple, obvious statements that identify and clarify his feelings are helpful. A typical sympathetic response would be, "You seem angry; you must have been upset." The interviewer can then attempt to link this to the immediate cause, saying, "Perhaps you were annoyed that I was late?" When this is solidly understood, he can begin to forge a link to the defensive behavior based upon it. This could be done with a comment such as, "You must have been angry all the time you were going over the list you brought to the session." In such a manner, the patient is given an awareness of the continuity of his emotional life, which has been fragmented by his defensive isolation. Identifying the patient's feelings and linking them to their cause is particularly useful when they involve the physician. For example, the patient feels angry when the interviewer questions his need to shake hands; his anger should be clearly linked to the physician and not explained away by his feeling irritable because he is getting sick. If he is angry because the interviewer will not allow him to use his notes, his reactions must be associated with the interviewer's behavior and expressed directly rather than displaced onto someone outside the interview.

At times the patient may be overtly angry and begin shouting at the doctor. This is not the time to remark, "You seem angry." Instead, the doctor should allow the patient to ventilate his rage and then comment, "You feel I have let you down," or, "I guess you are disappointed in me." Such responses accept the patient's anger in a non-defensive way without agreeing that his rage is justified. On occasion, the patient's anger may be realistically provoked by an error on the part of the interviewer. Rather than offer a simple apology, he can advise the patient that his resentment is justified, that he feels regretful that the patient was hurt, and that he will try to prevent future recurrences.

The patient will initially perceive the interviewer's confrontations as unreasonable, hostile, or provocative. In fact, it is this misinterpretation that most often allows him to bring forth his anger in a more direct manner. He is prone to feel disapproval and condescension from others, and any interference with his defenses will lead to these feelings. When the physician does not respond to his anger with anger or with attempts to suppress or deny it, the patient will be in unfamiliar territory; he may become guilty, fearing that he has been unfair, and attempt to appease with an apology. For the same reason that it is inappropriate to retaliate against the patient's anger, it is equally inappropriate to accept his apologies or to forgive his guilt feelings. Again, the feeling should be identified and linked to the behavior, and the defenses he has erected should be explored. "Were you afraid that you had offended me by your comment?" "Perhaps you agreed to come early next week because you thought you had been unreasonable before?" The patient may feel that the interviewer should be angry at him, and the unexpected response may be perceived as encouraging his transgressions. As the interviewer searches for areas of pleasure in the patient's life and points out his need to postpone pleasure, the patient may react by feeling that he is being corrupted into hedonism, with an abandonment of his conscientiousness and high moral standards.

When the patient has openly expressed his feelings, he is in a position to discover their origins and to learn new ways of coping with them. His defensive isolation has been penetrated; he has been helped to recognize his anger and fear, and he has experienced his characteristic modes of interaction with the doctor, who has accepted this without anger or retaliation. The interview has revealed the patient's characteristic conflicts and defenses, both to the interviewer and to the patient, and has laid the foundation for further exploration and treatment.

REFERENCES

Freud, S.: Character and anal erotism. Standard Edition of Complete Psychological Works of Sigmund Freud, Vol. IX. London, Hogarth Press, 1958, pp. 107–175.
Freud, S.: Notes upon a case of obsessional neurosis. Standard Edition of Complete Psychological Works of Sigmund Freud, Vol. X. London, Hogarth Press, 1958, pp. 153–320.
Levy, D.: Developmental and psychodynamic aspects of oppositional behavior. In Rado, S., and Daniels, G. (eds.): Changing Concepts of Psychoanalytic Medicine. New York, Grune and Stratton, 1956, pp. 114–134.
Rado, S.: Obsessive behavior. In Arieti, S. (ed.) American Handbook of Psychiatry, Vol. 1. New York, Basic Books, Inc., 1959, Chap. 17, pp. 324–344.
Salzman, L.: The Obsessive Personality. New York, Science House, 1968.

4 THE HYSTERICAL PATIENT

Psychopathology and Psychodynamics

The term "hysteria" is one of the oldest in psychiatric literature. Nevertheless, there is still much confusion and disagreement concerning the definition and usefulness of this concept. Terms such as "anxiety hysteria," "conversion hysteria," "hysterical character," "histrionic character," "hysteroid," "dissociative reaction," and "hysterical psychosis" have been used to describe conditions that may be similar, widely different, or overlapping. Laymen use the term "hysterical" to describe uncontrolled emotional displays. Although such reactions may be a manifestation of hysterical psychopathology, they also occur in other situations.

This chapter will consider the patient who exhibits predominantly hysterical styles of behavior. Both the phenomenology and the dynamics of these styles will be discussed, as well as the problems faced by the interviewer. Patients who are diagnosed as having a dissociative reaction or hysterical psychosis are considered *for the purpose of interviewing* to be schizophrenic. The problems of interviewing patients with overt conversion symptoms, e.g., sensory-motor disturbances, pain, "hysterical seizures," or other simulations of organic disease, are considered in Chapters 11 and 12. Some, but by no means all, patients with conversion symptoms have predominantly hysterical character traits, and therefore also present interviewing problems that are discussed in this chapter.

HYSTERICAL CHARACTER TRAITS

Hysterical and obsessive character traits fall at opposite ends of the same spectrum. The psychodynamic patterns that are closest to consciousness in one are deeply repressed in the other.

Some patients have mixtures of obsessive and hysterical character traits. They are often better integrated and more mature than those who display exclusively hysterical mechanisms. This leads to frequent disagreements concerning diagnosis, healthier hysterics being seen as obsessive or mixed neurotic characters and sicker hysterics as borderline or schizophrenic. The authors utilize the term "hysterical character" to describe those persons who display predominantly hysterical mechanisms and who do not have prominent schizoid or paranoid trends. Women more often display hysterical mechanisms; men utilize predominantly obsessive defenses. Hysterical patients exaggerate the traits and mechanisms that characterize normal femininity.

There has been much debate concerning the occurrence of male hysterical characters. Some male patients with hysterical personalities have a prominent admixture of obsessive traits, whereas others show strong feminine identifications, as in grossly effeminate men or passive homosexuals. In certain other cultures or subcultures of our own society, hysterical personalities are as common in males as in females.

Because of their vivaciousness, warmth, imagination, and charm, the hysteric is a favorite patient for the psychiatrist. The full clinical description only fits the most extreme cases, and there are many patients with more subtle manifestations of hysteria in their make-up. In general, they are attractive people who add much to their surrounding environment through their charm and sensitivity.

SELF-DRAMATIZATION

The speech, the physical appearance, and the general manner of the hysterical patient are somewhat dramatic and exhibitionistic. Communication is expressive and recollections of the past emphasize feeling and inner experience. Language patterns reflect a heavy use of superlatives; emphatic phrases may be used so repetitively that they acquire a stereotyped quality. The listener finds himself drawn in by the patient's view of the world. The patient exaggerates in order to dramatize a viewpoint and is unconcerned about rigid adherence to truth if a distortion will better accomplish the drama. These patients are usually attractive and may appear younger than their age. In both sexes there is a strong interest in style and fashion, which immediately calls attention to their physical appearance. In the woman there is an overdramatization of femininity; in the man there may be a quality of foppishness or excessive "masculinity" in some social classes.

EMOTIONALITY

Although the hysteric has difficulty experiencing real feelings of love and intimacy, his superficial presentation is quite to the contrary. This patient is charming and relates to others with apparent warmth, although his emotional responses are labile, easily changeable, and at times excessive. His seeming ease at establishing close relationships quickly causes others to feel like old friends, even though the patient may actually feel uncomfortable. This becomes clearer when further intimacy fails to develop after the first few meetings. Whereas the obsessive attempts to avoid emotional contact, the hysteric constantly strives for personal rapport. In any relationship in which the hysteric feels no emotional contact, he experiences feelings of failure, and often blames the other individual, considering him to be boring, cold, and unresponsive. He reacts strongly to disappointment, showing a low tolerance for frustration. A failure to elicit sympathetic responses from others can often lead either to depression or to anger, which may be expressed as a temper tantrum. His charm and verbal expressiveness create an outward impression of poise and self-confidence, but usually the patient's self-image is one of apprehension and insecurity.

SEDUCTIVENESS

The hysteric creates the impression of using her body as an instrument for the expression of love and tenderness, but the motivation stems from a desire to obtain approval, admiration, and protection rather than a feeling of intimacy or genital sexual pleasure. Physical closeness is substituted for emotional closeness. The attractive and seductive behavior serves to obtain the love or approval of others rather than to give sexual pleasure to the patient. Hysterics respond to others of the same sex with competitive antagonism, particularly if the other person is attractive and utilizes the same devices to obtain affection and attention.

DEPENDENCY AND HELPLESSNESS

Since Western society has different attitudes toward manifest patterns of dependency in men and in women, there are striking differences between the superficial behavior of male and female hysterics, but these disappear at a deeper level. The male hysteric is more likely to exhibit pseudo-independent behavior, which can be recognized as defensive because of the accompanying emotional responses of excessive fear or anger.

In the interview situation, the hysterical woman presents herself as helpless and dependent, relying on the constant responses of the physician in order to guide her every action. She is possessive in her relationship to him and resents any competitive threat to this parent-child relationship. The physician is viewed as magically omnipotent and capable of solving all of her problems in some mysterious fashion. The doctor, as a parent surrogate, is expected to take care of the patient, to do all of the worrying and assume all responsibility, the patient's obligation being to entertain and charm this person. In working out solutions to her problems, she acts helpless, as though her own efforts did not count. This leads to major countertransference problems in the doctor who enjoys the opportunity to enter an omnipotent alliance. Hysterical patients also adopt a particularly helpless posture when in the presence of their mothers. They are frequently regarded by their families as lovable, cute, ineffective, and "still a child."

These patients require a great deal of attention from others, and are unable to entertain themselves. Boredom is, therefore, a constant problem for hysterical patients, as they consider themselves dull and unstimulating. External stimulation is constantly pursued, and the histrionic, seductive, overly emotional, and helpless dependent behavior of the hysteric is designed to subtly involve others so that their continued interest and affection is assured.

The hysteric denies responsibility for the plight in which he finds himself, complaining, "I don't know why it always has to happen to me." He feels that all of his problems stem from some impossible life situation. If this were to be magically changed, he would have no complaint. When dependent needs are not met, these patients typically become angry, demanding, and coercive. However, as soon as it becomes apparent that one technique for obtaining dependent care is not likely to succeed, the patient will abandon it and abruptly switch to another approach.

Non-compliance

In this important group of character traits, the hysteric again appears to be the antithesis of the rigid obsessive character, showing disorderliness, a lack of concern with punctuality, and difficulty in planning the mechanical details of life. Whereas the obsessive patient feels anxious without his watch, the hysteric prefers not wearing a watch. She trusts that there will be a clock in the window of a jewelry store or on top of a billboard, or that she can ask a passing pedestrian the time. Management of the time during the session is delegated to the interviewer. This problem is less common in the male hysteric, since it is so closely related to overt dependency.

Record keeping and other mundane tasks are viewed by the hysteric as burdensome and unnecessary. The obsessive must always keep his checkbook stubs filled out, but the hysteric doesn't bother to fill out any stubs because the bank keeps a record of the money and will notify him if he is overdrawn. For an obsessive person, such an occurrence would be a shameful humiliation.

Hysterical thinking has been described as impulsive, with the patient relying on quick hunches and impressions rather than critical judgments that arise from firm convictions. The patient is typically not well-informed on politics or world affairs. His main intellectual pursuits are in cultural and artistic areas. He does not usually persevere at routine work, considering it unimportant drudgery. When confronted with a task that is exciting or inspiring and in which the patient can attract attention to himself as a result of his achievement, he reveals a capacity for organization and perseverance. The task can be done particularly well if it requires imagination, a quality that rarely is found in the obsessive character.

Suggestibility

Although it has been traditionally said that hysterics are overly suggestible, the authors agree with Easser and Lesser that the hysteric is suggestible only as long as the interviewer supplies the right suggestions, those that the patient has subtly indicated that he desires.

Self-indulgence

The hysteric patient's intense need for love and admiration creates an aura of egocentricity. The narcissistic and vain aspects of his personality are manifested in a concern with external appearance and with the amount of attention received from others. His needs must be immediately gratified, a trait that makes it difficult for the hysteric to be a good financial planner, as he buys impulsively. Whereas the hysteric is extravagant, the obsessive is penurious. It is often observed that the hysteric and obsessive marry one another; each seeking in the partner what is lacking in himself. The hysteric provides emotional expressiveness; the obsessive offers control and regulations.

Sexual and Marital Problems

The hysteric usually has disturbed sexual functioning, although there is considerable variation in the form this takes. In the woman, partial frigidity is a reaction to the patient's fear of her own sexual feelings. This fear is reflected in her hostile, competitive relationships with women and her desire to achieve power over men through seductive conquest. She has great conflict over these goals, with resulting sexual inhibition. Other patients are sexually responsive, but their sexual behavior is accompanied by masochistic fantasies. Promiscuity is not unusual, as the patient uses sex as a means of attracting and controlling men.

The man whom the hysteric woman loves is quickly endowed with the traits of an ideal, all-powerful father who will not make demands upon her. However, she always fears losing him as she lost her father, and consequently she selects a man whom she can hold because of his dependent needs. She may marry "down" socially or marry a man of a different cultural, racial, or religious background, both as an expression of hostility to her father and as a defense against her Oedipal strivings. In this way she substitutes a social taboo for the incest taboo. The group who marry older men are also acting out Oedipal fantasies, but have a greater need to avoid sex. Another dynamic mechanism that often influences the choice of a mate is the defense against castration fear, expressed by selecting a man who is symbolically weaker than the patient.

The male hysteric also has disturbances of sexual functioning. These include potency disturbances, Don Juanism, and homosexuality. In all of these conditions, there are strong unconscious homosexual fantasies or an intense neurotic relationship with the mother. Like the female patients, they have been unable to resolve their Oedipal conflicts.

Typically, the husband of the female hysteric is obsessive, with strong passive-dependent trends. These latter traits are not recognized by either party, and particularly not by the patient, who sees him as a selfish, controlling tyrant who wants to keep her a prisoner. There is usually some degree of validity in this perception, as the husband views her as a status symbol because of her attractiveness, seductive behavior, and appeal to other men. Unconsciously, he views her more as an ideal mother who will gratify both his sexual and dependent needs while he remains passive. The courtship may be stormy, and marriage soon leads to mutual disappointment. Interpersonal conflicts have a characteristic pattern: The wife is angered by her husband's cold detachment, penuriousness, and controlling attitudes. He becomes irritated with his wife's demanding behavior, extravagance, and refusal to submit to his domination. In their arguments, he attempts to engage her through intellectualization and appeals to rational logic. She may initially engage in his debate, but soon becomes emotional, displaying her anger or her hurt feelings of rejection. The husband either withdraws, feeling bewildered and frustrated, or erupts in a rage reaction of his own. Both parties compete for the role of the "much-loved child." Since she has selected a man who will not desire her as a woman and an equal partner, she has no choice but to shift alternately between being his mother and his child.

The female patient usually reports that her sexual life deteriorated after marriage, with loss of desire for her husband, or frigidity, or extramarital affairs. The relationship with her husband leads to disillusionment as she discovers that he is not the ideal man of whom she had dreamed. In her frustration and depression, she retreats to romantic fantasies. This often leads to the fear of impulsive infidelity, which, if it occurs, further complicates her life with added guilt and depression. Flirtatiousness and seductive charm are reparative attempts which fail to enhance her self-esteem, leading to additional disappointment.

Similar patterns occur with the male hysteric who becomes disillusioned with his partner and either develops potency disturbances or pursues new and more exciting partners.

Somatic Symptoms

Somatic complaints involving multiple organ systems usually begin in the patient's adolescence and continue throughout life. The symptoms are dramatically described and include headaches, backaches, conversion symptoms, and, in the female, pelvic pain and menstrual disorders. In patients with more serious ego pathology, there may be frequent hospitalizations and surgery—gynecological procedures are common in women. It is unusual for these patients to feel physically well for a sustained period of time. Pain is by far the most common symptom and often involves an appeal for help.

MECHANISMS OF DEFENSE

The mechanisms of defense utilized by the hysteric are less fixed or stable than those employed by the obsessive. They shift in response to social cues, which partially explains the difference in diagnostic impression among different psychiatrists seeing the same patient. Hysterical character traits and symptoms provide more secondary gains than most other defensive patterns. The derisive attitude that typically characterizes both medical and social reaction to this group of people is related to the fact that the secondary gains and special attention received are not only great, but also transparent to everyone but the patient. Successful hysterical defenses, unlike most other neurotic symptoms, are not in themselves directly painful, and therefore they potentially offer great relief of mental pain. However, lack of mature gratification, loneliness, and depression develop as a result of the patient's inhibition. In the case of conversion symptoms, the secondary loss is reflected in the painful and self-punishing aspect of the symptom.

REPRESSION

Hysterical symptoms defend the ego from the reawakening of repressed sexuality. Although repression is the basic defense in all neuroses, it is most often encountered in pure form in the hysteric. Memory lacunae, hysterical amnesia, and lack of sexual feeling are clinical manifestations of repression. Developmentally, the erotic feelings and the competitive rage of both the positive and the negative Oedipal situations are dealt with by this mechanism. When repression fails to control the anxiety, other defense mechanisms are utilized. Any therapeutic resolution of the other hysterical defenses is incomplete until the initial repression is interpreted as well.

DAYDREAMING AND FANTASY

Daydreaming and fantasy are normal mental activities that play an important role in the emotional life of every person. Rational thinking is predominantly organized and logical, and prepares the organism for action, based on the reality principle. Daydreaming, on the other hand, is a continuation of childhood thinking and is based upon primitive, magical, wish fulfillment processes which follow the pleasure principle.

Daydreaming is particularly prominent in the emotional life of the hysteric. The content centers around receiving love or attention, whereas in the obsessive, fantasies usually involve respect, power, and aggression. Daydreaming and its derivative character traits serve a defensive function. The hysteric prefers the symbolic gratification provided by fantasy to the gratification available in his real life, since the latter stimulates Oedipal anxiety. The central role of the Oedipal conflict in the genesis of the hysterical personality will be discussed under Developmental Psychodynamics.

Most patients consider this aspect of their mental life particularly private, and it is seldom revealed during initial interviews. The hysteric is no exception as far as the conscious disclosure of his fantasies is concerned. However, the content of the hysteric's daydreams are revealed indirectly. His infantile fantasies are projected on the outside world through the use of histrionic behavior. Emotionally significant persons in the patient's life are involved as participants. When the hysteric is successful, these persons interact with the patient so that his real world conforms to the daydream, with the patient as the central character in the drama. The self-dramatization and the overt daydreaming defend the patient against the imagined dangers associated with mature involvement in the adult world. At the same time, the patient is assured that his narcissistic and oral needs will be supplied. By acting out daydreams, the patient reduces the loneliness of the world of fantasy and yet avoids the Oedipal anxiety and guilt associated with mature adult behavior. The dissociative reaction is an extreme example of this process.

Misrepresentation or lying also defends against real involvement in the world by attempting to substitute the world of fantasy. Elaborate falsehoods often contain factual elements, which have psychological significance in terms of the past and which reveal both the Oedipal wish and the defense.

For example, a young woman frequently exaggerated or confabulated experiences concerning her cultural and artistic activities. She reported a feeling of elation while recounting such stories. She would begin to believe the story herself if it were told often enough. In the attempt to turn her daydreams into reality, fact and fantasy had become intertwined. In analyzing these stories, it was learned that the patient's father was a patron of the arts, and that her most frequent and intense contact with him in childhood involved discussions of music and art. In acting out the mother's role, she feigned knowledge and understanding in order to better please her father. The present-day confabulations symbolized past experiences of closeness to her father, while repression and denial blocked her awareness of the erotic feelings. This elation was the affectual residue that escaped into consciousness and represented the feeling of magical rapport that she had achieved with her father. In daydreams, the patient symbolically defeated her mother by sharing her father's interests to a greater degree than her mother did. At the same time, she avoided real competition with the mother.

When the interviewer attempts to challenge such confabulations, the patient will often indignantly cling to her distortion and even confabulate further to escape detection. Intense emotional reactions of guilt, fear, or anger may occur when the falsehood is finally acknowledged. The nature of the emotional response will tell the interviewer how the patient has experienced the confrontation. In the above example, responses of guilt or fear would reveal the patient's expectation of punishment, whereas a response of anger would indicate that she was enraged at the thought of having to relinquish her father.

Daydreaming assumes its greatest psychic importance during the Oedipal phase of development and may be associated with masturbatory activity. As hysterics come from families in which sexual activity is associated with great anxiety, it is no surprise that they often recall either real or imagined maternal prohibitions against masturbation during childhood. The child, striving to control his masturbatory temptations, utilizes daydreaming as a substitute means for obtaining pleasurable self-stimulation. In the Oedipal phase, the child's sexuality is focused on his erotic desire toward his parents. This desire cannot be directly gratified and is displaced to the masturbatory activity. Therefore, the fantasies that accompany or substitute for masturbation offer a symbolic gratification of the child's Oedipal wishes.

EMOTIONALITY AS A DEFENSE

The hysteric utilizes intense emotionality as a defense against deeper feelings. Seductiveness and superficial warmth with the opposite sex permits the avoidance of deeper feelings of closeness, with consequent vulnerability to rejection. Affective outbursts may serve as a protection from sexual feelings or from the fear of rejection. These dramatic emotional displays also relate to identification with an aggressive parent. Play acting and role playing ward off the dangers inherent in a real participation in life. This explains the quick development of transference as well as the pseudo-intensity and transience of the relationships that these patients develop. This mechanism also leads to the self-dramatization and labile emotionality that is so readily observed.

IDENTIFICATION

Identification plays a prominent role in the development of hysterical symptoms and character traits. First, the hysteric may identify with the parent of the same sex or a symbolic representative in a wishful attempt to defeat that parent in the competitive struggle for the love of the parent of the opposite sex. At the same time, this identification also maintains the child's relationship to the parent of the same sex. An example of identification with a symbolic representative is the man who developed cardiac conversion symptoms after seeing a man his own age collapse with a heart attack. Although this person was a complete stranger, the patient imagined that the heart attack had occurred because the man was driving himself too much in his work. The patient's father also had succumbed to a heart attack at a young age, and he identified with his father and feared punishment by death for his competitive Oedipal desires.

Second, the hysteric can identify with the much desired parent of the opposite sex or his symbolic representative. This occurs when the patient feels less chance of success in the Oedipal competition. Although on the surface the patient relinquishes the parent of the opposite sex, he unconsciously maintains the attachment through identification. In either of these two cases, the symbolic representative of the parent could be an older sibling.

A third type of identification is based on envy. Here the other person's significance to the patient lies in the fact that some experience in this person's life stimulates envious feelings in the patient. A common example occurs at any rock and roll show. One young lady will scream ecstatically, and immediately several others will emulate her as they unconsciously seek the sexual gratification symbolized by her behavior, in addition to attracting attention.

Identification is as important a mechanism as conversion in the production of hysterical pain. The identification through pain includes both pre-Oedipal and Oedipal components. The pain provides the symbolic gratification of the Oedipal wish as well as the compromise of healthy functioning and punishment for the associated feelings of guilt.

Identification is a complex mechanism that is utilized by everyone. Although many persons may identify predominantly with one parent, there are always partial identifications with the other parent as well as with other significant figures. In the mature adult, these partial identifications have fused, but in the hysteric this does not occur. This lack of fusion is particularly important in understanding the hysteric patient. Through successful treatment, the patient's partial identifications become fused into a new self-image.

SOMATIZATION AND CONVERSION

Hysteric patients express repressed impulses and affects through somatic symptoms. Conversion is not merely a somatic expression of affect, but a specific representation of fantasies that can be retranslated from their somatic language into their original language.

The process of conversion, although it is not thoroughly understood, has its origin in early life and is influenced by constitutional factors as well as by the environment. The fundamental step in this mechanism can be briefly explained as follows: Thinking represents trial action and later abortive action. For the young child, speaking in his mind is accompanied by actual talking and associated communicative behavior. Gradually there is a less fixed relationship between mental talking and the related motor activity. The child thereby learns that both his behavior and his thoughts have a symbolic as well as a concrete meaning. When the child's actions are prohibited or rewarded by his parents, he equates this with prohibition or reward for the related thoughts and affects. Therefore, the inhibitions of action that result from parental restriction usually are associated with repression of the accompanying thought and affect. In the infant, affect expression is directly accompanied by motor, sensory, and autonomic discharge. Since the parental prohibitions involve both the sexual and aggressive feelings of the child, it is the conflicts over the expression of these impulses that are dealt with through the conversion process.

Later, partial repression leads to a separation, so that the affect may remain repressed but the motor, sensory or autonomic discharge may break through. The term "conversion symptom" refers to the selective malfunction of the motor or sensory nervous system; the persisting abnormal autonomic discharge has been called "somatization." The impairment has features of inhibition as well as pathological discharge, the relative proportion varying with different symptoms. For example, conversion paralysis reflects a greater degree of inhibition, and a "hysterical seizure" manifests a greater discharge of the unacceptable impulse. Blushing demonstrates both inhibition and release through the autonomic nervous system.

In the case of sexual symptoms, the affected organ is an unconscious substitute for the genital. For example, a woman developed hysterical blindness when exposed to the temptation of an extra-marital affair. During the course of treatment, she revealed that as a child she had been caught watching her parents' sexual activities. A traumatic confrontation ensued, with the result that the patient repressed both her visual memory and the accompanying sexual arousal. For her, visual perception and genital excitement were equated, with the result that the conversion symptom had served as a symbolic compromise for sexual gratification and punishment for that forbidden pleasure.

In another instance, the sexual excitement is repressed but the accompanying cardio-respiratory discharge breaks into consciousness or perhaps an itching sensation affects the genital area. The protracted nature of these symptoms is explained by the fact that a vicarious means of discharge has a limited value in contrast with more direct expression.

The patient's particular choice of symptoms is influenced by many factors, including both physical and psychological determinants. The physical factors include organic predispositions or the direct effect of illness or injury on a particular organ system. Psychological factors influencing organ choice include historical events, the general symbolic significance of the affected organ, and the particular meaning it has to the patient because of some traumatic episode or because of identification with persons who have had a related physical illness. Conversion symptoms tend to reflect the patient's concept of disease. Gross symptoms are, therefore, more common in individuals with less medical sophistication. Patients who are in a health profession may simulate complex syndromes, such as regional ileitis, on a conversion basis. Conversion operates with varying degrees of effectiveness in binding the patient's anxiety, which accounts for the controversial opinions concerning the classic "la belle indifférence" or apparent lack of concern. In the author's experience, this attitude is relatively uncommon, since depression and anxiety usually break through the defense. The exception would be patients with a gross conversion reaction, and even then depression soon becomes apparent. "La belle indifférence" may be seen with those minor somatic complaints that form part of the character structure of the hysteric.

REGRESSION

In the hysteric, there is a selective regression in ego functions and a return to the period of the patient's life during which his inhibitions were established. The conflicts over his emotional experiences caused him to treat certain aspects of his body and its sensations as ego-alien. The selective regression from conflicts over genital sexuality may lead to an oral or anal level of adaptation although the same conflict will be expressed in the regressed symptom. Features of primitive incorporation are common, as has been shown by the prominent role of identification in hysteria. This can be seen directly in one patient who had globus hystericus, in which there is an unconscious wish to perform fellatio. As treatment progressed, the pregenital incorporative aspect became clear in the patient's associations of a penis with her mother's breast and her fantasy of oral impregnation by her father.

DENIAL AND ISOLATION

Hysterics deny awareness of the significance of their own behavior as well as the behavior of others. This unawareness is greatest in the areas of seductive and manipulative behavior and the secondary gain associated with their symptoms. They also deny their strengths and skills, further contributing to the façade of helplessness. These patients also deny painful emotions, with the result that isolation develops as a defense against depression, and if it is unsuccessful they will resort to distortion and misrepresentation to escape facing their unhappiness.

EXTERNALIZATION

Externalization, the avoidance of responsibility for one's own behavior, is closely related to denial. The patient feels that his own actions don't count, and views both success and suffering as being caused by other people in his life.

DEVELOPMENTAL PSYCHODYNAMICS

The developmental patterns of hysterical patients are less consistent than those of the obsessive. One common feature is that the patient occupied a special position in the family, such as being the youngest child. Physical illnesses that led to special indulgence are often described, and frequently another family member suffered from ill health, offering the patient an opportunity to observe the privilege accorded to the sickly.

When the future female hysteric enters the infantile struggles with her parents over sleeping, feeding, and being held, she discovers that crying and dramatic scenes lead to getting her own way. Her mother gives in, albeit with some annoyance. Her father is more likely to withdraw, often criticizing the mother's behavior and occasionally intervening with even more indulgence "because the poor child is so upset." The child is soon aware of the conflict between her parents, and she learns to play each against the other. This pattern interferes with the normal development of conscience, as she learns to escape punishment by indicating that she is sorry or "feels bad." The mother responds either by making no attempt to punish the child, or by not enforcing the punishment. The child never experiences the consequences of misbehavior, and is left with unresolved feelings of guilt as a result of escaping punishment.

The typical mother of the female hysteric is competitive, cold, and either overtly argumentative or subtly resentful. She unconsciously resents being a woman and envies the masculine role. Overprotection and overindulgence of her daughter compensate for her inability to give real love. Her most tender warmth is expressed when the child is depressed, sick, or upset, which helps to establish depression, physical illness, and tantrums as means of obtaining dependent care. The patient's need to maintain a dependent relationship with her mother makes it difficult for her to mature. She fails to develop an internalized ego ideal, as is clinically evidenced by the hysteric's continued reliance on the approval of others in order to maintain her own self-esteem.

The girl soon recognizes the feeling, shared by both parents, that special privileges and status are accorded to men. The female hysteric reacts with competitive envy, which may be expressed through symbolically castrating behavior, through imitation, as expressed in being a tomboy, or in competing directly with men, although retaining her feminine identity. The tomboy pattern is more likely if older brothers provide a readily available model. The hysteric may emulate her mother during childhood, but in early adolescence their relationship is marked by open strife. At that time she does not like or admire her mother as much as she does her father, and this also furthers her identification with men.

Since the hysteric is unable to obtain adequate nutrient warmth from her mother, she turns to her father as a substitute. He is most often charming, sensitive, seductive, and controlling. Mild alcoholism and other sociopathic trends are common. During the first three or four years of her life, she and her father are usually close to each other. If he feels rejected by his cold and competitive wife, he turns to his daughter as a safe and convenient source of gratification for his failing masculine self-esteem. He thereby rewards and emphasizes his daughter's flirtatiousness and emotionality. During her latency period, he becomes increasingly uncomfortable with her femininity and may, therefore, encourage her tomboyishness. As she becomes older, she finds her father a difficult man to please, since he is easily manipulated on one occasion, but may capriciously dominate her on another. At puberty, the romantic and erotic aspect of their relationship is denied by both father and daughter, as both are threatened by their incestuous feelings.

Her transient rejections by her father leave the patient feeling that she has no one, since she already feels alienated from her mother. She may express her rage with emotional outbursts and demanding behavior, or she may intensify her seductive and manipulative efforts. Self-dramatization, hyperemotionality, simulated compliance, seductiveness, and physical illness serve to reestablish control in her relationship with her father. She is unwilling to relinquish her attachment to him, and consequently all sexuality must be inhibited. Her Oedipal fears make her unable to experience sexual desires for any other man.

At puberty, as her sexuality unfolds, trouble begins. The father moves away from his daughter, sometimes finding a mistress, but at the same time jealously guarding his daughter from young suitors. The girl feels that she must inhibit her sexuality and remain a little girl in order to retain Daddy's love and at the same time to ward off threatening, exciting impulses. In the more healthy patient, the defense against the Oedipal conflict is the most significant factor. Fear of maternal retaliation for her success with her father and the fear of incestuous involvement lead to regression to a more infantile level of functioning. The less healthy patient, with more prominent conflicts at an oral level, already views her father more as a maternal substitute.

Variant patterns of hysterical development exist in which the daughter has a greater degree of overt dependence on the mother as well as a father who is more aloof and less seductive. At puberty, the mother makes a strong bid to keep her daughter dependent upon her, and thereby defeats the child in the struggle for her father's love. These girls inhibit their basically hysterical character traits, and this personality organization may only emerge later in life or during the course of psychotherapy.

In some patients, the real mother is absent, and maternal deprivation may stem from a foster mother who fails to provide closeness. The child learns to simulate emotionality. The father, although erratic, often provides the genuine experience that offers the child a chance at further development.

Beginning in the teenage period, the less well-integrated female hysteric has poor relationships with other girls, particularly attractive girls. She is too jealous and competitive with them to be accepted. She is not comfortable with her budding femininity and fears sexual involvement. Therefore, she may have only platonic relationships with boys. Everyone in the high school knows who she is, but she is not usually elected to class office. She is often pretty herself and is preoccupied with her appearance. Unattractive girls are less likely to develop hysterical patterns, as they are less successful in using them. The hysteric prefers girlfriends who are both unattractive and masochistic—an arrangement that offers mutual neurotic gratification. As she progresses through the teen years, she shifts her attention to men, but classically overvalues them, and selects men who are in some way unattainable. Disappointment, frustration, and disillusionment are inevitable, and she reacts with depression and anxiety.

In the case of the male hysteric, the situation is somewhat different, as the problem is often complicated by overt homosexuality. Although a predominance of hysterical character traits in men is unusual in our culture, there are a number of men who have a significant proportion of these traits mixed in with their obsessive ones. In these cases there is a strong identification with the mother, who was obviously the "aggressor" in the family.

She typically had many hysterical traits herself, whereas the father tended to be more withdrawn and passive, avoiding arguments and attempting to maintain peace at any price. The father often expressed his own inhibited aggression through being hyper-critical and overly controlling with his son. At times the father was relatively absent in the home or was disinterested in his son, or perhaps he was excessively competitive with his son. In either case, the boy fears castration as a retaliation for his Oedipal striving. Being unable to give up his attachment to his mother, he must repress all sexual desire for women. In adolescence he has less masculine self-confidence than the other boys and is fearful of physical competition. His feeling of masculine strength has been acquired through an identification with the aggressiveness of his mother, and consequently it is more likely to be manifested in intellectual rather than physical pursuits. The lack of a strong father figure with whom he can identify leads to faulty super-ego development and an inadequate ego ideal. When this constellation of factors continues into adolescence, the patient becomes predisposed to perverse sexuality.

The boy, in his quest for paternal love and affection, adopts techniques utilized by his mother for gaining the attention and affection of men. The greater the weakness, disinterest, or absence of the father, the more overtly effeminate the boy will become.

CHIEF COMPLAINT
AND PRECIPITATING STRESS

The female hysteric usually arrives at the physician's office after being disappointed or disillusioned by her husband or lover, resulting in an intensification of fantasy and the fear that an impulsive loss of control of sexual impulses will occur. The psychiatrist is sought as a safe substitute and an inhibiting force. Chief complaints involving depression or generalized anxiety occur in patients of either sex. On some occasions, particularly with male hysterics, somatic symptoms may be in the foreground and the patient is referred for psychiatric help when no adequate organic basis can be found to explain his suffering. The somatic symptoms often screen depressed feelings, particularly if pain is prominent. Suicidal gestures may lead to the initial psychiatric contact in other cases.

Concern over sexual symptoms is expressed early in treatment. The patient may quickly acknowledge some degree of frigidity or impotence, although this did not lead to seeking treatment until it threatened a love relationship. In healthier patients, there are also complaints of social anxiety and inhibition. These are discordant with the patient's actual performance in social situations. This same phenomenon occurs during the interview, in which the patient may conduct himself with apparent poise and composure, but feels subjective discomfort.

Management of the Interview

The beginning psychiatrist finds the hysterical patient one of the easiest to interview; the experienced psychiatrist finds him one of the most difficult. This is because it is so necessary for the patient to elicit a favorable response from the doctor in obtaining help in overcoming his problems. The interviewer is usually pleased with his new patient, especially if the patient is young, attractive, and of the opposite sex. He may experience the vague aura that accompanies a new romance. Attempts on the part of the interviewer to explore the patient's role in his problems will threaten the patient's feeling of acceptance because of his strong need to feel that the doctor likes him. Too vigorous an effort in this direction will drive the patient away, and yet he cannot be helped unless the difficulties are first brought into the open. The interviewer must develop a relationship that will permit the patient to continue in treatment as well as encourage the unfolding of his problems.

THE OPENING PHASE

INITIAL RAPPORT

The hysteric establishes "instant contact" at the beginning of the interview. He quickly develops apparent emotional rapport, creating an impression of a strong commitment to the interviewer, although feeling little involvement. The patient's first comments are frequently designed to please and flatter the interviewer, complimenting the doctor's office or remarking, "I'm so glad you were able to see me," or, "What a relief finally to have someone I can talk to." A reply to such comments is unnecessary and instead the interviewer can shift the focus by asking, "What seems to be the problem?"

DRAMATIC OR SEDUCTIVE BEHAVIOR

The hysteric is obviously relieved by the opportunity to describe his suffering and does so with a dramatic quality. Before the interviewer can inquire about the chief complaint, the patient may begin by asking, "Shall I tell my story?" The drama unfolds as he describes his difficulties in vivid, colorful language, using many superlatives. The patient's behavior is designed to create an impression, and the interviewer begins to feel that the scene has been rehearsed and any questions will be an intrusion.

The hysteric usually prefers a physician of the opposite sex. The female hysteric is disappointed if she finds that her new doctor is a woman. The disappointment is concealed, although the patient may remark, "Oh, I didn't expect a woman doctor!" There is no point in exploring the patient's disappointment in the first part of the interview, as it will only be denied.

Even the inexperienced interviewer quickly recognizes the most common stereotype of the female hysteric. The patient is stylishly dressed and has a seductive manner, ranging from social charm to overt sexual propositions. Body language provides clues in understanding the patient. The patient who dresses up when coming to see the doctor employs a form of body language that lends itself to exploration early in treatment. The most frequent example of the use of the body is the female patient who sits in a provocative posture, exposing a portion of her anatomy in a suggestive way. This behavior is designed to engage and attract the interviewer sexually.

Self-dramatization can be interpreted relatively early in treatment, although not in the first few sessions. Premature interpretations cause the patient to feel rejected and are usually made because the doctor is anxious. When the male interviewer comments on the female patient's seductiveness and her tendency to sexualize every relationship, she will protest that her behavior is not sexual. She might say, "I just want to be friendly, but they always have other ideas." The interviewer should maintain his opinion without getting into an argument with the patient, who has difficulty accepting the idea that a pretty woman cannot initiate a casual conversation with strange men.

Early interpretations are often useful when the patient directs the interviewer's attention to her behavior in the initial interview. For example, an attractive young lady pulled up her dress and asked the psychiatrist to admire her suntan. He replied, "Yes, you have a nice tan," and then added, "Perhaps you fear that I won't admire what I will find beneath the surface?" This general, but supportive, interpretation is preferable to silence early in treatment, as it is less of a rejection for the patient.

The dramatization of roles that are less obviously sexualized is more difficult to recognize. For example, a young woman arrived for an interview without make-up, hair carelessly arranged into a pigtail, and the remains of chipped polish on several fingernails. She wore a messy housedress and slippers—a caricature of the harried housewife, interrupted in the middle of scrubbing the floor. The interviewer asked about her problem, and she replied, "Well, I've been depressed for months, and a week ago I had a big fight with my husband, and got furious, and that's when I took the pills." The patient did not appear to be depressed, and she related her story with histrionic flourish. When the interviewer inquired about the pill episode, the patient answered, "First I started popping in the aspirin, and then I went for the urine test pills, and that's when he hit me and I got this lump on my head." The interviewer requested further details about the fight and the patient said, "Actually he did not hit me, he shoved me against the wall and I bumped my head." Rather than the result of a depressive spell, the suicidal episode was the culmination of a dramatic free-for-all involving the patient, her husband, and her children.

On several occasions, this patient casually, but abruptly, introduced highly charged material, which is typical hysterical behavior. Early in the interview, she gave the ages of her five children as 12, 10, 6, 5, and 1. No explanation was given when, in the next sentence, she indicated that she had been married only seven years. Later in the interview, she was asked about her relationship to her inlaws, and she replied, "Well, it is not too bad now, but at first they were not happy about Bill marrying a divorcée with two children." Dramatic remarks are made frequently during the interview. For instance, the same patient, when volunteering that she was a housewife, added, "That's a glorified term." The above description easily identifies the patient as a hysteric because the features of diagnostic significance have been abstracted from the interview. However, many interviewers do not recognize this behavior when it is mixed with non-hysterical material and the patient is not the typical pretty, seductive, young woman.

Another patient may dramatize indifference on arriving 10 minutes late, showing no awareness of the time. This patient, unconcerned about small amounts of time, will feel that the doctor is picayune to terminate the session on time even though the patient is in the middle of his story. The patient remarks with annoyance, "Can't I even finish what I'm saying?" or, "I had so much to tell you today." The interviewer can reply, "Yes, we had a late start," and let the matter drop. The interviewer wants the patient to become responsibly interested in the lateness and the motivation behind it.

Some hysterics will dramatize obsessiveness in the initial interviews, leading to errors in the doctor's understanding of the patient. This occurs more often in males and competitive phallic females. An example would be the patient who brings a pad to the session and jots down notes about the doctor's remarks, and then loses the notes or never reads them. Beginning interviewers often mistake any of the patient's remarks that involve performance or competitiveness as evidence of an obsessive character. Although the hysteric can be just as competitive as the obsessive, the object of the struggle is love or acceptance, whereas the obsessive is more concerned with power, control, and respect. The hysteric may express anger over the doctor's fee or some other issue, but the subject is dropped when the emotional tone changes, but the obsessive remains inwardly angry for a much longer time, using intellectualization or displacement in order to keep his anger out of consciousness.

DISTORTIONS AND EXAGGERATIONS

When the first interview is almost over, the interviewer suddenly realizes that he has little historical data and almost no chronological sense of the patient's development. Instead, he has become immersed in the interesting and lively details of the present illness and senses that he has already lost his neutrality. At some point in the first or second interview, the physician must intervene in order to obtain more factual information. As he succeeds in getting behind the rehearsed façade, the patient will reveal feelings of depression and anxiety, which can then be explored sympathetically.

Initially, the hysteric ascribes his suffering to the actions of others, denying any responsibility for his own plight. He tells what was said and done by the other person but leaves his own behavior a mystery. Rather than interpret these defenses in the initial interview, the physician can simply ask the patient what he himself said or did in each situation.

The patient's response to this confrontation will usually be vague and expressive of his disinterest in his own role. The interviewer must be persistent if he is to obtain the information he seeks. In addition to gathering information, he subtly communicates that he considers the patient's role important and that the patient has the power to influence his human environment rather than merely being influenced by it. After the first few interviews the interviewer can comment, each time the patient leaves his own behavior a mystery, "You don't tell me what you contributed to this situation—don't you consider your own behavior important?" or, "In describing each situation, you emphasize what the other person does, but you leave yourself out!"

Frequently the patient will contradict details of his story or add further exaggeration when telling the story for the second time. The therapist should be alert to these occurrences, as they provide excellent opportunities to interpret the patient's misrepresentation. Usually it is the patient's desire for extra sympathy that underlies these distortions. The interviewer can then comment, "It appears that you feel you must elaborate your problems or I won't appreciate your suffering." It is through these openings that the therapist encourages the patient to share feelings of sadness and loneliness.

EARLY CONFRONTATIONS

EXPLORING THE PROBLEMS

It is common for a hysteric to complete the initial interview without revealing the major symptoms that caused him to seek help. The patient frequently uses generalizations in describing his problems. These are accompanied by expressive emotionality, but specific difficulties are not defined. Intense affect conceals the vagueness of what is said. The interviewer finds that his questions are answered superficially and that the patient seems mildly annoyed when asked for further details. For example, a patient described her husband as a "wonderful person." The interviewer replied, "Tell me some of the ways in which he is wonderful." The patient hesitated briefly and then said, "Well, he is very considerate." The interviewer, realizing that he had actually learned nothing, asked for some examples. What emerged was that her husband never tried to force his attentions when she was not in the mood for sex. The interviewer could now ask the patient if she had difficulty with her enjoyment of sex. Without this step, it would have been easier for the patient to deny that she had a sexual problem.

Often the hysteric will discuss feelings of depression or anxiety without any outward manifestation of these emotions. The interviewer can indicate to the patient that he does not appear to be depressed or anxious. This confrontation invites the patient to share his true feelings rather than merely enlist the interviewer's sympathy with a sad story. The patient's fear of rejection leads to his attempt to gain sympathy without really sharing himself.

The prominence of physical symptoms in the interview, to some extent, reflects the interest of the interviewer. It is a rare hysteric who does not suffer from some mild physical complaints, such as fatigue, headaches, backaches, and menstrual or gastrointestinal symptoms. The patient does not consider such symptoms to have important psychological determinants, and the interviewer should avoid challenging this view early in treatment. He can best inquire about the patient's physical health as part of his interest in the patient's life, without implying that he is seeking to find a psychological basis for such symptoms.

With the patient who has an extensive history of physical complaints, the interviewer must not interpret the secondary gain in the first few interviews, even though it may be quite transparent and is seemingly acknowledged by the patient. For example, a patient says, "My family certainly suffers because of my frequent hospitalizations." The interviewer can reply, "Yes, I'm sure that it is very hard on all of you," thereby emphasizing the patient's secondary loss rather than his secondary gain. The hysteric will occasionally state early in treatment that his physical symptoms are psychosomatic or are "all in my mind." The experienced interviewer recognizes this as a resistance, since the patient is making a glib statement that really has little meaning.

THE DENIAL OF RESPONSIBILITY

RESPONSIBILITY FOR THE PATIENT'S FEELINGS.   The hysteric attempts to avoid responsibility for his emotional responses. The female hysteric finishes describing a fight with her husband and then asks, "Wasn't I right?" or, "Wasn't that a terrible thing for him to say?" The patient will not be helped to better understand herself if the interviewer merely agrees with her. Initially, he could address himself to the patient's self-doubt and guilt by a comment such as, "You must not feel very sure of yourself." However, as such incidents recur, the therapist should sharpen his focus on the problem by replying, "Are you looking for an ally against your husband?" The patient's need for an ally is legitimate, although underneath the patient has the feeling that she is not entitled to what she seeks. In the transference, the patient has reconstructed the triangular relationship that once existed with his parents, except that the therapist and the spouse now represent these parental objects in the patient's unconscious.

Frequently, the patient will create a very negative picture of someone close to him. If the interviewer attempts to be supportive and comments that the patient's relative seems to be unfair or selfish, the patient will often repeat the interviewer's remark to the other person, stating, "My doctor says that you are unfair!" This can be avoided by remarking, "From your description, your mother sounds like quite a selfish person," or, if the patient's remarks are sufficiently critical, "That is quite an indictment."

RESPONSIBILITY FOR DECISIONS.   The hysteric will, whenever possible, attempt to have the physician assume responsibility for his decisions. The wise physician will not accede to these helpless appeals. Instead, he suggests that the patient explore the conflict that prevents him from making the decision for himself. The patient responds by seeming not to understand what factors are involved in making a decision. Even if the hysteric explores the psychological meaning of the decision, when all the discussion is over, he is likely to confront the doctor with, "Now, what should I do?" It is as though the discussion were something quite separate from the actual decision. In other situations, the patient has already made the decision in his own mind, but he wants the doctor to share the responsibility for the consequences.

An example of one patient's helplessness occurred when the physician changed the hour of an appointment. The patient trusted his memory and came at the wrong time. Then he said with annoyance, "How do you expect me to remember these things?" The physician replied, "You are right, it is difficult, and I could never manage either if I hadn't written it in my appointment book!" The physician should refrain from writing the time down for the patient, as this will only indulge his helplessness and reinforce the pattern. One patient telephoned to inquire if she had missed an appointment on the previous day. When the interviewer replied that she had, the patient sounded distraught and said, "I had so much to talk about; isn't there anything you can do?" The patient hoped that the doctor would take pity on her and find some way to squeeze her into his schedule. When he replied, "We can talk about it next time," she insisted, "There must be something you can do!" The interviewer answered, "I don't think a make-up appointment would be desirable." At this point it was clear that the manipulative effort had failed and the patient said with a tone of resignation, "All right, I'll see you at the regular time tomorrow."

Another way in which the hysteric manifests attitudes of helplessness is the use of rhetorical questions. He exclaims, "What should I do about this problem?" or, "Can't you help me?" or, "What do you think my dream means?" Stereotyped replies such as, "What do you think?" are of little help to the patient. Often no reply is necessary, but early in treatment the interviewer could remark on the patient's feeling of helplessness. A different approach is for the doctor to demonstrate his honesty and humility with a statement such as, "I don't know."

INTERPRETATION OF THE PATIENT'S ROLE

As the therapy progresses, the unconscious role that the hysteric lives out in life will emerge. The role that is most common and closest to consciousness is that of the injured party or the victim. Although the origins of this role lie in the distant past, the patient perceives it as a reflection of his current life situation. Other roles, such as that of Cinderella or a princess, are typically related to the patient's narcissism and grandiosity. The patient may elevate her self-esteem through exaggeration of her social status. The achievements of her more successful relatives or friends are inflated to create an overall impression of greater culture, romance, or aristocracy than is accurate. This attitude may manifest itself as a feeling of superiority to the physician or veiled reference to the lesser intellectual backgrounds of other people with whom she is involved.

This defense is not interpreted during early interviews. As the psychiatrist pursues the origin of these grandiose fantasies, he will find that they are Oedipal. The female patient's father led her to believe that she was his little princess, and she dared not grow up. She compensates for her apparent helplessness in the adult female role through her pride in being a more feeling and sensitive person than those upon whom she is dependent, who symbolically represent her mother. The hysteric feels that she has subtler tastes and finer sensibilities and appreciates the better things in life. She feels that it is herself rather than her husband whom their friends see as the interesting and attractive person. This attitude toward her husband also defends against sexual involvement with him. He is considered a crude and insensitive person who merely responds to basic animalistic drives.

During therapy, there are shifts in the role that the patient dramatizes. These shifts reflect changes in the patient's current self-image as well as her style of recreating part object identifications from the past. Often the changes in role are in response to the patient's successful attempts to elicit the interest of the interviewer.

THE PATIENT RESPONDS

EMOTIONALITY AS A DEFENSE

Hyperemotionality, one of the hysteric's most important defenses, occupies a prominent position in the treatment. The emotionality influences the interviewer to empathize with the patient's feeling; however, the physician is unable to gratify all of the patient's demands and instead offers interpretations, which serve to block some of the gratifications that the patient receives through his symptoms. As a result, the patient inevitably experiences frustration, and may utilize an initial response of anger to conceal his hurt feelings.

For instance, a male hysteric elicited a feeling of sympathetic understanding while describing the "impossible situation" of a family business in which he was constantly put in the position of the baby. He went into considerable detail describing his father's tyrannical and excitable behavior. As the interviewer persisted in his questions, it became apparent that the patient had temper outbursts at work. At such times his family would cater to him because he was upset. The patient's need to play the role of injured child because of his fear of the adult male role was interpreted. As would be expected, the patient reacted with an outburst of anger and depression. The next session the patient stated, "I was so upset after our last session, I felt much worse. I couldn't stop churning inside, but I finally felt better when I ate something on the way back to work." The interviewer then inquired, "What was it that you felt so badly about?" After the patient described his feeling of unhappiness, the physician interpreted, "The food seems to provide a form of comfort and security." The patient revealed that he had been given food and extra privileges during his childhood when he felt bad or had been punished by his parents. The indulgence was associated with feelings of being loved by his parents or having been forgiven for his transgressions.

In his adult life, the same experience was unconsciously represented by buying himself food. Rather than gratifying the patient's bid for love, the therapist offered only an interpretation, which blocked this area of gratification and required the patient to seek a new solution to his injured pride. However, in working with this defense, the physician must convince the patient that his traditional solutions are only psychological first-aid and offer no permanent resolution of the underlying problem, which is the patient's feeling of helplessness and damaged self-esteem. The physician must then show the patient that the hyperemotional response that led to the purchase of food also warded off a deeper and more disturbing emotion. At this point, the patient frequently becomes angry and asks, "Why should I have to change?" or, "Why can't anyone accept me the way I am?" No comment is required on the part of the interviewer. Once again the hysteric utilizes his hyperemotional anger as a defense against his fear of the adult role.

In due time, the patient will recognize that other people have less intense emotional reactions. It is then that the interviewer can point out the pride with which the patient regards his hyperemotional responses. This pride reflects a compensatory sense of superiority to the parent. The hyperemotionality is also a reaction to the emotional response expected by the parents. The reactions of feeling sorry, appreciative, or frightened were expected by the parent and produced by the child in order to gain parental approval. Later, these same processes operated intrapsychically as the ego attempted to obtain approval from internalized objects.

The interpretation of the hysteric's defensive patterns frequently leads to depression. If kept within reasonable limits, this emotion provides the motivation for therapeutic change, and the psychiatrist should not be overly concerned about alleviating mild depressive moods early in therapy.

REGRESSIVE BEHAVIOR

Those hysterical patients who have more serious ego defects are particularly prone to regressive behavior as the psychiatrist begins to interpret their defensive patterns. The patient may become even more helpless, depressed, and preoccupied with physical illness, or may threaten suicide. These symptoms are associated with considerable secondary gain. When such infantile behavior emerges, it should occupy the central focus of the interviewer's interpretations. Thus, it is not appropriate to interpret the female hysteric's fear of Oedipal competition while she is depressed and threatening suicide. Instead, the doctor interprets her feeling of deprivation and need for dependent care. After the patient has improved and is experiencing the desire to compete in the adult feminine role, the therapist can explore her Oedipal fears as a source of her inhibition.

INVOLVEMENT AND PSEUDO-INVOLVEMENT

The female hysteric is usually pleased with her psychiatrist during the early phase of treatment. She eagerly anticipates her sessions and is prone to feel romantically involved with the physician. She sees him as a strong and omnipotent figure who could provide the protection and support that she feels she needs.

The hysteric's enjoyment of treatment is accompanied by a flare for psychological thinking. The patient is likely to acquire intellectual knowledge about emotional problems from books, friends, or from the doctor himself. Even the most experienced psychiatrist may find himself pleased with the patient's early enthusiasm for treatment and the effort he applies to the work. Because of his emotionality, insights are related with feeling, in contrast to the intellectualization of the obsessive or schizophrenic patient. The inexperienced interviewer is convinced that this is true emotional insight, as contrasted with intellectual insight. However, after a year or two he discovers that the daily successes do not add up to long-term progress.

It requires experience to recognize when the hysteric is not really involved in changing his life and is only playing the role of psychiatric patient. There are certain clues that are helpful in recognizing this process. For example, in his enthusiasm for analysis, the patient may bring in material about a spouse, mistress, lover, or friend. He may ask the psychiatrist for advice concerning the other person's problem, or he might offer his own insights, hoping to win the interviewer's approval. If the patient receives any encouragement, he might bring in a friend's dream and request the doctor's aid in interpreting it. The interviewer, rather than responding directly, can say to the patient, "I'm not able to see how this is relevant to your problem," or, "How is this going to be helpful to you in resolving your difficulties?"

Another instance is the patient who enlists the aid of auxillary therapists. This process may take the form of reading books on psychology and psychiatry, or it may involve the discussion of his problems with friends. On some occasions, the interviewer can point out that the patient has obtained a contradictory opinion from a friend by not describing the situation in the same way as he had presented it to the therapist. On other occasions, the physician can interpret the patient's feeling that the therapist is not providing enough help, and that outside assistance from books and friends is necessary as he feels unable to work out his own answers.

Another example of the hysteric's style of involvement in treatment is his pleasure in watching the doctor "at work," while maintaining an emotional distance from the process. For instance, the patient asks, "Could you explain what you meant last time when you were talking about my mother?" His tone makes it clear that he is not asking for clarification of something he did not understand, but that he wishes the physician to provide sustenance in the form of interpretations. When the doctor supplies this gratification, the patient may seem to become interested and involved, but he does not extend the perimeters of the physician's explanation. He might even remark, "You seem so wise and understanding," indicating that he is responding to the doctor's strength rather than the content of the interpretation. At these times, the physician can say, "I get the feeling that you enjoy listening to me analyze you."

A more subtle clue to the incomplete involvement is provided by the patient's tendency to omit crucial data from his current life situation, such as the fact that he has started a new romance or that he is in danger of losing his job. When such omissions occur, the interviewer can interpret them as indications of the patient's partial involvement in treatment.

RECOGNIZING THE PATIENT'S PAIN

The hysterical patient's emotional display is not always a drama. When the interpretations of the defensive pattern are successful, the patient will experience genuine feelings of loneliness, depression, and anxiety. At such times it is essential that the interviewer allow the patient to feel that the doctor cares, that he is able to help and will permit some measure of dependent gratification. The mature interviewer is able to accomplish this without abandoning his professional stance. The interviewer who fears being manipulated when the patient genuinely feels bad will miss appropriate opportunities for sympathy, kindness, and understanding. This failure will prevent the development of trust and insight. The interviewer may on occasion have an opportunity to share the patient's real pain before the end of the initial interview, but with many patients this does not occur for weeks or even months.

TRANSFERENCE AND COUNTERTRANSFERENCE

Transference is prominent in the behavior of the hysteric from the first interview. The transference is usually positive in the first few interviews, and often assumes an erotic quality when interviewer and patient are of opposite sexes. Overtly sexual fantasies about the doctor at the very beginning of treatment often suggest borderline psychopathology.

The following paragraphs refer to the transference and countertransference phenomena seen between a female patient and male interviewer, but a similar relationship also develops between the female interviewer and the male hysteric patient. The patient soon refers to the interviewer as "my doctor," or "my psychiatrist." She may make flattering references to the physician's clothing or the furnishing of his office. She is solicitous if he has a cold and takes pains to learn about his interests from clues provided by his office furnishings, books, magazines in the waiting room, and so forth. She is likely to bring newspaper or magazine articles or books that she feels might interest him. She will be particularly interested in the other women patients in the waiting room, with whom she feels intensely competitive. Her traits of possessiveness and jealousy are easily uncovered by exploring remarks that she makes concerning these competitors for the physician's love.

Body language often reveals early indications of transference. For example, the female hysteric may take out a cigarette and look expectantly to the interviewer for a match, or rummage through her pocketbook in search of a tissue, or put the interviewer in the position of having to help with her coat. Such behavior is difficult to interpret in an initial interview, although it provides important clues about the patient. On one occasion the interviewer indicated that he had no matches, and the patient responded by bringing a large supply to the next interview, as a deposit. The interviewer did not accept this offering, as it would have assured the patient that the doctor would provide gratification of her dependent needs upon demand. In refusing, the interviewer remarked, "If you are able to bring your own matches today, I think you should be able to manage other times." Each interviewer must rely on his own personal background and personality style with regard to social formalities such as opening doors, shaking hands, and so on. Behavior that would be natural for a European-born doctor might be forced for an American.

The hysteric makes intrusions on the doctor's time. There may be requests for extra sessions or telephone calls to the physician's home if the patient is "upset." After several months of treatment, a patient related a dream of visiting the doctor and his family at home. She was particularly interested in the doctor's wife, and in the dream the patient was disappointed that the doctor did not seem as strong in his home as he did in the office. The dream was told late in the session, and the doctor's comments were limited to the patient's disappointment in him. A weekend intervened before another session, and the patient became upset and telephoned the doctor at home. In the following session, the telephone call was interpreted as an acting out of the wish in the dream, i.e., to compete with the doctor's wife for his affection. With much embarrassment, the patient revealed that, shortly before she had become upset, she had met a woman friend in the park who knew the doctor's wife, and that the patient had made inquiries about her competitor. The patient was soon able to relate this behavior to the situation of her childhood home.

It is common for the hysteric to ask the doctor questions such as, "Are you married?" or, "Do you have any children?" Rather than answer these, the interviewer could reply, "What are you curious about?" or, "What did you have in mind?" If the interviewer does elect to answer these questions, he must realize that he will eventually have to draw the line, as the patient will say at some point, "Tell me about your wife."

A borderline patient, having learned from the doorman that the doctor lived in the same building as his office, waited outside all day in order to discover the identity of his wife. If such behavior persists or becomes troublesome to the doctor, it often suggests a countertransference problem, since the patient receives subtle encouragement from either the doctor's anxiety or his enjoyment of the patient's interest.

The hysteric evokes guilt in the interviewer by continually placing him in the position of having to choose between being an indulgent parent and a depriving, punitive one. Even the most skillful interviewer cannot always avoid this dilemma. The physician can use a combination of sympathy and interpretation. The hysteric soon asks, either directly or indirectly, for special privileges. He may request a glass of water or an aspirin, or to use the physician's telephone. The female patient might ask to change her clothes in his bathroom, or to have her friends meet her in his waiting room. One hysteric, who noted that a plant in the physician's office was dying, brought a new one. Another patient who came into the session drinking a Coke remarked, "I didn't have time enough for lunch today." The interviewer is put in the position of choosing between denying the patient lunch or permitting her to eat during the session. The physician could remark, "I agree that you are entitled to lunch, but is it necessary to have it right now?"

In general, the interviewer should explore the underlying motivation rather than grant these requests. Hysterical patients with more serious ego defects might be treated more indulgently early in the treatment. The physician will be more successful if he avoids an unreasonable, rigid approach. For example, if the patient explains that there were people waiting at the only public telephone near his office and requests the use of the telephone for a personal call, the doctor should grant the request and refrain from interpreting the behavior unless he learns that the patient distorted the situation, or that the call could easily have waited until later.

Sometimes the patient will mention that he has discussed his treatment with a friend. On other occasions, the patient may indicate that a friend made some particular comment about the patient's treatment or the patient's therapist. For example, the patient might say, "My friend does not agree with what you told me last time." The therapist inquires, "What did you tell your friend I said?" In this way, the therapist will learn the nature of the patient's distortions of his remarks. The interviewer can interrupt the patient to ask, "Is that what you thought I said?" Often the patient will be able to recall the physician's actual statement, but then add, "But I thought you meant . . ." or, "What I repeated is almost what you said." It is important to demonstrate the distortion before attempting to analyze its meaning. A series of such experiences with the patient will quickly reveal the nature of the transference. An alternate method is to explore why the patient wants to discuss his treatment with someone else.

When the hysterical patient and the physician are of the same sex, competitive behavior is more prominent in the transference. The female hysteric expresses feelings of envy about the woman physician's "stimulating professional life." At the same time, she looks for opportunities to imply that the physician is not a good mother, dresses in poor taste, or is not very feminine. The patient usually experiences disappointment that her therapist is a woman, and this can be interpreted quite early in treatment.

The major countertransference problems involve the physician's erotic response to the patient's seductive charm and helplessness, his enjoyment of the patient's capacity for apparent insights, and his anger at the patient's demanding behavior. Few therapists can avoid personal emotional responses to this patient. Beginning therapists have particular difficulty, as they alternate between inappropriate indulgence and angry rigidity.

The warmth and seductive behavior of the female patient is frightening because of its sexual implication, with the result that the male interviewer becomes aloof, cold, and business-like, allowing no engagement in the interview. The physician can look for opportunities to initiate engagement with the patient instead of merely responding to the patient's attempts at control.

As the interviewer acquires experience and professional maturity, he finds it easier to be firm with the hysteric and at the same time to be kind and understanding. The hysteric always responds to the doctor's understanding by feeling loved. This feeling is followed by unreasonable demands. The physician cannot gratify these demands and the patient then feels rejected. The treatment of this patient typically alternates between these two extremes.

One of the easiest ways to avoid being manipulated in the matter of decisions is to admit to the patient that the interviewer does not know what would be best for the patient. At the same time, this challenges the patient's image of the physician as an omniscient figure of authority. If the patient does succeed in manipulating the doctor, it is possible to use the experience constructively instead of becoming angry with the patient. The interviewer could ask, "Do you feel that this is the way that I can best help you?" or, "Why is it so important to manipulate me in this way?" The patient will often misinterpret the firmness or control on the doctor's part as a rejection and as an attempt to inhibit the patient's spontaneous feelings. This misperception stems from the patient's inability to experience a subjective sense of emotional freedom and at the same time successfully regulate and control his life. This is why the female hysteric has an obsessive partner. He manages practical matters that require order and organization; she expresses emotion both for herself and her partner.

In summary, the hysteric is one of the most enjoyable patients to treat. Although there are many stressful periods for the patient and the doctor, the experience is rarely boring. As treatment progresses, the patient will eventually develop his capacity for genuine emotional responses and also manage his own life. His emotional swings will become less marked as he gradually is able to understand and accept his deeper feelings and repressed sexual wishes. The physician will usually feel some personal enrichment from this therapeutic experience in addition to the satisfaction customarily derived from helping his patient.

REFERENCES

Abse, D. W.: Hysteria. In Arieti, S. (ed.): American Handbook of Psychiatry, Vol. 1. New York, Basic Books, Inc., 1959, Chap. 14, pp. 272–291.

Blinder, M. G.: The hysterical personality. Psychiatry, 29:227, 1966.

Chodoff, P., and Lyons, H.: Hysteria, hysterical personality, and "hysterical" conversion. Amer. J. Psychiat., 114:734, 1958.

Easser, B. R., and Lesser, S. R.: Hysterical personality: A re-evaluation. Psychoanal. Quart., 34:390, 1965.

Easser, B. R., and Lesser, S. R.: Transference resistances in hysterical character neurosis—technical considerations. In Goldman, G., and Shapiro, D. (eds.): Developments in Psychoanalysis at Columbia University. New York, Hafner, 1965, p. 69.

Freud, S.: Fragment of an analysis of a case of hysteria. Standard Edition of Complete Psychological Works of Sigmund Freud, Vol. VII. London, Hogarth Press, 1953, pp. 3–122.

Freud, S., and Breuer, J.: Studies on hysteria. Standard Edition of Complete Psychological Works of Sigmund Freud, Vol. II. London, Hogarth Press, 1955.

Guze, S. B., and Perley, M. J.: Observations on natural history of hysteria. Amer. J. Psychiat., 119:960, 1963.

Halleck, S. L.: Hysterical personality traits—psychological, social, and introgenic determinants. Arch. Gen. Psych., 16:750, 1967.

Reich, W.: Character-Analysis. New York, Orgone Institute Press, 1949.

Zeigler, F. J., Imboden, J. B., and Meyer, E.: Contemporary conversion reactions. I. Clinical Study. Amer. J. Psychiat., 116:901, 1960.

Zeigler, F. J., and Imboden, J. B.: Contemporary conversion reactions. II. A conceptual model. Arch. Gen. Psychiat., 6:279, 1962.

Zeigler, F. J., Imboden, J. B., and Rogers, D. A.: Contemporary conversion reactions. JAMA, 186:91, 1963.

5 THE PHOBIC PATIENT

Psychopathology and Psychodynamics

Although the psychodynamic basis of phobic behavior seems relatively simple at first glance, the beginning psychiatrist continues to have difficulty in interviewing the phobic patient. The obsessive or hysterical neurotic may seem to be more complex, but the doctor soon finds that the phobic patient presents tenacious problems in the interview. He quickly develops magical expectations of the physician, which become a major source of resistance.

Phobic behavior is found in a wide variety of neurotic and psychotic syndromes. The phobic person copes with his inner emotional conflict and anxiety by attempting to repress his disturbing thoughts and impulses. When this repression fails, he displaces his conflict to a place or situation in the outside world, and tries to confine his anxiety to that situation. The external situation now symbolically represents his inner psychological conflict; if he can avoid this situation, he can decrease his anxiety. It is this avoidance that is the essence of the phobia. The specific symptom is usually a symbolic condensation that includes aspects both of the forbidden wish or impulse and of the unconscious fear that prevents its direct gratification. Phobic defenses lead to a general constriction of personality as the patient relinquishes freedom and pleasurable activity in order to avoid conflict and anxiety.

147

The term "phobia" is sometimes misused. The "cancer phobic," for instance, suffers from an obsessive fear, or perhaps a hypochondriacal idea, but not a true avoidance. Another misuse is illustrated by the phrase "success phobia," which refers to a psychodynamic formulation explaining an unconscious fear of success. The patient with "cancer phobia" may avoid going to hospitals, and the patient with a "success phobia" may avoid vocational advancement because of an unconscious fear. This overt avoidance then becomes a phobic symptom, psychodynamically based on fear, although in its clinical usage the term is not a synonym for fear.

PHOBIC SYMPTOMS

The phobic individual is characterized by his use of avoidance as a primary means of resolving problems. In the classic phobic reaction, neurotic symptoms dominate the patient's existence. His mental life centers on unrealistic and distressing fears—open spaces, heights, subways, dirt, and so on. The phobia always involves something that the patient can and does encounter frequently. He offers rational explanations for his fear, but usually recognizes that these only partially account for his feelings. However, although he perceives his fear to be inappropriate, he feels that avoidance of the phobic situation is the only reasonable choice in view of his intense fear. The patient will agree that it is irrational to be afraid of the subway, but he is convinced that since he is afraid, he has no alternative but to keep away!

Phobic symptoms frequently progress and extend from one situation to another. A woman who is first afraid of buses becomes fearful of crossing streets and finally even hesitates to venture outdoors. A man who is frightened of eating in restaurants overcomes this fear, but is then unable to ride on subways. Patients will not readily volunteer the details of their initial symptoms, and it may require many interviews to uncover the fear that precipitated the first episode. Such persistence is worthwhile, as it is in the original context that the major psychodynamics will be exposed. This, of course, accounts for the patient's propensity to obscure the matter.

The typical phobic patient attempts to conquer his fears. As he does so, shifts in symbolization or displacement result in the substitution of new phobias for the old ones. The new symptoms may be less distressing to the patient, or may involve more secondary gain, but they are always aimed at avoiding the same basic conflict.

PHOBIC CHARACTER TRAITS

Far more common than the symptomatic phobia is the use of avoidance and inhibition as characterological defenses. This is present in all patients who have phobic symptoms, but is also widespread in other individuals. The psychodynamics of phobic character traits are similar to those of phobic symptoms. In both, the patient avoids a situation that represents a source of anxiety, but in the phobic character the fear is usually unconscious and the avoidance is explained as a matter of taste or preference. Often interest or intrigue are mixed with fear, representing the emergence of the forbidden wish, and the patient envies people who can comfortably enter the phobic area. To illustrate, a young woman who did not like speaking in front of groups envied her husband's ability to do so, and felt that this ability meant that he was totally free of all anxiety. Other patients may be unaware of the neurotic basis of their avoidance, but accompanying symptoms of anxiety will reveal the underlying emotional conflict. An attorney who avoided all athletic activity was a devoted follower of newspaper accounts and telecasts of sports events. On occasion he would feel palpitations and faintness during the violent moments of football games. The anxiety that prevented him from participating in his childhood emerged directly when he was a spectator in adult life. If the denial is more extensive, there is simply a lack of interest in the entire area. This is recognized as defensive avoidance only when the person's life situation exposes his inhibition as maladaptive. For example, a housewife living in a large city can explain her inability to drive a car as a reasonable choice, but when she moves to the suburbs and still refuses to drive, the neurotic basis of the preference is exposed.

Phobic traits can be basic to the character structure. The individual is preoccupied with his security and fears any possible threat to it, constantly imagining himself in situations of danger while pursuing the course of greatest safety. This person is familiar as the man who spends his vacations at home, pursues the same interests, reads the same authors, and works at the same tasks, year in and year out. He has a limited number of friends and avoids new experiences.

Perhaps the most common example of phobic character traits is the young woman who is married to an older man. She lives near her mother and speaks to her by telephone several times daily. Her children have also developed phobic symptoms and are excused from school gym classes because of minor physical difficulties. The family members are familiar visitors to their general practitioner's office. The woman looks younger than her age and is quite charming with men, although not quite as popular with her female friends. At times she may seem impulsively exhibitionistic, as her seductiveness emerges in protected social settings. The man with a similar defensive pattern is more prominently concerned with assertion than with sexuality. His boyishness is often mixed with so much bravado that he may seem more foolhardy than frightened. This defensive assertiveness is more likely to be aimed at a powerful superior than at a peer, and he hopes he will be seen as a self-confident and promising young man, but does not expect to be seen as an adult.

The phobic individual usually values sexual behavior primarily for the accompanying sense of warmth and security. He is often reluctant to initiate sex, thereby hoping to avoid any responsibility for acting on forbidden impulses.

RELATIONSHIP TO OTHER PERSONALITY TYPES

Phobic defenses are often seen in patients whose personality types are predominantly obsessive or hysteric. The resulting clinical picture reflects both the phobic avoidance and the more basic character structure. This patient's conflicts are revealed through exploration of his phobic defenses. He often has no awareness of their content, which may involve dependency, sexuality, or aggression.

The obsessive-phobic individual is most often concerned with the avoidance of aggression. He may be fearful of knives or of driving a car. These fears may extend to symbols of control and power. A successful businessman with a strongly obsessive character refused to touch any money, a symbol of social power. The obsessive spends hours ruminating about his phobia, and his constant preoccupation is often more disabling than the actual symptom itself. Every obsessive patient, even if he does not have phobic symptoms, will reveal some characterological inhibitions that involve defensive avoidance. For example, one may see an aversion to contact sports rather than a symptomatic fear of handling knives or sharp objects. In this case, aggressive impulses are avoided through an inhibition of activity, rather than by a neurotic symptom relating to symbols of aggression.

The conflicts of the hysterical patient with phobic defenses are most likely to involve sex or dependency. Symptoms are frequently elaborated and dramatized. It may require many interviews to determine the content of the patient's phobias. To illustrate, in an initial interview a woman described her fear of walking in the street alone. She denied awareness of what she feared, admitting only that she might become "upset." Several interviews later, she added that she feared that a man might make sexual advances. Her fear that she might not decline such overtures was only revealed after years of treatment. The hysteric-phobic patient is frightened by her own emotionality, and avoids experiences that produce overwhelming emotions. Either her sexual responses are inhibited or her sexual behavior is almost non-existent. Some fears involve physical sensations that are similar to those of sexual excitement. The avoidance of roller-coasters is an example; both the popularity of such experiences and the common phobias of them are explained by the exciting sensations accompanying the ride.

It is common for several conflicts to be represented symbolically by a single phobia. An agoraphobic woman who insists on being accompanied on the street by her husband avoids sexual temptation, and her husband's presence also reassures her that he has not been injured. Her interest in other men and her fears for her husband's welfare are both related to her repressed anger toward her husband, and this anger is more directly expressed by her excessive demands, which restrict his life as well. Her phobic symptom enables her to obtain gratification of infantile dependent wishes, while at the same time avoiding direct expression of her sexual and aggressive feelings. The denial and avoidance of these impulses stem from an early fear of the parental disapproval that would result from their recognition and gratification.

Phobic defenses are only partially effective, and the phobic individual continues to experience anxiety. Therefore, phobic patients typically experience the emotional and physical symptoms of anxiety, e.g., palpitation, dyspnea, dizziness, syncope, sweating, and gastrointestinal distress. These may form the basis for hypochondriacal preoccupation and fears of death or insanity in more severely phobic patients.

The psychiatrist's reassurance and simple explanation of the psychological basis of these physiological symptoms may seem to be readily accepted by the phobic person; however, he is prone to continue his worries about somatic illnesses, and often pursues other medical treatment without telling the psychiatrist. When he obtains evidence of an organic disease, or when some medical treatment leads to improvement, he has further support for his own belief that his problem is really physical and that emotional conflicts are of little importance.

MECHANISMS OF DEFENSE

DISPLACEMENT AND SYMBOLIZATION

For avoidance to be effective, the conflict within the mind of the patient must be displaced to the outside world. When displacement occurs without symbolization, the patient shifts his attention from an emotional conflict to the environment in which that conflict occurs. For example, the child who is fearful of competitive relations with his classmates avoids going to gym. More elaborate displacements may be based upon symbolic representation. This is seen in Freud's case of "Little Hans," whose fear of horses was traced to a fear of his father, who had been represented by the animals. Every mechanism of symbolic representation may be involved, and the interpretation of phobic symptoms is as complex as the interpretation of dreams. Displacement can also be based on some accidental connection between the emotional conflict and a particular place or situation. This is readily seen in a man who took refuge in a movie theatre during the bombing of his city, and then later developed a strong aversion to movies.

In most clinical phobias, all of these mechanisms are involved. For example, the common fear of subways in young women is often traced to the symbolic sexual significance of the subway, which is a powerful vehicle that travels through a tunnel and vibrates in the darkness. The ride may also recall provocative experiences of previous subway trips, and the patient's emotional responses to these.

PROJECTION

Phobic avoidance often involves projection as well as displacement and symbolization. The analysis of a subway phobia may first reveal a fear of attack, then a fear of sexual attack, and finally a fear of loss of control over sexual impulses. The patient's impulses are projected onto the other riders in the subway, and this projection allows the patient to rationalize the fear.

The link between phobic defenses and projection relates to the link between phobic and paranoid traits. Like the paranoid, the phobic patient uses relatively primitive defenses, with denial playing a prominent role. He thinks concretely, focuses on the external environment rather than his inner feelings, and keeps secrets from the interviewer. However, in contrast to the paranoid patient, the phobic maintains reality testing. He denies the inner world of emotions more than the outer world of perception. The phobic patient displaces his anxiety to the environment and projects his impulses onto others, but rarely onto anyone emotionally important to him. He maintains firm object relationships in order to insure continued gratification of his dependent needs. Therefore, the initial interviews are conducted with an aura of goodwill. The patient represses his hostile or negative feelings and often exhibits an infantile confidence in the doctor's magical ability to alleviate his distress.

AVOIDANCE

The defensive utilization of avoidance is the essential characteristic of the phobic individual. The ancillary defenses of symbolization, displacement, and rationalization serve to make the avoidance possible. Phobic defenses are effective only when anxiety can be confined to a specific situation that the individual is able to avoid, so that his psychological conflicts will no longer disturb him. This sequestration of anxiety to an external situation is rarely effective, and therefore the phobic individual must also avoid thinking about his internal conflicts. It soon becomes apparent in the interview that a phobic individual does not, cannot, or simply will not discuss certain topics. The central problem in interviewing or treating a phobic patient is to lead him, even at times to urge him, to move into the areas that he avoids, into areas of thought in the interview, and into areas of action in his daily life. The patient must be encouraged to do something that he does not want to do, but the interviewer must not make the patient phobic of the interview itself. This usually means allowing the patient to establish a dependent relationship and then using it to reward him for entering frightening situations.

The phobic patient shows a striking intolerance to anxiety, and it is this fear of anxiety that usually motivates him to seek help. He may be able to avoid the object of his phobia, and even be able to avoid thinking of his conflicts, but he is not able to avoid the anticipatory anxiety of what would happen if he were to enter the phobic situation. His usual goal in treatment is to become immune to anxiety, even in circumstances that would frighten anyone. During the treatment, the physician must inquire not only into what is so frightening about the phobic situation or the forbidden impulses, but also into the patient's intolerance of anxiety.

THE PHOBIC PARTNER

The patient's fear of anxiety is highly contagious, particularly for other individuals with unconscious phobic tendencies. The partner of the phobic patient, who accompanies him whenever he ventures outdoors or across the street, has accepted the patient's belief that anxiety must be avoided at all costs. If the patient improves with treatment, the partner can become a major obstacle to therapy as his latent phobias become more manifest. Questions such as, "Are you sure she's ready to try it by herself, Doctor?" are common. The patient will often attempt to enlist the interviewer into the partner role. He does this by dramatizing his anxiety and suggesting that the interviewer's help is all that is needed to conquer the problem. This infantile magical orientation toward treatment may feed the interviewer's omnipotent fantasies, but it only reconstructs the pattern of relationships which created the phobia.

COUNTERPHOBIC BEHAVIOR

Counterphobic patterns are an interesting developmental variant in which the patient denies his phobias. His behavior dramatizes his disregard of realistic fears, and he seems to prefer situations in which there is a danger of disastrous consequences. This patient has also displaced his anxiety to an external situation, and has symbolized his unconscious fear by a realistic external danger. However, whereas the phobic person then avoids the external situation, the counterphobic individual tries to master the realistic danger and thus conquer his unconscious fear. Both defensive patterns involve magical thinking. The phobic patient usually selects a situation in which there is some realistic danger, however slight, and then magically believes that it will certainly happen to him. The counterphobic person selects a setting in which danger is possible, or even probable, but never certain. His magical feeling is, "It can't happen to me." The individual who is fearful of asserting himself with women, and yet participates in high-risk athletic activities, is a common example.

Mixtures of phobic and counterphobic defenses are common, and detailed investigation of counterphobic persons often reveals widespread patterns of inhibition in other areas of life. For example, the same individual who risks life and limb racing cars might be uncomfortable speaking in public. Counterphobic defenses may provide greater secondary gain and social usefulness, and, as with all symptoms, it is necessary to separate their adaptive value from their neurotic origins. They may also allow relatively direct gratification of the forbidden impulses, but with little flexibility or spontaneity of behavior. The counterphobic individual rarely seeks help for this pattern, but the dangerous or self-destructive aspects of his behavior may alarm others.

DEVELOPMENTAL PSYCHODYNAMICS

Phobic symptoms are universal in children. In fact, although initially they are frequently denied, the existence of childhood phobias will eventually emerge in the history of almost every neurotic patient. The widespread phobic symptoms of children

no doubt reflect the normal tendency toward primitive and magical thought in the developing child.

The phobic individual learns as a child that the world is a
frightening and unpredictable place. His parents may reinforce
this view through either their timidity or their explosive or violent
outbursts. In some families, the mother is herself somewhat
phobic, and the father unpredictably irritable and angry. The
whole family is frightened of his spells, and tries to avoid them.
Other patterns are common; for example, the father may share
the mother's fearfulness, and the threat of aggression may come
from outside the family circle. There is an important difference
between the typical childhood experiences of the paranoid and
of the phobic. Both involve the fear of rage and even violence,
but the family of the phobic offers some hope of safety, so that
the child does develop a sense of potential security, though at a
price of anxiety and diminished self-confidence. In contrast, the
paranoid person learned that the only security from external
dangers that his family could provide involved a total loss of his
sense of identity, and that his only chance for both independence
and safety resided in constant lonely vigilance.

The phobic person overestimates both the dangers of the
outside world and the inner emotional danger of anxiety. The
fears of outer dangers have often been learned directly from his
parents. At times these may be reinforced by actual increases in
danger, either because the child is vulnerable, as in the chronically
ill, or because the family lives in a neighborhood that presents
realistic dangers. The exaggerated fear of anxiety is related to
the mother's inability to perceive her child's emotional state and
her consequent defensive overprotection. The infant needs both
adequate exposure to external stimuli and protection from over-
stimulation. The appropriate balance between these is a function
of the mother's sensitivity to her child's signals of distress. If she
responds indiscriminately to all such signals, the child does not
have an opportunity to develop a normal tolerance for anxiety.
In other words, the mother's anxiety and consequent difficulty in
responding to her child can lead to the later development of
intolerance to anxiety in that child.

The mother's insensitivity to and overevaluation of the
child's anxiety continues through the subsequent stages of development. She responds to his normal separation anxiety by refusing
to allow him out of her sight, she handles his stranger anxiety by

limiting his contacts with new people, and she teaches him to deny sexual or aggressive impulses that may lead to conflict with his parents or with his developing super-ego. At each stage of development, the child fails to conquer his anxiety and must learn to deal with it in some other way. He copies not only his parents' fears of the world, but also their unusual sensitivity to fear and their mode of coping with it. His fear increases his dependency on his parents and makes any expression of anger toward them all the more dangerous.

Normal anxieties seem intolerable, and he defends himself from them with phobic symptoms. One result is that his symptoms replace his emotions, and the phobic individual will describe his responses in symptomatic rather than affective terms.

The developmental history of the phobic patient typically reveals that he was afraid of the dark, of being alone in his bedroom at night, of nightmares, and the "bogey man." The door to his room was left open, or his light was left on. He was comforted by these reassurances that his family was close at hand. His parents emphasized the dangers of traffic in the street, bullies in the playground, evil men lurking in the park, or the hand of fate in the form of terrible illness. He was warned never to cross the street or to ride his bike after dark, although his peers had long engaged in these activities. Parental prophecies about bullies were accurate, as his timidity provoked bullying behavior from his classmates. If he did not want to go to camp, or became frightened of school, his family reacted to these fears by allowing him to avoid the situations that caused them.

The phobic patient frequently utilized one of his parents as a partner during his childhood. By agreeing to accompany and protect the child, the parent not only encouraged the development of phobic defenses, but also revealed his own underlying phobic character. The child was led to feel that his own adaptive skills were inadequate, and that magical reliance on his parent would somehow help to compensate for this. If he was helpless, his parents might be able to protect him. He learned to conceal his forbidden thoughts and wishes and to dramatize his fear and need for parental assistance, so that they would guarantee his security. This device continues into later life, as the individual uses his symptoms in order to placate external authorities and his own super-ego, and thus to gain permission for the gratification of his impulses.

The combination of little self-confidence, low tolerance for anxiety, a dependent mode of adaptation, a tendency for magical thinking, early exposure to models who use phobic defenses, and the use of symptoms and suffering as a means of dealing with authorities, leads to the development of the phobic character.

Management of the Interview

The phobic patient relates easily during the initial portion of the interview. He comes seeking relief, and is polite and eager to talk about his problems. Silence and resistance arise later in the interview, but the opening moments are marked by an aura of goodwill. As the interview progresses, it becomes apparent that the patient's agreeableness continues only if the interviewer cooperates with the patient's defenses; that is, if he helps the patient avoid anxiety by not pursuing certain topics and by promising magical protection. The task of the interviewer is to direct the discussion into these forbidden areas, but at the same time to maintain the rapport necessary to sustain the relationship through the painful exploration of the patient's psychological problems.

EARLY COOPERATION

The phobic patient is frequently accompanied to the first appointment. He may come with a member of his family or with a friend. If he comes alone, he often expects to be picked up afterward, or his companion is waiting in the car. If the interviewer has reason to suspect that the patient is phobic, it is advisable to see the patient alone, speaking to his companion only afterwards, if at all. If the diagnosis is not apparent until both are in the doctor's office, the doctor should use the first convenient opportunity to dismiss the companion in order to speak with the patient alone. The companion's presence protects the patient from anxiety by inhibiting thoughts and feelings that are disturbing. Since the doctor wants to explore these thoughts and feelings, he is more likely to be successful if the companion is not present. There is no purpose in interpreting the defense at this point, and a simple "Could you wait outside while I speak with your brother?" or, "Can we talk alone while your husband waits outside?" will suffice. The request should be addressed to the individual who the interviewer senses is least likely to object.

Some phobic patients have an almost exhibitionistic eagerness to relate their distress and describe their inability to overcome irrational fears. Others are more ashamed of their problems, and may conceal their symptoms. The interviewer will learn to recognize the latter group by the overt anxiety and the extensive use of avoidance in the patient's life and in the interview itself. Whether the patient presents his symptoms as a chief complaint, or reveals them only reluctantly, he is more eager to obtain the doctor's reassurance than to investigate his own emotional life. The interviewer, however, wants to discuss the patient's problems and symptoms and thereby gain some understanding of the patient's psychological conflicts. In view of these discrepant goals, the natural starting point for the interview is a discussion of the symptoms.

Early in the interview, the patient may ask, "Will you be able to help me?" The timing of the question suggests that it is a request for magical reassurance. The interviewer can use this as a lever to initiate a more thorough investigation of the problems, replying, "I can't give you an answer to that until you've told me more about yourself." He offers the promise of future help in return for enduring present anxiety. Although many patients experience relief from simply talking about their problems, this process makes the phobic patient more anxious. He needs a direct promise of the benefit before he will participate in the treatment process.

EXPLORING THE SYMPTOMS

The problems encountered in interviewing a phobic patient are often encapsulated in the exploration of his phobic symptoms. Obsessive and hysteric patients also have symptoms, but their discussion is seldom a central focus of resistance. The phobic patient responds differently. His characteristic defenses often emerge in the discussion of his symptom, just as they did in its formation. When the interviewer tries to talk about the patient's behavior, the patient shifts the discussion to a neutral topic, or asks the doctor for help while avoiding exposure of his problems.

His displacement of inner conflicts to the outside world may appear as a concentration on the external arrangements of treatment, on the doctor's behavior, on medication, or on any other issue that is removed from his inner thoughts and feelings.

His symptoms are associated with considerable anxiety, and may be offered as the chief complaint or mentioned early in the interview. The doctor asks for a detailed description of the symptom, the situations which evoke it, the history of its development, and the therapeutic measures that the patient has attempted on his own behalf before coming to the psychiatrist.

UNRAVELLING THE DETAILS

The interviewer carefully listens to every aspect of the patient's description of his symptoms in order to understand their psychological significance. For example, one woman who is afraid of crowds may emphasize her concern about the people who brush against her; another will speak of her feeling of being "alone in the midst of strangers." The first description would suggest concern about sexual feelings; the second connotes anxiety over separation from the sources of dependency gratification. Of course, the interviewer would not interpret this to the patient until the advanced stages of treatment.

The consequences that a patient fears if he were to enter the phobic situation may involve the projection of a repressed wish or the fear of its expression and the retaliation that would ensue. The patient may be able to elaborate detailed fantasies of what he fears, with no awareness that he is describing a wish. This is valuable information for the doctor, but again, it cannot be shared with the patient early in treatment. For example, a woman who was afraid to go out on the streets was able to portray in vivid detail the sexual assault she feared. However, it was many months before she was aware of her own sexual desires. The phobic symptom may represent the unconscious fear far more clearly than the forbidden wish. A woman described her fear of restaurants, and the doctor inquired, "What would happen if you did go into a restaurant?" The patient replied, "I would get upset," expecting the interviewer to stop at this point. Instead he asked, "And what would happen if you did get upset?" The patient was surprised and answered with annoyance,

"I might faint and have to be carried out on a stretcher." The interviewer continued, "And what if that happened?" Now the patient felt justified in her anger, and she replied, "How would you like to be carried out on a stretcher, Doctor?" The interviewer answered, "We both know that you have a dread of such a situation that is different from the distaste that the predicament would hold for others, and I would like to help you with it." The patient relaxed, saying, "Well, my dress might come up —people might notice the rash on my legs, or they might say, 'Look at that one, she must be on her way to the booby hatch.' "

The interviewer had uncovered the patient's fear of going crazy as well as her shame about her appearance. Further exploration revealed a mixture of exhibitionistic and aggressive impulses, and her self-punitive need to be controlled and humiliated in retaliation for them.

The Initial Episode

The initial episode of the symptom is particularly enlightening. A middle-aged woman who was afraid of eating meat could offer no explanation for this behavior, but was able to recall that it had first occurred at the dinner table during an argument between her husband and daughter. She later revealed that a frequent battle in her childhood centered on the religious proscription against eating meat on Fridays. The symptom was related to her fear of the open display of aggression both in her current life and in her childhood.

Physiological Symptoms

In describing their symptoms, some patients discuss their subjective sense of anxiety, whereas others, utilizing more extensive denial, emphasize the physiological concomitants of anxiety, such as trembling, palpitation, or chest pain. The interviewer can lay the groundwork for future interpretations by linking these physical responses to the appropriate subjective states. He might say, "When you get giddy and faint, there must be something frightening you," or, "That tightness in your chest is the kind of feeling people get when they are anxious." Some phobic individuals experience anxiety as a diffuse bodily sensation that borders on depersonalization. If hyperventilation plays an important role in the production of symptoms, the patient may loosen his collar, complain that the room is stuffy, or ask to have the window opened.

A common physiological manifestation of anxiety, which the phobic patient tries to ignore, is the gurgling of his stomach. When this occurs during the interview and the patient reacts with discomfort, the interviewer can remark, "It seems as though you're embarrassed about the noises your body makes." This indicates that the interviewer is comfortable discussing such matters, and that the patient's feelings about his body are an appropriate topic for the interview.

IDENTIFICATION

If the patient has ever known anyone with a similar symptom, the exploration of this relationship can offer further insight. Phobic patients frequently employ relatively primitive modes of identification, and phobic symptoms are often based on a specific model. It is unusual not to uncover a phobic parent or grandparent, or some other individual who offered a phobic pattern for the patient to imitate. Furthermore, the patient usually has great empathy for other phobic persons, and may have surprising insight into the dynamic significance of the other person's symptom, although he is quite unable to see the same mechanism in his own behavior.

CHANGES IN THE SYMPTOMS

It is revealing for the interviewer to detail the shifts and developments in the history of the symptom. A specific conflict that is difficult to identify in any given symptom becomes obvious when this historical pattern is viewed as a whole. For example, a man presented a fear of eating in restaurants. When more details were elicited, he revealed that this was a recent symptom, and that previously he had been afraid of traveling on trains. The history soon revealed a long string of apparently unconnected phobic symptoms, all of which occurred in situations in which he could not be reached by phone. He harbored great unconscious resentment of his mother, and his aggressive impulses toward her were manifested by a fantasy that she would become ill and be unable to contact him. His resulting guilt and anxiety were controlled by the phobic symptoms.

AVOIDANCE

THE PATIENT SENSES DANGER

At some point, the interview progresses to a more general discussion of the patient's life. The interviewer may ask "What are your other worries?", or inquire into the patient's mode of dealing with problems in his life. The patient is skillful at shifting the topic to comfortable subjects, and the interviewer's task is to frame the questions so that the patient cannot escape dealing with the real issues. When this is successful, the avoidance mechanism will be seen in its purest form as the patient says, "I'd rather not talk about that," or, "That is very upsetting to me." This is a critical point in the interview, for it allows the interviewer to establish that anxiety is not a valid reason for avoidance. He can reply "I appreciate that it is difficult for you, but I know that you want help, so let's go ahead and see what we can do," or, "Try to do the best you can." In this way, he bargains with the patient, withholding the promise of help until the patient is willing to move into the phobic area, at least in his thinking.

It is difficult to provide the needed reassurance and at the same time to avoid condescension or the suggestion that the patient is an infant. However, with sicker or more dependent patients, the interviewer's direct assurance of protection from anxiety may be necessary—"I've treated other patients with this symptom, and I don't think that any harm will come to you." This is a magical maneuver, and it encourages a dependency adaptation on the part of the patient. It may solve the immediate problem only to create more serious future ones, but with a severely phobic patient the exchange of avoidance for magical dependency may represent a major improvement.

THE PATIENT'S SEARCH FOR TREATMENT

Phobic patients actively seek treatment. They consider it a form of insurance, and may collect therapies and remedies in the same way that other people collect insurance policies. There is a feeling of security that stems from having a doctor, and it is this security, rather than the therapeutic effect, that seems to motivate the patient's search.

Often the patient conceals his treatment from others, and it is helpful to ask the phobic patient who knows that he is seeing a psychiatrist. He may feel that he will get more support and reassurance from other people if they are not aware that a doctor is caring for him. He does not trust the physician to provide adequate assistance, and therefore feels safer if he is able to keep other channels open. At times this patient may see two doctors simultaneously, keeping one a secret from the other. One woman requested tranquilizers from the doctor because she feared that she might become anxious during his vacation. When he refused to supply them, she obtained a prescription from her gynecologist, not informing him that she was also seeing a psychiatrist. When the latter returned from his vacation, she wanted him to renew the prescription. She knew he didn't approve of the medication, but explained that she could get it from the other doctor anyway. She was indignant when the psychiatrist refused, feeling that he was inconsiderate of her many household obligations and the expense and inconvenience he would cause her if she had to return to the other doctor.

Phobic patients try to treat themselves. They develop magical rituals that partially alleviate their difficulties, and frequently conceal these from the doctor until they find out whether his "magic" is an adequate substitute. It is necessary to systematically but sympathetically explore the treatment techniques that the patient has utilized before coming to the psychiatrist. Useful questions include, "What do you do when you get anxious?", "Whom have you seen for help?", and "What kind of advice have other people given you?". The patient has usually consulted a number of doctors or other therapists before coming to the psychiatrist.

The patient's self-treatment often involves the substitution of one phobia for another, trying to maximize his secondary gain and minimize his realistic inconvenience and secondary pain, but still defending himself from anxiety. He may report with great pride that he has forced himself to ride in an airplane, as long as it isn't a jet, or to go out in crowds, as long as it is not at night. By bargaining with himself in this way, he achieves a subjective sense of trying to deal with his problems while continuing to avoid their psychological roots.

SECONDARY GAIN

The secondary gain is important to the interviewer because it aids in understanding the patient's psychodynamics and also because it provides one of the strongest resistances to change. The interviewer can ask, "What can't you do because of your symptoms?" This may seem to be a blunt inquiry into their psychodynamic meaning, but there is usually sufficient denial that the patient has no awareness that the answer reveals emotional conflicts. Other useful questions include, "What is the effect on your family if you are unable to go outdoors?" or, "How do you manage to get things done if you can't take the subway?" The patient often reveals discomfort in describing the impositions that he makes upon his family and friends. The interviewer can use this opportunity to sympathize with the embarrassed portion of the patient's mature ego.

For example, with a woman who reveals discomfort while describing her need to be accompanied to the neighborhood store by her husband, the interviewer can comment, "You are unhappy about asking him to go with you." The patient will either respond with further expression of her guilt or with an attack on her husband for his exploitation of her, justifying her own behavior. In either event, the comment has led to a shift from a discussion of the overt behavior to its emotional significance. It is true that the symptom may stem from hostility toward her husband, but this is too strongly repressed to be interpreted in an initial interview. It is more useful to reinforce the patient's conscious unhappiness with the secondary effects of her symptoms. This also avoids repeating the struggles with friends and family that every phobic patient has had before he comes to the doctor, and begins to cement an alliance between the therapist and the healthy portion of the patient's ego.

Those social acquaintances who recognize a psychological basis for the patient's difficulties usually interpret the secondary gain as providing the basic motivation. Their view is that the patient is manipulating his environment in order to obtain certain benefits. The patient responds with injured indignation, feeling that he is accused of enjoying painful symptoms over which he has no control. The interviewer can avoid this unfortunate struggle by maintaining his position of neutral inquirer into the patient's behavior, attempting to understand rather than to judge it. For example, if a patient's family thinks that she acts frightened of going outside in order to avoid her responsibilities, the interviewer can ask "How do you feel when they say things like that?" If she reveals her anger, he can support it, and if she denies it he can give her permission to express her feelings by commenting, "It must be annoying to be blamed for something over which you feel you have no control."

AVOIDANCE IN THE INTERVIEW

The defensive avoidance that characterizes the phobic symptom is also a critical resistance in the interview. It may appear as an inadvertent omission, a tendency to steer the conversation away from certain subjects, a request for permission not to talk about uncomfortable topics, or an outright refusal to speak.

This patient frequently omits crucial data about important areas of his life, and then denies responsibility for this omission. A phobic woman spoke at great length about her plans for marriage, but only inadvertently revealed that her fiancé was Oriental. She explained, "You never asked me about that," a characteristic phobic response. The interviewer replied, "Did you think I might have something to say about it?", addressing himself to the avoidance behind the patient's denial.

Another patient, a young psychologist with phobic character traits, first revealed that he had congenital heart disease when, after months of treatment, the therapist pursued a reference to his scar. The patient explained that the scar resulted from a childhood surgical procedure to correct the defect. The surprised therapist inquired, "Why have we never discussed this before?" The patient explained, "I didn't realize that it had any psychological significance." The interviewer responded with a direct confrontation, "It is hard for me to believe that, with your training, you could think that such a childhood experience was unimportant."

PRINCIPLES OF TREATMENT

THE NEED FOR REASSURANCE

After relating his difficulties, the phobic patient will seek reassurance. He may ask, "Do you think you can help me?" or, "Is there any hope?" Other patients may seek the same reassurance more indirectly, asking, "Have you ever treated any cases like mine?" The interviewer translates the meaning by responding, "I guess you wonder if I'll be able to help you." The phrasing of the patient's question has prognostic significance; the patient who is more optimistic and who expects to play an active role in his own treatment has a more favorable prognosis.

The doctor can reply to these requests for reassurance by saying, "The more we talk about your problems, the more I will be able to help you deal with them." This answer shifts some responsibility for the cure to the patient, while offering the doctor's assistance and at the same time indicating the first step that the patient must take.

The phobic patient also characteristically asks, "Am I going crazy?" His fear of anxiety leads him to perceive his symptoms as evidence of total emotional collapse, with the loss of all control over his impulses. He wants the doctor to take over, to tell him that he's not going crazy, and to assume the responsibility for his emotional controls. The question about going crazy provides an opportunity for exploring the content of the patient's fear. The doctor asks, "What do you mean, crazy?" or, "What do you think it would be like to be crazy?" He can further inquire whether the patient ever knew anyone who was crazy, and how that person behaved. Finally, he can offer reassurance coupled with an initial interpretation of the patient's inner psychological conflicts: "You must be frightened about the feelings you have bottled up inside. You've never lost control in the past, so why should it happen now?"

Often the patient will not be reassured by the content of what the doctor says, but he will detect the doctor's calm and lack of anxiety. Phobic patients frequently try to provoke anxiety in others, particularly in parental surrogates such as physicians. The way in which the doctor handles his own anxiety and his attitude toward his patients will serve as a model for the patient and, particularly in early interviews, is more important than any interpretation of the patient's behavior.

EDUCATING THE PATIENT

The phobic patient avoids far more than he is aware of, and one goal of the early interview is to explore the scope of the avoidance and to educate the patient about it. The initial interventions are aimed not at providing the patient with insight into his symptoms, but at expanding his awareness of neurotic inhibitions. The therapist might comment, "It is striking that you haven't said anything about the sexual aspects of your marriage," or, "Do you ever feel angry at anyone?" The patient will probably reply that he has no problems in these areas, that he has nothing to say about them, or that this has no bearing on his symptoms, but the groundwork for future interpretations is established.

One goal of treatment is to facilitate understanding of anxiety. Phobic patients often think that other people do not experience anxiety, and their goal is to become immune from it themselves. Early attempts to interpret this are bound to be superficial and ineffective. In time, the interviewer can indicate that anxiety is a normal emotion, and that the patient's anxiety is often appropriate, but only disproportionate to the stimuli that trigger it.

Questions concerning the patient's perception of other people's reactions are useful in increasing the patient's knowledge about anxiety. After a patient reported an anxiety attack following a "near miss" accident, the interviewer asked, "How did your friend feel at the time?" The patient answered, "He was a little upset, but not as upset as I." This provided an opportunity to explore the patient's overevaluation of his anxiety, and the fact that his responses were qualitatively similar to those of others. The interviewer replied, "Could it be that you were just more aware of your own feelings than you were of his?" The patient answered "No! He doesn't feel like I did. He isn't afraid of fainting or having a heart attack or feeling 'way out.' " The doctor then said, "It sounds as if you and your friend were afraid of different things, and his anxiety was only related to the danger and the accident." This provided an avenue for the exploration of the unconscious determinants of the patient's fear.

The phobic patient often needs assistance in recognizing his emotions. This has already been discussed in relation to anxiety, but it is also true of other feelings. Feelings are replaced by symptoms, and in time the doctor will learn the pattern this follows. When the patient describes a headache, the doctor can point out, "The last few times you complained about a headache you were angry at someone; are you angry again?"

MEDICATION

The phobic patient's search for treatment often emerges as a request for tranquilizing drugs. He asks the doctor for something to calm his nerves, or tells the doctor that he has already obtained such medication from someone else and wants to know whether he should take it. The question frequently comes at the end of the interview, as the patient is leaving the office, and there is no time for discussion. The patient's manner suggests that it cannot wait until the next appointment.

The doctor is tempted to dispose of the problem by the easiest response, i.e., providing a prescription for tranquilizers. This sets a pattern for the type of assistance that the patient will expect. The opposite response, telling the patient that the question will have to be discussed at the time of the next appointment, may lead the patient to feel that the doctor doesn't understand the urgency of his problem. The dilemma is created by taking the question at face value. The patient is not simply asking for a pill; he wants assurance that the doctor has powerful magic that offers protection from anxiety and provides safety and security. The doctor can sometimes alleviate the patient's anxiety by simply identifying it, saying, "You seem concerned about whether I'll be able to help you." The doctor can then add, "Whether to use tranquilizing medication is an important decision that we cannot make in just a few minutes. I know you don't feel well, but I think we should discuss medication next time, when we can talk about it more fully." The discussion of medication at the end of the session can be prevented by early systematic inquiry into what treatments the patient has considered in the past. If he does not mention medication, the doctor can ask about it, and specifically ask why the patient has not tried it, without implying that he should have done so. The phobic patient who has not experimented with tranquilizers is more likely phobic of the medicine than desirous of solving his problems through other routes. Often the patient has received a prescription from a previous physician, but has not yet used it. The interviewer should discuss this carefully, since the fears that prevented the patient from following the former doctor's advice are usually still active, and offer an opportunity for early exploration of an important resistance.

Although the use of tranquilizing drugs in the treatment of phobic syndromes cannot be fully discussed in a book on interviewing, certain aspects of the strategy of drug treatment illustrate a major point in the interview of phobic patients. The patient wants relief from his anxiety, and the drugs seem to promise such relief. Any reluctance on the part of the doctor to provide these drugs will seem to be cruel and unreasonable. The doctor can make use of the magical comfort that the drugs represent by linking it to the patient's entry into the phobic situation. If the patient will try to enter the situation that makes him anxious, the assurance provided by the medicine may speed his progress. If, on the other hand, he takes tranquilizing drugs to alleviate his normal anxiety, without increasing his range of activity, he will grow dependent on the drug with no net improvement in his condition. Phobic patients who are given medication on a P.R.N. basis, for use only when they enter the situation that makes them anxious, frequently report that they never actually use the drug. The insurance of having it available is all that is necessary.

The Role of Interpretation

The early activity of the interviewer is aimed at encouraging the patient to tell his story, to describe the details of his symptoms, and to discuss his personal life. The patient doesn't want to talk about his sexual, aggressive, or competitive feelings, but it is important that he be urged to do so. The interviewer demonstrates that he is not phobic of these areas of life, and that he expects the patient to follow his lead.

In these early phases of contact, it is seldom helpful to challenge the patient's avoidance in the outside world, but the doctor quickly interprets the avoidance that appears in the interview, such as the omission of important material or the refusal to discuss some area of life. Premature direct suggestions or interpretations concerning the psychological meaning of a phobic symptom will increase the patient's defensiveness and interfere with the interview. The interviewer characteristically understands far more than he interprets to the phobic patient.

When a phobic symptom is analyzed, anxiety and avoidance are discussed before symbolization or displacement. The patient must first realize that he is anxious, and that he avoids the source of his anxiety, before he can begin to explore the conflicts that underlie it. Projection is usually interpreted after the other defenses have been thoroughly analyzed.

The specific secondary gains associated with the patient's symptoms may offer clues as to what type of bargain will be most effective in getting the patient to relinquish his phobia. In time, the doctor will offer to replace these secondary gains, but will require as a precondition that the patient enter the feared area. Medication, magical reassurance, and supportive interest and concern can be used as substitutes for the secondary gratifications that the patient obtains from his symptoms. For example, if the secondary gain involves the gratification of dependency needs, the doctor may develop a relationship in which the patient can obtain this gratification within the transference. The doctor can also support the direct expression of the patient's aggressive feelings, particularly when they occur without the rationalization provided by the symptom. For example, when the patient becomes angry and then makes a guilty apology, the therapist could say, "You have the right to get angry," or "Aren't you allowed to feel angry?"

The bargain aspect of treatment occurs when it is necessary to associate the therapist's support and gratification explicitly with the patient's relinquishing his symptom. Needless to say, this is a technique that is employed only after extensive treatment. An example occurred when a phobic man arrived for his session and stated, "I know I won't be able to talk about anything today; I'm just too anxious." The therapist, who knew from previous experience that the man meant what he said, replied "Well, perhaps it would be better if we stopped now." The patient became quite angry, but he didn't want to leave, and so he was forced to talk about his feelings.

When the phobic patient seeks help from others, he often

seeks rules for life, formulae that will serve as safeguards against anxiety. This emerges in the psychiatric interview as an interest in general formulations that suggest guides for conduct without involving the details of his life. The phobic patient will ask if he needs more rest, or suggest that his trouble is that he worries too much. He wonders if he should just take it easy, and clings to any suggestion from the doctor in this area. The doctor can reply to these requests by interpreting the patient's avoidance. He can say, "I guess that you don't like the idea that your symptoms are related to emotional problems." On other occasions, the patient may ask, "Do you think I should try to take the subway?" The therapist could reply, "I guess you're wondering whether I'll push you before you're ready."

After the meaning of a phobic symptom has been explored in detail, it still may seem necessary for the doctor to play an active role in encouraging the patient to enter the feared situation. However, this clinical problem may represent the patient's fear of assuming the responsibility for acting on his new insight—in a sense, he is phobic of giving up his phobia. He is fearful of the new and unknown feelings and also of the mature adult role involved in deciding to make a major change in his behavior. Frequently, the patient will accuse the doctor of becoming impatient or fed up with him, projecting his own self-contempt onto the therapist. The doctor now shifts from analyzing the dynamics of the specific symptom to discussing the transference relationship, and the patient's attempt to avoid any personal responsibility for his own improvement by attributing it the doctor's power. If this is successful, the doctor's active intervention may no longer be necessary.

DEPRESSION

Phobic patients often become depressed during treatment. They fear that giving up their symptoms will necessitate relinquishing infantile dependency gratifications. Depression is a sign that treatment is progressing, and the therapist should provide the support and encouragement that the patient needs at this phase. It is often a critical point in treatment, for the patient is not asking the doctor to protect him from imagined danger, but to help him with the problems he has when he faces the real world.

COUNTERTRANSFERENCE

The phobic patient elicits two major countertransference problems, condescending infantilization and frustrated anger. The patient seems to want to be treated as a helpless child. If the therapist goes along with this, he inevitably adds the condescension that reflects his feelings about adults who want to be treated as infants. The presence of this response may reflect the therapist's difficulty with his own feelings of dependency, but it may also suggest that he is overresponding to the patient's demands.

If the therapist initially accedes to the patient's demands, accepting the omnipotent idealization of the doctor as reality rather than transference, he will eventually grow irritated and angry. If the doctor then reveals this anger, the patient will feel that his transference fears have been confirmed, and that treatment is another strange and frightening situation in which he is helpless when confronted with a powerful and arbitrary parent.

The phobic patient has more overt anxiety and is more effective at eliciting responsive anxiety in the interviewer than the patient with any other major neurotic disorder. This anxiety often leads to contradictory short- and long-range goals—the soothing, calming effects of reassurance and support may be antitherapeutic. The problems of sensing the amount of anxiety that the patient can tolerate at any given stage and of timing interventions appropriately are a major challenge to the art of the psychiatrist.

REFERENCES

Freud, S.: On the grounds for detaching a particular syndrome from neurasthenia under the description "Anxiety Neurosis." Standard Edition of Complete Psychological Works of Sigmund Freud, Vol. III. London, Hogarth Press, 1962, pp. 87–117.

Freud, S.: Analysis of a phobia in a five-year-old boy. Standard Edition of Complete Psychological Works of Sigmund Freud, Vol. X. London, Hogarth Press, 1955, pp. 3–149.

Ovesey, L.: The phobic patient: A psychodynamic basis for classification and treatment. In Goldman, G. S., and Shapiro, D. (eds.): Developments in Psychoanalysis at Columbia University. New York, Hafner, 1966.

6 THE DEPRESSED PATIENT

Psychopathology and Psychodynamics

Depression refers both to a symptom and to a group of illnesses that have certain features in common. As a symptom, depression describes an affective tone of sadness accompanied by feelings of helplessness and diminished self-esteem. The depressed individual feels that his security is threatened, that he is unable to cope with his problems, and that others cannot help him. Every facet of life—emotional, cognitive, physiological, behavioral, and social—may be affected.

In early or mild depressive syndromes, the patient actively attempts to alleviate his suffering. He solicits aid from others, or attempts to solve his problems by magically regaining a lost love object or enhancing his strength. As the depression becomes more chronic or more severe, the patient gives up. He feels that others cannot or will not help him, and that things will never improve. The clinical syndromes of depression range from severe psychoses to mild neurotic and adjustment reactions.

The depressed person not only feels bad, but typically he is his own worst enemy, and he may use that specific phrase in describing himself. Self-destructive or masochistic and depressive tendencies frequently coexist in the same individual. Suicide, a dramatic complication of serious depressions, is a phenomenon of crucial importance in the understanding of the psychological functioning of the depressed person.

174

A patient does not think of himself as depressed unless he is aware of subjective feelings of sadness. However, the psychiatrist refers to some individuals as suffering from "masked depressions" or "depressive equivalents." These patients have the other signs and symptoms typical of depression, but the affective component is warded off or denied. The diagnosis is justified, however, by symptoms other than the patient's conscious affect and by the frequency with which depression is uncovered if the patient's defenses are penetrated. One common syndrome involves prominent somatic symptoms coupled with denial of affective disturbance, and these patients are often seen by non-psychiatric physicians.

This chapter will consider the clinical and psychodynamic aspects of depression, the problems of masochistic behavior and suicide, and the developmental origins of depressive patterns of adaptation.

CLINICAL FEATURES

Depressive syndromes involve a characteristic affective disorder, retardation and constriction of thought processes, slowing and diminished spontaneity of behavior, impoverished social relationships, and physiological changes that are magnified by hypochondriacal preoccupation.

Affect

The depressed person feels a lowering of his mood. He describes this as sadness, gloom, or despair, or uses any of a number of other words. Laymen who use the word "depression" are referring to this mood with or without the other clinical features of depressive syndromes. The patient may emphasize one particular aspect of depressive feeling, talking of anguish, tension, fear, guilt, emptiness, or longing.

The depressed patient loses his interest in life. His appetites diminish before his overt behavior is affected, and in mild depressions he goes through the motions of eating, sex, or play, but with little enthusiasm. As his depression progresses, he finally becomes indifferent to what had previously been major sources of pleasure. The patient may smile slightly and sadly at someone else's humor, but he has little of his own, unless it is a cynical or sardonic mask covering his self-contempt.

Anxiety, a common feature in certain depressive syndromes, is the psychological response to danger, and is often seen when the individual feels that there is an ongoing threat to his welfare. At times, anxiety, and the closely related picture of agitation, may become a chronic feature, as in the so-called "involutional depressions," which are described in greater detail below. In severe or chronic depressions, the anxiety may disappear and be replaced by apathy and withdrawal. This is the common picture in patients who have given up and feel hopeless. The apathetic patient makes no attempt to help himself, and elicits little sympathy or assistance from others. However, his withdrawal does protect him from the pain of his own inner feelings, and the patient may grow accustomed to his symptoms, so that he again feels more comfortable.

Depersonalization may play a similar defensive function in more acute depressive conditions. The most familiar aspects of the patient's personal identity seem strange. He no longer experiences his body or his emotional responses as part of his self, and thereby protects himself from painful feelings. Often the sense of emptiness and unreality is itself experienced as unpleasant. Depersonalization is a complex symptom that is also seen in other conditions, and that does not always have defensive significance.

Anger is also prominent in the affect of depressed patients. It may be expressed directly, as the patient complains that he is unloved and mistreated. In other cases it is more subtle, and the patient's suffering makes the lives of those around him miserable. For example, a woman would constantly tell her husband what an awful person she was and how difficult it must be for him to put up with her. Her self-abuse was far more disturbing to him than the faults for which she berated herself. Furthermore, if he failed to reassure her that her self-accusations were not true, she would complain that he too must feel she was awful.

Thought

The depressed person is preoccupied with himself and his plight, worrying about his misfortunes and their impact on his life. He ruminates about his past and is filled with remorse, as he imagines magical solutions to his current problems that involve the intervention of some omnipotent force, although he has little hope that these solutions will occur. His stereotyped thoughts lend a monotonous coloration to his conversation. The mildly depressed individual may fight his depression by consciously directing his thoughts elsewhere, a defense that is particularly common in obsessive patients. However, this usually becomes another self-preoccupation as his previous ruminations are replaced by new ones: "How can I get my mind off my problem?" instead of, "Why did it have to happen to me?"

The psychotically depressed patient may brood over minor incidents of his youth, which are recalled with guilt and fear of severe punishment. One middle-aged man thought that the local newspapers would expose an adolescent homosexual episode, humiliating him and his entire family. In the final stages of psychotic depression, the patient attempts to explain his feelings by finding a hidden meaning in them. This may involve projection, as in the patient who interpreted his plight as a punishment inflicted by a distant relative who was jealous of him. For other patients, the explanatory delusional system may reflect grandiose displacement, as in world destruction fantasies or nihilistic delusions that the universe has come to an end. Still others employ concrete symbolization, becoming convinced that their body is diseased and rotting away, although they may deny emotional distress. These defensive patterns are related to those seen in paranoid patients, and are discussed in detail in Chapter 8.

The topics that do not enter the patient's mind are as important as the thoughts with which he is preoccupied. He has difficulty remembering the joys of the past, and his view of life is gray with periodic spells of black. The interviewer must bear in mind that there is considerable retrospective falsification as the patient describes his life. It is not unusual for the patient to portray his mood as long-standing and gradual in onset, whereas others describe the symptoms as relatively recent and abrupt. In a sense the patient is right; he has simply been concealing his depression from others, and perhaps from himself. As he improves, this process may reverse itself; in the early phases of recovery the depressed patient sometimes sounds much better than he really feels. This may lead to premature optimism on the part of the therapist, and is one of the factors that contributes to the increased risk of suicide as the patient starts to improve.

Not only is the thought content of the depressed patient

disturbed, but his cognitive processes are distorted as well. His thoughts are diminished in quantity, and although he may be responsive, he shows little initiative or spontaneity. He answers questions, but does not offer new data or topics, and his mental life has little variety. He understands what is said, and replies appropriately, although his thinking is slowed and his speech may be halting or uncertain.

BEHAVIOR

Slowness characterizes the depressed patient's entire life as well as his thought processes. His movements and responses take longer, and even if he seems agitated and hyperactive, purposeful or intentional behavior is diminished. Thus the patient who paces the floor wringing his hands may require many minutes to dress himself or carry out simple tasks. For the retarded patient, the change in tempo may be almost bizarre, and in extreme cases it is as though one were watching a slow-motion film.

The patient may participate in life if he is urged, but left to his own devices, he is likely to withdraw. Those activities that he does select are passive and often socially isolated. One man with an early depressive syndrome first tried to seek social contact with friends. As this failed to alleviate his suffering, he retreated to sitting alone and reading, but in time even this required energy and attention that he could no longer command, and he simply sat staring at the television screen, scarcely noticing the program.

PHYSICAL SYMPTOMS

The depressed person's preoccupation with himself is often expressed concretely as a concern with his body and physical health. Hypochondriasis or frank somatic delusions are a more serious manifestation of the same process. These symptoms are related to those seen in paranoid syndromes, and are discussed in Chapter 8. Depression is also associated with actual changes in physiological functioning. The patient's metabolic rate is lower, his gastrointestinal functioning abnormal, and his mouth dry, and there are shifts in almost every bodily function that is under neuro-hormonal control.

The most common complaints include difficulty falling asleep, early morning awakening, fatigue, loss of appetite, constipation (although, occasionally, early depressive syndromes are marked by diarrhea), loss of libido, headache, neckache, backache, other aches and pains, and dryness and burning of the mouth with an unpleasant taste. The specific choice of somatic symptoms has symbolic meaning to the patient. The common symptoms concerning the mouth and digestive system are associated with the importance of oral motives and interests in depressive individuals. Other symptoms may have more individual significance. The headaches of the college professor or the pelvic pain of the menopausal woman are both closely related to the patient's self-concept. One man complained of an "empty gnawing" in his bowels, which further discussion traced to the feeling that he was being eaten up from within by a tumor.

SOCIAL RELATIONS

The depressive person craves love from others, but he fails to reciprocate in a way that rewards the other person or reinforces the relationship. He may become isolated, feeling unable to seek out others, or he may actively search out friends and companions, only to alienate them by his clinging and self-preoccupation.

Fearing rejection, the patient makes undue efforts to win the favor of his acquaintances. One man always brought gifts to friends when he visited them, and remembered the birthdays of even casual acquaintances. Unfortunately, the message he conveyed was more of self-sacrifice and desperation than of spontaneous warmth and comradeship. Similar behavior may be seen in obsessive individuals, since both obsessive and depressed persons are concerned with concealing their aggression and winning the favor of others. However, each often alienates others by the very behavior with which he hopes to attract them.

In early or mild depressive states, there may be an increase in social activity, with the patient seeking out others to ease his pain. In his eagerness to be accepted and loved, the mildly depressed person can be a faithful, reliable companion, but he will subordinate his own interests and desires to those of the other person. Although he has feelings of envy and anger, he does his best to conceal them, usually by turning them inward, deepening his despair.

As the depression worsens, the patient stops trying. He cannot face his friends, and consequently withdraws into himself. Anticipating that he would be a burden to others, he suffers in bitter silence and guilty self-reproach. The hostile aggressive aspect of his behavior is apparent to those who are close to him, although the patient is himself unaware of it. If others reject him, it confirms his feeling that he is unlikeable and unwanted.

PSYCHOTIC AND NEUROTIC
DEPRESSION AND NORMAL GRIEF

The psychotically depressed individual's contact with the real world is impaired. Gross social withdrawal, perceptual alterations, or mental preoccupation that interferes with normal cognitive functioning may be involved. He regresses to a level at which his more mature and autonomous ego functions may be sacrificed, if necessary, to maintain his failing self-esteem. Some measure of comfort is gained if he can avoid the painful realities of the world by retreating to a less threatening delusional substitute. Unlike other diagnostic groups, the distinction from neurotic reactions often seems to be a quantitative one. The clinician considers the external precipitants, the duration of the patient's symptoms, and their severity in making his diagnosis. The interviewer feels far more estranged from the psychotically depressed patient. He finds himself observing the symptoms with a feeling of emotional distance, rather than participating empathically in the patient's suffering.

Psychotic depressive syndromes, particularly the involutional type, are frequently subclassified as "agitated" or "retarded." These terms refer to familiar clinical pictures. The agitated patient paces the floor, wringing his hands and bemoaning his fate. He approaches every stranger, pleading for help in a stereotyped and often annoying way. He may sit down at the table for a meal, but immediately gets up and pushes his plate away. He creates an overall impression of intense anxiety, but the lines of his face and the content of his thoughts reveal his depression.

The retarded patient, on the other hand, shows inhibition of motor activity, which may progress to stupor. He sits in a chair or lies in bed, head bowed, body in a posture of flexion, eyes staring straight ahead, indifferent to distractions. If he does speak or move, the act is slow, labored, and of brief duration.

The neurotically depressed patient continues to function in the real world, and his depressive feelings either are mild or seem appropriate to the external precipitants. If the depression is severe, the precipitating trauma has been extreme, and the interviewer can easily empathize with the patient's distress. He continues to recognize the realities of the world around him, and gradually improves over a span of weeks or months. For example, a neurotically depressed young widow felt that she could never enjoy her life alone, nor could she conceive of remarriage. However, she was able to take solace in her relationships with her children and in her job. A year later, she looked back on her husband's death with sadness, but she had begun to date other men, was enjoying life, and was contemplating remarriage. Another woman, who developed a psychotic depression following a similar stress, quit her job, was unable to care for her children, and withdrew to her bed, certain that a terrible physical illness had developed. She became morbidly preoccupied with her widowhood and, although after a year her pain was less intense, her only interest in life was in pursuing her numerous medical treatments.

The spectrum runs from the normal grief reaction through neurotic depression and on to psychotic depression. The grieving individual responds to a real and important loss with feelings of sadness and a temporary withdrawal of interest in other aspects of life. His thoughts are focused on his loss, and it may be weeks or months before his interest in the world returns to its former level and he is able to develop new relationships that might fill the gap. There are several features that differentiate this normal syndrome from pathological depression. The grief-stricken individual does not suffer from a diminution of self-esteem. He is not irrationally guilty, and it is easy for the interviewer to empathize with his feelings. He may have some insomnia, but somatic symptoms are mild and transient. He may *feel* that his world has come to an end, but he *knows* that he will recover and cope with his problems. Finally, grief is a self-limited condition, rarely lasting more than six months, and usually subsiding rapidly within a few weeks. If the reaction is disproportionate to the loss, either in terms of severity or duration, or if the person feels guilty or personally inadequate, we speak of a depressive syndrome.

PRECIPITATING FACTORS

BIOLOGICAL AND PSYCHOLOGICAL THEORIES

Exogenous or reactive depressions are seen as a response to traumatic precipitating experiences in the patient's life; endog-

enous depressions are viewed as the expression of a constitution-
ally determined reaction pattern that is relatively unaffected by
external events. The term "endogenous" connotes a more severe
or psychotic picture, such as manic depressive psychosis.

There is, however, a danger to the concept of endogenous
depression. It is helpful for the depressed patient to realize that
his symptoms have meaning. The discussion of the trigger for
the episode, whether or not it is the major etiological factor, often
helps the patient to understand himself. A simplistic use of the
concept of endogenous depression may interfere with this process.
In the authors' experience, most depressive episodes, psychotic
as well as neurotic, can be traced to some external precipitating
cause. Neurotic depressions can be traced to specific precipitating
factors more easily than any other type of neurotic symptom.

Constitutional or biological models of depression are often
seen as being opposed to reactive or psychodynamic concepts, but
there is no contradiction between these two frames of reference.
The ability of depressive syndromes to communicate helpless
dependency and to elicit nurturing care suggests that depressive
mechanisms may have adaptive value, and that the capacity to
develop them may have been selected in the course of evolution.
This is in contrast to most biological theories of schizophrenia,
which emphasize the maladaptive aspects of the illness. For
depression, biological and psychodynamic explanations are not
only compatible, but interdependent.

SPECIFIC STRESSES

Loss.   The loss of a love object is the most common precipitant of depression. This loss is usually the death of or separation from a loved one. In other instances, it is an internal psychological loss resulting from the expectation that one will be
rejected by his family and friends. The loss may have actually
occurred, or it may be imminent, as in the depressive reactions
that appear in anticipation of the death of a parent or spouse. Of
course, not all losses lead to depression. The loss must involve
someone important to the patient, and there are certain necessary
predisposing characteristics of the patient's psychological functioning and his relationship to the lost object which will be discussed later.

There is sometimes an interval of days, weeks, or even years between the actual loss and the depressive response. In these cases the patient has denied the loss, or its impact on him, and therefore has avoided his emotional response. When something—often an event that symbolizes or exposes the initial trauma—renders this denial ineffective, depression follows. One woman showed relatively little response to the death of her husband, but became deeply depressed two years later when her cat was killed in an accident. She explained, "I suddenly realized that I was really alone." Mourning can also be delayed, as in the adolescent boy who seemed relatively unaffected by his father's death. Five years later, his mother found him crying in his room on the night before his graduation from college. When she asked what was wrong, he said, "I keep thinking how Dad would enjoy it if only he were here."

The so-called anniversary depressions are based on a similar mechanism. A specific season or date is unconsciously associated with a feeling of loss in the patient's earlier life. The anniversary of a parent's death is a common example. The frequent depressions during Christmas holidays are in part related to the tendency for feelings of deprivation and impoverishment to be heightened when others are happy. The child whose depression was aggravated when his friends were happiest in later years finds himself inexplicably depressed during the holiday season.

In one sense, all adult depressive reactions are delayed responses, with the immediate precipitant in adult life exposing feelings that can be traced to early childhood. Since every child experiences loss and feelings of inadequacy and helplessness, every adult has the capacity for depressive responses.

THREATS TO SELF-CONFIDENCE AND SELF-ESTEEM. Every individual has internal mental representations of the important people in his life, including himself. Self-representation, like object representation, may be highly accurate or grossly distorted. We use the term "self-confidence" to describe one aspect of this self-representation, a person's image of his own adaptive capacity. In other words, someone who is self confident perceives himself as able to obtain gratification of his needs and to insure his survival.

In addition to his self-representation, or mental image of what he is actually like, each person has an image of what he would like to be, or what he thinks he ought to be—his ego ideal. The degree to which his self-image lives up to that ego ideal is a measure of his self-esteem. That is, if a person feels that he is close to the way he would like to be, he will have high self-esteem; conversely, if he falls short of his own goals and aspirations, his self-esteem will be lowered.

Diminution in self-confidence and self-esteem are cardinal symptoms of depression. The self-esteem of most depression-prone individuals has been based upon continuing input of love, respect, and approval from significant other figures in their life. These may be figures from the patient's past who have long since been internalized or real external figures of current importance. In either event, the disruption of a relationship with such a person poses a threat to the patient's source of narcissistic supplies, love, and dependent gratification. This endangers the person's self-esteem, and therefore may precipitate a depression. Depression may also follow the disruption of a relationship with a person who, while not a source of these narcissistic rewards, had become a symbolic extension of the patient's self-image. In this case, the loss of the object is equivalent to an amputation of part of the patient's own ego. The loss of a child frequently has this meaning to the parent.

It is possible for the patient's self-image and self-esteem to be shattered by blows other than the disruption of object relationships. For many individuals, self-esteem is based upon self-confidence; that is, as long as they feel able to cope with their own problems independently, they have a good opinion of themselves. A direct threat to this person's adaptive capacity, such as a major injury or illness, may render him helpless and destroy his self-confidence and self-esteem. This is the basis of some depressions seen in association with incapacitating traumatic injuries or chronic illness.

The direct threat to one's adaptive capacity and the loss of love and respect from important people are closely related clinically. For example, the college student who fails an examination may revise his image of his intellectual capacity sharply downward, and for this very reason may feel that his parents will have less love and respect for him.

SUCCESS. Some people become paradoxically depressed in response to apparent success. Thus, occupational promotion, or any sudden reward that carries increased responsibility and status, may lead to a depressive syndrome. When these paradoxical depressions are studied, one of two common underlying dynamics is usually found. In the first, the patient feels that he does not deserve this success, in spite of objective evidence to the contrary. He believes that the increased responsibility will expose him as inadequate, and therefore he anticipates rejection from those who have rewarded him. For example, a physician who had an outstanding record was asked to direct a clinical program. He first rejected the offer, and then accepted it, but became increasingly mistrustful of his clinical judgment and administrative skills. When he spoke to his superiors about this, they reassured him, but this only made him more convinced that they did not really understand him. Finally, in order to escape from the danger of injuring his patients because of his fantasied incompetence, he made a serious suicide attempt. When provided an opportunity for success, he feared that he would be expected to function independently and would no longer qualify for dependent care.

The second psychodynamic theme underlying depressive responses to success stems from the fear of retaliation for assertion and aggression. This patient has often struggled to get to the top, but successful assertion is equated with hostile aggression, and he feels guilty about any behavior that furthers his own advancement. He views competition in terms of Oedipal or sibling conflicts, and success involves a transgression, for which punishment will follow. He escapes by regressing to an oral dependent level of adaptation, rather than risking the danger of retaliation.

PSYCHODYNAMIC PATTERNS

The depressed patient has suffered a blow to his self-esteem. This can result from the disruption of a relationship with either external or internalized objects or from a direct blow to his adaptive capacity. In either event, the patient experiences a deflated self-image, and attempts to repair the damage and to defend himself from further trauma. This section will discuss several psychodynamic mechanisms that are related to this sequence: identification, the relation of anger to depression, the role of isolation and denial, the evolution of manic states, and the relationship of depression and projective defenses.

IDENTIFICATION AND INTROJECTION

When death or separation lead to the loss of a loved one, the emotionally charged mental representation of the lost one remains a permanent part of the self. This mechanism is called introjection, whereas identification is a less global and more subtle process in which the individual modifies his self-image in accordance with his image of the important person whom he has lost, but does so only in specific selected areas. Both of these defenses serve to recapture or retain the lost object, at least in terms of the patient's psychological life. They are crucial mechanisms in normal development. The child's character is molded by his identifications with parents and parental surrogates from his early years, and the Oedipal complex is resolved by the introjection of the parent, with this introject forming the basic framework for the adult superego.

Clinical manifestations of identification as a defense against grief are common. One young man who had been born and raised in the United States developed speech and other mannerisms similar to those of his recently deceased father, a European immigrant. A woman developed an interest in religion, for the first time in her life, after her deeply religious stepmother died. A woman whose husband was away in the armed forces began to attend baseball games, his favorite pastime, in which she had previously had little interest.

Introjection is vividly illustrated when the depressed person's anger toward his lost love object continues after that object has been introjected. We speak of "ego introjects" when the patient attacks himself with accusations that bear little relation to his own faults, but that clearly refer to the faults of the lost person. The introject has become allied with the patient's ego, and is being attacked by his punitive superego. "Superego introjection" is demonstrated when the voice and manner of the patient's self-criticism can be traced to criticisms that had been expressed by the lost loved one, but that now originate in the patient's superego.

Depression and Anger

Depression is a complex emotion, and it commonly includes admixtures of anger. Perhaps the simplest psychodynamic basis for this is the patient's anger at the lost love object for abandoning him. This is dramatic in small children, who frequently attack or refuse to speak to their parents following a separation from them. It is also demonstrated by the man who, following the death of his mother, destroyed all of her photographs and letters, rationalizing this as a desire to avoid painful reminders of his loss.

The depressed patient displaces his anger to substitute persons who he hopes will replace his loss and continue to gratify his needs. This coercive hostility is frequently expressed toward the therapist. The patient wants the doctor to replace the loss personally, not merely to facilitate the healing process. When, as is inevitable, the doctor fails to do so, the patient is disappointed and bitter.

The patient feels guilty about his hostile feelings toward others, and is also afraid to express his anger directly. He feels inadequate, and is convinced that he cannot survive without the love and care of others. Therefore, any outward expression of hostility is dangerous—he might destroy what he most needs. He therefore turns it against himself in the form of self-accusation and condemnation, a cardinal feature of depression. The self-love and self-respect of the normal person protect him from destructive self-criticism. These supporting factors are seriously deficient in the depressed person, and he may torture himself mercilessly, suffering extreme shame and guilt.

ISOLATION AND DENIAL

The depressed individual often struggles to keep his feelings out of awareness and to ignore their origins in the outside world. These defensive maneuvers protect him from psychological pain. When the patient is successful, one sees depression without depression, that is, the clinical condition without the subjective affect. Usually some aspect of the emotional complex emerges. Often, the somatic symptoms are most apparent, and some psychiatrists speak of "somatic equivalents" of depression. These patients look and act depressed. They come to the doctor because of physical symptoms and hypochondriacal complaints, which are usually refractory to treatment. However, when asked if they feel depressed, they say "No," but add that they have been run down, tired, and worried about their physical health. Others reserve the term "depression" for conditions in which the subjective clinical affect is present and see these equivalent symptoms as premorbid conditions.

Isolation and denial are characteristic defenses of the obsessive personality, and an underlying depression is commonly exposed as one analyzes the defenses of the obsessive. This patient has high expectations of himself, and he often feels that he can not live up to them. He maintains his self-esteem by turning his neurotic traits into highly regarded virtues. When this is interpreted and his underlying feelings are brought into the open, the patient becomes depressed.

MANIC SYNDROMES

The manic patient clinically appears to be the opposite of the depressed one. His affective display is elated or euphoric, and he is overly active, physically and mentally, as he races from one topic to another, unable to keep his mind on a continuous train of thought. In spite of this superficial elation, mania is best understood as a defense against depression. It is the product of denial and reversal of affect.

There is often clinical evidence that the patient's underlying feelings are not as gay as they first appear. His humor is infectious, unlike that of the autistic schizophrenic, but it is often barbed and hostile. If he is being interviewed in a group, he may make embarrassing and provocative comments about the others, perhaps focusing on one person's unusual name or another's physical defect. Although the group may laugh with the patient at first, the discomfort of his victim will quickly win their sympathy. The patient seems to have little compassion, although he may switch to a new target. This behavior reveals his defensive projection; he focuses on the weaknesses of others to avoid thinking of his own. At times, his underlying depression may emerge openly, and in a private interview, in response to warmth and sympathy, he may lose control and break into tears.

Depression represents the reaction to a feeling of narcissistic injury and loss, with the ego fearing the punitive and disapproving superego. Mania can be seen as the ego's insistence that the injury has been repaired and the superego conquered, and that the individual has incorporated all of the narcissistic supplies that he might need. There is a triumphant feeling of omnipotence; since the ego has defeated the superego, it is no longer necessary to control or inhibit impulses. The manic patient insists that he has no restraints, that he is exactly what he wants to be. He is supremely self-confident, undertaking projects and acquiring possessions that would normally seem out of reach. In spite of this apparent victory, his underlying uneasiness is readily apparent. Superego fears may persist in the manic episode, and the patient's frantic, driven quality in part represents his flight from punishment.

This psychodynamic constellation is related to the hallucinatory wish fulfillment of the hungry infant and the cyclic periodicity of mania and depression has been compared to the infantile cycle of hunger and satiation. The manic patient has gratified his appetite by ignoring reality and insisting that he has what he so dearly wants. However, this illusory gratification is only transient, and the feeling of depression returns, just as the fantasies of oral gratification fail to quiet the hunger pangs of the infant.

PROJECTION AND PARANOID RESPONSES

Patients frequently alternate between paranoid and depressive states. The depressed patient feels that he is worthless, and tends to blame himself for his difficulties. He looks to others for help, and may be angry and resentful if it is not forthcoming. If he utilizes the defense of projection to protect himself from his painful self-condemnation, he feels not only that others are failing to help him, but also that they are the cause of his difficulty. It is as if the patient said to himself, "It is not that I am bad; it is only that he says I am bad," or, "My unhappiness is not my fault; it is what he did to me." Projection is accompanied by shifts from sadness to anger, from looking for help to expecting persecution. The patient's diminished self-esteem changes to grandiosity as he feels, "I must be very important to be singled out for such abuse."

However, one pays a heavy price for paranoid defenses. This patient's ability to appraise the outer world realistically is seriously impaired, and his social relationships are disrupted. Although his self-image may be inflated, his actual adaptive capacity is often more seriously impaired than it had been while he was depressed. These changes serve as precipitants of a new depressive reaction, and the cycle continues.

The interview with such patients may be marked by shifts from one pole to the other in response to the therapist's interventions. The relationship between paranoid and depressive syndromes is one reason that paranoid patients present suicidal risks —sudden intervening depressions can occur. It is also related to the prominent paranoid features in manic states.

MASOCHISM AND THE DEPRESSIVE CHARACTER

Human behavior is governed by the pleasure principle. The individual avoids pain and seeks pleasure. Masochistic behavior is an apparent exception to this rule; the patient seems to avoid pleasure and may even seek painful experiences, or he may only allow himself pleasure if it is associated with pain. Masochism is a central character trait of depressive individuals. A mild form involves the inability to avoid misfortune. The patient files applications after their deadline or is careless about routine preventive health measures. In more severe conditions, actively self-destructive behavior appears, culminating in overt suicidal acts. The explanation of masochistic behavior has been one of the most perplexing problems in psychoanalytic theory, and the treatment of patients with strong masochistic tendencies is a frustrating and difficult clinical problem.

Several psychodynamic mechanisms operate separately or in concert to produce masochistic behavior. We will discuss pain as a condition for pleasure, pain in the service of fantasies of omnipotent control, pain as providing the security of the familiar, and the secondary gain of masochism.

For some individuals, pain is a necessary prerequisite in order to enjoy pleasure. Pain has become a means of assuaging the superego and expiating guilt. The patient atones for his real or fantasied wrong-doing by his masochistic behavior. He avoids, or at least lessens, the pangs of conscience by arranging punishment in the real world. At times, the punishment may be designed to compensate for a crime that has not yet been committed—the patient may be building up "credits" so that he can enjoy future pleasures more comfortably. This is ritualized in some religions, in which a period of fasting, deprivation, and prayer is followed by feast and revelry and, in more primitive religions, orgiastic ceremonies that suspend the usual barriers to sexual expression. The same mechanism is demonstrated by the girl who "accidentally" cuts her hand shortly before a date with a boy of whom her family disapproves. In one variant of this dynamic, the patient engages in forbidden acts or fantasies, but he experiences them as unpleasant episodes that are forced upon him and he therefore avoids responsibility for them. This is particularly common in the masochistic sexual fantasies of women whose conscious fear of attack or rape is a disguise for their unconscious wish for sexual activity.

A second mechanism of masochistic behavior is related to the infantile desire to maintain omnipotent control of the universe. Pain and frustration challenge the child's view that he is in control of the world and of his own subjective experience. The child who goes on to become masochistic can resolve this problem by rationalizing that his unhappiness is not the inevitable consequence of things over which he has no control, but rather the result of his own behavior. An example is the unattractive girl who dresses drably and claims that she has no interest in men, but only in her academic pursuits. She maintains a subjective sense of absolute autonomy at the cost of suffering repeated painful experiences. This type of individual will break off relationships if there is a threat that others might leave first, will quit a job lest he be fired, and will volunteer for unpleasant tasks rather than risk being drafted for them. He may be aware of this trait, but he usually views it with pride rather than despair, considering it evidence of strength rather than pathology.

A third mechanism of masochistic behavior relates to the safety and comfort provided by the familiar. The child whose life is marked by frequent punishment may feel loved only if abused, and may feel insecure if he goes for any length of time without punishment. He learns to seek out situations that recreate his early experiences, and is uncomfortable if he cannot re-establish the role of victim. One man would play the clown with his friends, eliciting the same sarcasm and verbal abuse from his contemporaries that he had received earlier from his family. This dynamic is seen in the patient who clings to his familiar neurotic defensive patterns, no matter how clearly he sees their maladaptive nature.

Masochistic behavior can have great secondary gain. People feel sorry for the miserable or unfortunate, and the patient may get satisfaction from the sympathy of others. A sense of moral superiority is associated with suffering for a good cause, and the patient may feel the exaltation of the martyred saint. Suffering can also be a heavy burden for those who are involved with the sufferer, and aggression directed against the self can be a most effective means of attacking others. For example, a patient arrived for a session although she obviously had a severe cough. She repeatedly apologised, saying, "I didn't know whether to come or not. I felt miserable and didn't want to give you the flu, but I know every session is so important."

The interviewer can become an unwitting participant in the patient's masochism. An example is the patient who listens to an interpretation, quickly accepts it, and then berates himself for the behavior that the doctor attempts to examine. The result is that psychotherapeutic efforts make the symptoms worse. This poses an extremely difficult problem for the doctor. Caution is required in the phrasing and timing of interpretations, and close attention must be paid to the patient's mode of dealing with them. If insight seems to make the patient worse, supportive therapy may be effective, but further uncovering therapy should await exploration of the patient's mode of handling interpretation.

Not all masochistic patients are clinically depressed. Masochism can serve as a defense against depression, and when this is effective, the patient may actually take pride in his plight. This is often associated with denial of the patient's own role in his difficulties and projection onto the outside world, adding a paranoid component to the masochistic picture. This is further discussed in the section called "Masochism and Paranoia" in Chapter 8.

SUICIDE

The exploration of suicidal thoughts and feelings is not only of critical importance in the practical management of a depressed person, but it also provides one of the most valuable routes to understanding him. The discussion of suicide, like that of any complex act, can be separated into a consideration of the motives or impulses and of the regulatory and controlling structures that interact with these motives.

The motivation for the seemingly irrational act of taking one's own life can be complex and varied. Some patients have no intention of killing themselves, and if the behavior is consciously intended as a dramatic communication rather than a self-destructive act, we speak of suicidal "gestures." However, these are subject to miscalculation and may lead to death. They also may be followed by more serious suicidal behavior, particularly if their communicative purpose is not successful. The distinction between a suicidal gesture and a suicide attempt is somewhat arbitrary, and most suicidal behavior involves communicative as well as self-destructive goals. The interview with the depressed patient is designed to provide other channels of communication, and this in itself may reduce the pressure for suicidal behavior.

The self-destructive aspect of suicidal motivation is itself complex and varied. For some depressed persons, suicide may provide an opportunity to regain some feeling of mastery over their own fate. There are schools of philosophy that suggest that it is only by taking his own life that an individual can truly experience freedom. Psychodynamically, it is clear that some depressed people feel they are unable to control their own lives in any other way. They are able to regain a sense of autonomy and self-esteem only by deciding to kill themselves. The often observed clinical phenomenon of an improvement in the patient's mood after he has decided to take his own life is related to this mechanism.

An impulse to commit suicide may be related to an impulse to murder someone else. Suicide can serve as a means of controlling one's own aggressions, as a turning of aggression against the self, or as a means of murdering another person who has been psychologically incorporated by the suicidal individual. Although these mechanisms are quite different, their effect is similar. A person who unconsciously wants to kill someone else may try to take his own life.

Life may seem intolerable under certain circumstances, and suicide can provide a means of escape from a painful or humiliating situation. This is often the case with culturally or socially sanctioned suicide. This motivation is the most comfortable one for a patient's friends, family, or even his physician to accept. However, in our society, suicidal behavior is relatively uncommon, even in those who are suffering from painful terminal illnesses and who are familiar with their diagnosis and prognosis. When it does occur, it is usually associated with pathological depression. The doctor must be careful not to convey to the patient that suicide is a reasonable act in view of the patient's problems.

Since no one has any personal experience with his own death, the psychological meaning of dying varies from person to person and is related to other experiences with which it is symbolically associated. Death may mean isolation and loneliness, peaceful and permanent sleep, or a magical reunion with those who have already died. More elaborate ideas may be based on religious or spiritualist convictions concerning life after death. Each of these meanings may be attractive under certain circumstances, and the motive for suicide may have more to do with these symbolic equivalents of death than with death itself. At the same time, most patients retain some realistic awareness of the meaning of taking their own lives side by side with their unconscious symbolic elaboration of death. This dichotomy is culturally instituted by those religions that emphasize the pleasant aspects of the next world but, at the same time, strictly forbid suicide as a sinful act.

The specific method of suicide that the patient contemplates or attempts often sheds light on the unconscious meaning of the act. For example, the person who takes an overdose of sleeping pills may be equating death with a prolonged sleep, and the use of firearms often suggests violent rage. Dramatic modes of death such as self-immolation usually involve attempts to communicate dramatic feelings to the world. The patient who uses multiple methods simultaneously, such as pills and drowning, is often struggling against his own desire to live and is trying to insure that he will not be able to change his mind at the last moment.

The strength and nature of suicidal impulses is only one of the factors that determine whether or not an individual attempts suicide. Most individuals have internalized strong prohibitions against murder, and furthermore, one's own narcissistic self-regard serves as a specific deterrent to suicide. However, if an individual has identified with a parent or other significant figure who himself committed suicide, the situation is different. The incidence of suicide in the children of parents who themselves committed suicide is several times higher than in the general population. These individuals may have failed to develop the usual inner restraints, and they cannot judge suicidal behavior harshly because to do so would be to reject their own parents.

If a person simply and unambivalently wanted to take his own life, he would probably not be sitting and talking to the doctor. Some patients want to place their lives in the hands of fate, acting in a way that courts danger but allows the possibility of escape. The behavior associated with such feelings ranges from Russian Roulette to taking overdoses of pills when one is likely to be discovered, or simply driving dangerously under hazardous conditions. In some respects this is the opposite of the desire for a sense of autonomy and mastery mentioned above. The individual denies all responsibility for his continued existence, thereby relieving himself of a weighty burden. If he is saved, he may interpret this as a magical sign that he is forgiven and will be cared for, and the intensity of his suicidal impulses will diminish.

Individuals who are prone to impulsive behavior in general are also more likely to act on suicidal impulses. The combination of depression and impulsiveness is related to the high incidence of suicide in alcoholic patients and in those with acute organic mental syndromes. In evaluating a patient's suicidal potential, his general impulsiveness is an important factor.

The patient who has suicidal thoughts and impulses has often evaluated his potential for acting on them himself, and he is usually willing to share his conclusions with the interviewer. These can provide an important source of information, but they cannot simply be accepted at face value. They must be considered in the light of his general capacity for self-observation and insight and the reliability of his previous predictions about how he would act in given situations. The patient's intention of maintaining a separation between impulse and action is also tested by the extent to which he has elaborated concrete plans for suicide and his preparations for carrying out these plans.

DEVELOPMENTAL PSYCHODYNAMICS

The depressed patient frequently comes from a family with a history of depression, and his high aspirations and low self-image have often been transmitted from generation to generation. The death or separation of a parent early in the patient's life is a common feature in the history. The patient not only suffers the separation and loss, but he also lives with the remaining parent through a period of grief and despair. The patient has often been the bearer of more than the usual amount of parental hopes and fantasies. Frequently the parents felt themselves to be unsuccessful, and they wanted their child to succeed where they had failed. The child becomes a vehicle for their hopes, and he feels that their love is contingent on his continued success. For example, the syndrome is common in the oldest child born of upward mobile immigrant parents. The overt climate of family life is usually one of protective and loving concern. As a consequence, the patient must suppress and deny any hostile feelings. He is pushed hard, not provided with the basis for self-confidence, and not allowed to complain.

The origins of depressive patterns can be traced to the first year of life. The young infant is the center of his own psychological universe. He sees himself as controlling his environment in his primitive state of omnipotent narcissism. However, even if his parents attempt to gratify all of his needs as quickly as possible, thereby maintaining his narcissistic state, frustration is inevitable. Reality forces him to modify his initial picture of the world and to accept his actual helplessness and dependency on others. This is the prototype for the later experience of depression. As an adult, any blow to this patient's self-esteem triggers a depressive reaction, recreating the feelings of the infant who realizes that he needs his mother and discovers that she is not available.

When the infant first relinquishes his original narcissistic self-image, it is only to delegate these same characteristics to his mother. He may be helpless, but as long as his mother is available, his needs are gratified and his life is secure. Separation from the mother is the most dangerous possible threat. Clinical studies suggest that depression-like pictures appear in infants who are separated from their mothers as early as the second half of the first year of life, when this delegation of omnipotence has presumably already occurred. These infantile depressions, like the adult syndrome, result from the separation from a love object, which leads to a threat to his security with which the infant cannot cope by himself. His early developing concepts of object constancy and of time leave him uncertain that this threat will ever end. He is helpless and hopeless.

This primordial depressive state is complicated by further developmental experiences. The child's oral fantasies include incorporative and destructive components. Making the mother part of himself involves cannibalistic or symbiotic impulses that threaten her existence as a separate individual. The child becomes fearful that his need for her will lead to her destruction. This mixture of dependent love and hostile aggression is the beginning of the ambivalent relation to objects that characterizes the depressive individual.

Later, family pressures may push him toward the denial of his dependency desires and the outward appearance of competence and independence. However, his craving for security and warmth from parent figures is intensified by every exposure to the outside world. He develops close psychological ties to his parents and loved ones, in effect making them part of himself. As internalized sources of love, they also become inner critics and censors, and the patient's ambivalence continues in relation to these introjected objects. When this pattern has been laid down, subsequent losses are followed by the internalization of the lost object, which is then regarded with intense ambivalent feelings. The result is clinical depression.

The patient who is prone to depression has little joy in life. His superego is punitive and sadistic, stemming from his own aggressive fantasies and the incorporation of demanding and perfectionistic parents. He allows himself little pleasure and constantly measures his performance to determine whether he has lived up to his inner standards, always finding himself lacking. Life is an examination, and if he takes time to enjoy himself, he feels guilty and knows that he will fail. His self-esteem depends on a combination of support from external objects, maintenance of his own adaptive capacity, and protection from unusual demands or expectations from others. The result is such a fragile balance that recurrent disruptions are inevitable, and life is a series of repeated depressions.

Management of the Interview

The interview with the depressed patient requires active participation by the physician. The patient wants the doctor to take care of him, and it is often helpful for the interviewer to provide the structure for the discussion as well as to gratify the patient's dependent needs in other ways. It is not enough to help the patient to help himself; he wants more, and subtly or overtly he communicates this to the interviewer. The very nature of his illness makes him pessimistic about the outcome of treatment, and he is more likely to be a passive or immobile object than a willing partner. In addition, his characteristic patterns of relating lead to technical problems in the interview. The doctor must make certain strategic decisions concerning the mode of therapy earlier than is necessary with most other patients, and he may have to do so feeling that an error would be not only antitherapeutic, but disastrous.

This section considers the chronological development of the interview with the depressed patient, his initial presentation, problems in communication, and the exploration of symptoms, including suicidal desires. The principles of psychotherapy will be presented with particular emphasis on their early impact on the patient. The interview with the family of the depressed patient, some special problems in dealing with manic patients, and the characteristic transference and countertransference problems that emerge in interviews with depressed patients are also discussed.

INITIAL PRESENTATION

The seriously depressed patient usually does not come to the doctor's office alone. He lacks the energy and initiative to get there, and his friends and family feel sorry for him because he seems so helpless and unable to care for himself. When the doctor enters the waiting room, it is the friend or relative who looks up first, greets the doctor, and introduces himself. The patient may observe what is happening, but he will not participate unless invited. The person who has accompanied the patient often speaks to the doctor as though the patient were incapacitated. The daughter of one elderly depressed woman started by saying, "I guess I'd better do the talking. My mother is hard of hearing, and she doesn't like to talk anyway." The patient's companion expresses an urgent wish that the doctor "do something to find out what is the matter." This introduction emphasizes the patient's role as a helpless child, an attitude that the physician should avoid reinforcing. He should introduce himself to the patient and invite him into the consultation room—unless the patient seems unable to speak, in which case the doctor can include the companion. The doctor should always talk with the companion of a seriously depressed patient at some time during the first interview. Important data concerning the precipitants of the problem, suicidal communications, and the severity of the depression are often obtained from the third party.

The less severely depressed patient may come alone, but his posture, grooming, facial expression, movements, and the physical qualities of his voice will reveal his problem before he has completed his first sentence. Initially, the patient's sadness and gloom is usually most obvious, but his anger may also emerge in the interview. His dependent attitude is reflected by his waiting for instructions before selecting a chair, or seeking permission before lighting a cigarette. The doctor is advised to respond realistically to such requests, and to avoid interpreting their deeper meaning, as this patient would experience any such interpretation as a rebuff and rejection.

Some patients conceal their depression, and the first suggestion of the patient's condition comes from the interviewer's own empathic response. Although this is not a manifestation of countertransference, it is so intimately associated with it that it will be discussed under that heading.

As the interview continues, the severely depressed patient will wait for the doctor to speak first. He lacks spontaneity, and may stare blankly into space or down at the floor. With this patient, it is preferable to begin the interview by commenting on his retardation and lowering of mood, rather than routinely inquiring about his reason for seeking help. This non-verbal behavior has already provided a chief complaint. The interviewer could say, "You seem quite depressed."

The patient is slow in answering, and his replies are brief and repetitious, revealing the constriction of his thought processes. In addition, his remarks are either complaining or self-flagellating, and are often worded in a rhetorical fashion, for example, "I can't go on, I'm no good to anyone, why must I suffer like this?" If the physician replies, "I know you feel badly, but if I can learn more about it maybe I will be able to help," this patient answers, "What's the use? Nothing can be done for me." The patient has stated his feeling, and the doctor can show concern and continue with the interview. He might ask, "How did it begin?"

The doctor's general manner should be serious and concerned, supporting the patient's mood rather than challenging it. Cheery or humorous comments, too rapid or energetic a pace, or even a smile, may give the patient the feeling that the doctor will not tolerate his gloom. The entire interview will be slow, and the physician must allow extra time for the patient to respond.

The patient with a milder or masked depression will speak spontaneously or respond to the doctor's initial inquiry. He often begins with a comment on his emotional pain, or the time when things were different and better. He might say, "I don't feel like my old self anymore," or, "I've lost interest in everything." At times the patient's self-deprecating tendencies will appear in his first words, as they did in the woman who said, "I feel so old and ugly." It is important to recognize that the patient who says, "I don't feel like my old self," has not yet described his feelings. The depressed patient wants to express his unhappiness, and the doctor must provide an opportunity for this before exploring his healthier state. After he has elicited the patient's description of his depression, he can ask, "What were things like before you became depressed?" or, "What was your old self?"

The withdrawn, depressed patient does not become emotionally engaged with the interviewer. His outward participation seems peripheral to his inner thoughts and feelings, and he may sit staring at the floor, answering questions monosyllabically in a voice that suggests reflex responses. This barrier is extremely difficult to overcome, and continuing with routine queries about the patient's symptoms or his living arrangements will only heighten it. The doctor can start by calling attention to the problem, saying, "Talking seems to be a great effort for you." The patient's conscious desire to be cooperative and agreeable is already demonstrated by his attempt to answer questions, and he may be able to participate more fully if he senses the doctor's sympathetic interest. On rare occasions, sharing silence with the patient will be helpful, but depressed people usually experience the doctor's silence as a form of disinterest, dissatisfaction, or frustration.

THE EXPLORATION
OF DEPRESSIVE SYMPTOMS

The doctor reaches out more than halfway in the first interview with the depressed patient. The patient is more comfortable when the interviewer leads him, and it is important for the physician to organize the interview and to provide the patient with continual support and approval for his participation.

If the doctor adopts a passive attitude, trying to force the patient into a more active role, the patient will feel incompetent, frustrated, and finally, more depressed. On the other hand, if the doctor gives the patient the feeling that, by answering questions, he is doing a good job, the interview will be therapeutic from the start.

The doctor must accept the patient's slowed sense of time in pacing his interview. The interval between comments is longer than usual, and topics that are usually discussed in the first few minutes of contact may be delayed for many hours. If the patient becomes unable to talk or loses the thread, the doctor can sympathize, review what has occurred so far, and try to continue at a slower pace.

Depressed people often cry. This is particularly true with the moderately depressed person early in the course of the illness. The more severely or more chronically depressed rarely cry. If the patient cries openly, the doctor waits sympathetically, perhaps offering a tissue. However, if the patient seems to ignore his tears, the doctor can refer to them, encouraging the patient to accept his feelings. A quiet, "What is it you feel bad about?" is usually sufficient. Sometimes a patient tries to conceal his crying. The doctor can comment on this defense without challenging or interpreting it by asking, "Are you trying not to cry?" The doctor permits the emotional display and treats it as an appropriate means of expressing feeling. He gently continues the interview when the patient seems able to participate; waiting too long can lead to further tears without any feeling of understanding, and proceeding too rapidly may leave the patient feeling that the doctor has no interest or patience. If the patient looks up at the interviewer, or gets out his handkerchief in order to blow his nose, it is usually time to continue.

The patient has established dependent relations with other individuals, and it is helpful to explore these early in the interview. Disruption of such a relationship is a common precipitant of depressive symptoms, and the pattern that they follow is indicative of the transference that the patient may be expected to develop. For example, the interviewer asked a depressed woman, "Who are the important people in your life?" She replied, "I'm all alone now. I moved to the city last year when I realized that I was in love with my boss, and that nothing could come of it. He was married and had a family." The doctor has acquired information about a possible precipitating cause, and might anticipate that similar feelings will develop in the therapeutic relationship.

The depressed patient may begin by talking about how unhappy he feels, or he may discuss what he sees as the cause of his unhappiness. For example, one patient said, "I can't stand it any longer—what's the use in trying, nobody cares anyway." Another tearfully related how she had learned that her husband was having an affair. The doctor can accept the patient's initial emphasis, but later in the interview it is necessary to explore other aspects of the problem.

Physical Symptoms

Although the depressed person may not relate his physical symptoms to his psychological problems, he is usually quite concerned about them, willing to discuss them, and grateful for any advice or assistance that the doctor may have to offer. Frequently the interviewer must actively pursue them, since the patient does not think they will be of interest to the doctor. For example, a man sought psychiatric assistance for his depressed feelings following his divorce, but neglected any mention of his insomnia and weight loss. When the doctor asks about disturbances of sleep, appetite, sexual drive, and so forth, the patient realizes that these all form part of a complex illness that the doctor has seen before. This raises the patient's hopes and enhances his confidence in the physician. At times the patient may not realize that he has had a change in physical functioning until the doctor inquires directly about it, and he may deny the extent of its impact unless detailed data are obtained. For example, a 50-year-old man with a moderately severe depression did not spontaneously mention sexual difficulties. When he was asked, he related that he had noticed a mild decline in his sexual interests, and it was only after specific inquiry that he disclosed that he had had no sexual interest or activity for six months.

The discussion of physical symptoms provides an opportunity for exploring the patient's style of coping with problems and their impact on himself and his family. If the doctor merely obtains a catalogue of physical complaints, this opportunity is lost, and the patient will feel that the focus is on establishing a diagnosis rather than understanding him. For example, if a patient says that he has insomnia, the doctor first determines the exact nature of the sleep disturbance. Is it difficulty in falling asleep or early morning awakening, or both; does the patient feel that he wants to sleep and can't, or is sleep so frightening that he fights it and tries to stay awake? Then the doctor goes on to inquire what the patient does when he can't sleep, what thoughts go through his mind, and what remedies he has tried. He can also inquire about the impact of the patient's insomnia on others and their response to it. The discussion of sleep difficulties is also an ideal time to inquire about dreams and the patient's view of their significance.

The depressed patient is often preoccupied with his physical symptoms, feeling that they are manifestations of a serious physical illness. If the physician inquires about these symptoms and makes no further comment about them, the patient is likely to become more alarmed. A simple, "That problem is common when someone is depressed," or, "That will get better as you start to feel like your old self," is often reassuring.

The interviewer does more than elicit the description of the patient's symptoms and their impact on his life; he also provides the patient with some understanding concerning their relation to his psychological problems. If the patient is severely depressed, this will be deferred until later interviews, but even then the doctor can lay the groundwork in his initial inquiry into the symptomatology. For example, in speaking with the depressed man who had lost his sexual interest, the interviewer inquired, "How did you feel toward your wife during this period of time?" This apparently simple question suggests that the patient's loss of sexual interest is not only a physiological side effect of his depression, but is also related to his emotional reactions to important people in his life.

The interview with the hypochondriacal patient is discussed in greater detail in Chapters 8 and 11. The depressed person is likely to discuss his hypochondriacal feelings as he does everything else, in a hopeless and self-demeaning way. One woman sighed and said, "I guess it's all my change of life. I'm just getting old and withered." A man suggested, "My bowels just don't work anymore. They're making me weak all over and giving me terrible headaches. It's affecting my whole body." Further exploration revealed that he was convinced that he had or was about to develop rectal cancer, a conviction that was later traced to his childhood misinterpretation of his father's recurrent complaints of hemorrhoids.

THE NEED FOR ACTIVE INQUIRY

There are some aspects of the depressed patient's behavior that he actively tries to conceal from the physician. The most prominent of these is his aggression. The man mentioned earlier, who became depressed following his divorce, was able to discuss his mood and his physical symptoms in considerable detail. However, he avoided revealing his violent temper outbursts, which had contributed to his wife's decision to leave, until a later interview. When he finally did describe these, he quickly became tearful and began to berate himself for driving his wife away.

It is usually easy for the experienced doctor to ascertain that a patient is depressed, to evaluate the depth of the depression, and to trace the clinical picture through the precipitating events in the patient's life to the underlying premorbid personality. In general, one of the most valuable allies in exploring a patient's life is his interest in and curiosity about anything he might learn about himself. However, there are problems that sometimes make this difficult with the depressed patient, whose preoccupation with himself centers on feelings of guilt and blame. He has little interest in broadening his self-knowledge, as he anticipates that each discovery will only confirm his inadequacy and unworthiness. In addition, he lacks the energy necessary for a project of self-discovery. This means that the doctor has to assume a larger than usual share of responsibility in mobilizing the patient's motivation. Interpretations around the patient's defensive lack of interest in understanding his problems are ineffective, and will be perceived only as criticism and rejection.

The so-called "parallel" history is frequently valuable. After obtaining the chronology of the illness, the interviewer inquires about the rest of the patient's life, and develops a longitudinal picture of the patient's experiences during the period in which the illness developed. Links that are obviously important and which were not mentioned by the patient are common. For example, a middle-aged woman who was mildly depressed said, "I have no right to feel so bad. I have no real problems." Later, in describing her recent life, she revealed that her youngest daughter had left for college, and that she had moved to a new apartment shortly before she began to get depressed. The interviewer later said, "It must be lonely with your daughter gone." This comment has the effect of an interpretation, but it is gentler and less disturbing to the patient than a direct confrontation.

The doctor notes to himself that the patient's reaction of severe loneliness reveals problems in her relations with husband and friends, but he specifically avoids commenting on this early in the interview. In retrospect, he is also aware that her initial denial, "no real problems," reveals that she has some beginning insight into her difficulty, but that she doesn't feel entitled to respond in the way she has. It is common for the depressed person initially to deny knowledge of the precipitant of his depression and, later, when confronted with it, to claim that it is too minor or trival a problem to cause a serious reaction. The patient is ashamed of what he feels is a weakness, and tries to conceal it.

Another example is the businessman who complained of several months of mild depression, with no awareness of the precipitant. Later, in discussing his occupational history, he mentioned that his immediate superior recently announced his retirement, and that he (the patient) was asked to replace him. When this was explored further, it became apparent that the patient began to feel depressed shortly after he learned of his pending promotion. This paradoxical response results from the patient's guilty reaction to the threat of success.

DISCUSSION OF SUICIDE IN THE INTERVIEW

The discussion of suicide is crucial in gauging the severity and danger of the patient's depression and in planning a treatment program. It also offers a unique but often overlooked opportunity for understanding the basic structure of the patient's personality. This latter function will be considered here; the evaluation of suicidal risk is discussed in Chapter 14.

The experienced interviewer knows that the discussion of

suicide aimed at increasing the doctor's understanding of the patient often is the most effective therapeutic measure against suicidal impulses. If the doctor can help the patient to express the same emotions in the interview that are represented by the act of suicide, the patient's own controls will be able to operate more effectively, and it may not be necessary for him to end his life. Often the doctor's air of concern and his response to the urgency of the situation are themselves therapeutic. A common sequence is illustrated by the young woman who came to a hospital emergency room because she was thinking of jumping off a bridge. An inexperienced first year resident spoke with her and felt that immediate hospitalization was imperative. The patient objected, but he told her that there was a definite risk and insisted that she accept his plan. He then summoned a more experienced colleague, who arrived to find the patient comfortable, in relatively good spirits, and convinced that the suicidal thought could not possibly lead to any overt behavior. The patient's statements seemed convincing to both physicians, and she was sent home to return for a routine appointment the following day. The young resident was thoroughly confused, and felt that he had missed some basic feature of the case. In fact, both doctors' initial impressions were accurate: The younger resident's response had been highly therapeutic, and his interest and concern had helped the patient through an acute crisis.

Suicidal behavior is a final common pathway, growing out of many types of thoughts, fantasies and impulses. The doctor inquires about suicide from two points of view. First, he wants to know how seriously the patient has considered it, what plans he contemplated, what steps he has taken toward realizing them, and his attitude toward these feelings. These questions consider the way in which the patient treats the idea of killing himself. At the same time, the doctor inquires into the meaning of suicide to this specific person. What are the unconscious significances of the suicidal act; what is its expressive or communicative function? For example, a woman in her fifties came to see a psychiatrist because of multiple somatic symptoms that several doctors had told her were psychological in origin. She cried during the first interview, saying, "Why does it all have to happen to me? I haven't slept for days; all I do is cry; doesn't anyone care? Won't anyone do something?" She admitted that she was depressed, but insisted that this was a reaction to her physical problems, not the reverse. The doctor asked her, "Have you ever thought of suicide?" She replied, "Yes, sometimes I think that it's the only way out, but I know that I'd never do anything like that." She had spontaneously provided a clue to the basic meaning of suicide to her (a "way out"), and her current attitude toward it (a thought that she could contemplate, but not act on). However, the doctor knew from other material in the interview that she tended to be impulsive, so he inquired further, "Have you ever felt that you might do something like that?" She hesitated, and then replied, "Well, yes, once. My back pains got so bad I felt it must be cancer, and before I went to see the doctor I promised myself that if it turned out to be the worst, I would spare both myself and my family the pain." The patient had again suggested that suicide is an escape from certain problems, and she had given a suggestion as to the kind of problems she had in mind. At the same time, it was clear that the controls that were apparently effective at that moment might break down if she felt that severe pain and sickness were imminent. She had also provided the doctor with an important clue as to a route for therapeutic intervention in this area should it later be necessary; she wanted to spare her family any suffering, and he could point out the suffering that her suicide would bring. In this episode the doctor learned something of the patient's attitude toward suicide and the meaning it had for her, and enlarged his view of her as a person. It was clear that there was no immediate suicidal risk, but he had some knowledge of the circumstances in which such a risk might appear, and the steps that would be available if it were to occur.

Experienced psychiatrists introduce the subject of suicide into the interview with a depressed patient. The beginner fears that he may give the patient an idea, or that the patient may take offense at the question. A carefully phrased but direct inquiry, such as, "Have you thought of taking your own life?" or, "Have you felt that you want to kill yourself?", can be of great value, even if the answer is, "No." It shows the mildly depressed person that the doctor is concerned and takes his problem quite seriously, and it can lead to a discussion of the positive features of his life, his hope for the future, and his areas of healthy functioning.

Every depressed patient has considered suicide long enough to reject it. In fact, it is the rare individual who has not thought of the idea of suicide at some moment in his life, but most people do not realize this. They are ashamed and want to hide what they think are strange feelings. A simple, direct question about suicide can alleviate this anxiety. If the doctor treats the subject as serious, but not bizarre, the patient will feel less ashamed. The patient can also be helped to trace the historical development of his ideas about suicide, giving him more sense of continuity with his past experiences. For example, when a patient indicates that he has been considering suicide, the doctor can, at some point, inquire, "Have you ever thought of suicide in the past?" If the patient answers, "No," the doctor can pursue this further, saying, "What were your feelings concerning the idea of suicide?" This shift from "suicide" to "the idea of suicide" allows a shift in the patient's mind from admitting impulses to contemplating abstract ideas. The patient may reply, "It always seemed horrible to me, such a cowardly thing to do." This will allow the doctor to inquire as to when the patient first had these thoughts, what his mental image of suicide is, and how it developed. Suicidal feelings do not arise *de novo* in adult life, but can be traced to earlier roots, important figures who talked about killing themselves or about the advantages of death, and family attitudes to which the patient was exposed as a child. For example, one woman revealed that her mother frequently said, "Someday it will all be over," obviously looking forward to death. Another patient's mother would say, "Someday I'll be gone and then you'll be sorry for how you treated me." The discussion of suicide can help to reveal the origins of the patient's problems in his earlier life.

The average person who has suicidal thoughts and comes to see a doctor is intensely ambivalent and struggling to control his behavior. The doctor can easily ally himself with the healthy portion of the patient's ego, and thereby keep the conflict of interests within the patient's mind, rather than between the doctor and the patient. The doctor is concerned and involved, but maintains his role of a neutral, understanding figure, rather than immediately trying to convince the patient to act in a particular way. If a person is anxious and uncertain, and an authority tries to push him toward a specific course of action, he will frequently respond by pushing back. For example, if a patient indicates that he has considered killing himself, and the doctor replies, "That wouldn't solve any of your problems," the patient is likely to reply with an argument. However, if after discussing the suicidal feelings, the doctor asks, "What are the reasons that have kept you alive?", the patient will be presenting the arguments that restrain his impulses.

For some individuals, death is not the end of life, but only the entry into another state that may be more pleasant than this one. The patient anticipates gratification of dependent needs and the reunion with lost loved ones. This kind of denial and magical thinking is reinforced by popular myths and religious beliefs. Some patients will offer these beliefs as rationalizations in favor of suicide. In treating such patients, the doctor does not challenge the patient's conviction of life after death. Rather, he explores the prohibitions against suicide that are usually associated with such beliefs and the patient's own doubt and ambivalence. It is helpful to inquire into the immediate reason for the patient's plan, and to point out that since his philosophical views have been long-standing, some more concrete event must have led to his suicidal thought. For example, a middle-aged woman became severely depressed after her husband was killed in an automobile accident. She spoke of killing herself, and said, "When I think that I could be with him again, I feel alive!" She had been active in a Fundamentalist sect and believed in a concrete life after death, and her suicidal feelings were combined with near-delusional episodes in which she felt that she communicated with his soul. The psychiatrist did not challenge her religious beliefs, or even her communication with the dead, but rather asked her what she felt her husband would have wanted her to do and what course of action her religion prescribed. She was able to give up her idea of suicide with the feeling that she was honoring her husband's wishes.

PRINCIPLES OF TREATMENT

The treatment of depressed patients is based upon two fundamental principles. First is the alleviation of suffering and guilt, the stimulation of hope, and the protection from self-injury; in short, supportive therapy. This can involve psychotherapy, drugs, or other organic therapies used separately or in combination. The second principle is that of psychodynamic exploration of the meaning and causes of the depression, with the aim of both solving the immediate problem and preventing recurrence in the future.

SUPPORTIVE THERAPY

PSYCHOTHERAPY.   The first basic goal in the treatment of depression is to alleviate the patient's pain and suffering. This can be done by psychotherapeutic and pharmacological techniques aimed at improving the patient's defensive functioning and providing substitute gratifications. The doctor attempts to enhance denial, projection, repression, reaction formation, or whatever defenses are most effective in protecting the patient from his painful feelings, and he offers himself as a replacement for the patient's lost love object, providing transference gratifications that temporarily substitute for the frustrations of reality.

The depressed patient feels hopeless, and he may have little motivation for treatment. Initially it is necessary to stimulate his hope and to develop motivation. When the patient can visualize a future in which he is not depressed, the doctor has begun to establish a therapeutic alliance. The interviewer attempts to convey hope from the initial contact. For example, although a depressed college student reported that he had been unable to attend classes, the doctor carefully scheduled his appointments so that when the patient was ready to return, he would not have a time conflict with school. The message was that the doctor expected the patient to be able to resume his activities. In other situations, the doctor might advise the patient to defer an important decision "until you are feeling better." This phrase is used rather than "because you aren't up to it." The patient is told not only that he is sick, but also that he will get well.

This brings up a second but related principle of treatment, the protection of the patient from self-injury. The most dramatic aspect of this is the prevention of suicide, but there are subtler forms of self-destructive behavior that are common in depressed patients. The law student who wants to quit school and obtain a lower status job as a police trainee and the businessman who relinquishes an opportunity for promotion as a result of depression are both examples. Initially, the doctor's role is to identify this behavior and use his authority to prevent the patient from doing serious or irreparable harm to himself. Later, he offers the patient insight into the meaning of his masochism and interprets its psychodynamic origins. For example, a woman who became depressed after her husband indicated that he planned to seek a divorce told her doctor, "What's the use, nobody cares about me anyway. I'm tired of working so hard for other people. I'm going to quit my job, and when I use up my money, I'll go on welfare." Her depression was mixed with conscious anger, which suggested a relatively good prognosis for the depressive symptoms. The doctor noted this, and realized that once she left her job she might have difficulty obtaining a comparable one. He told her, "You're angry at the world, but right now you're mad at yourself too. I'm afraid if you quit your job you might suffer more than anyone else. Perhaps you should wait until we can talk about it more and you can decide exactly what will be in your best interest."

This type of intervention creates a problem, since the doctor does not want to assume responsibility for the patient's executive ego functioning, thereby diminishing the patient's self-confidence and self-esteem and adding to his depression. In order to minimize this, the doctor implies that his offering of direct advice is only a temporary role. For example, another woman sought psychiatric help following a separation from her husband. Her physician asked about the practical legal aspects of the impending separation. She said "I told my husband to do whatever he wanted and just give me the papers to sign. I'm no good to anyone else; I might as well help him." The doctor indicated concern at her failure to protect her financial and legal interests, but she said she just didn't care. He explored her feeling that she didn't deserve anything, and finally said, "It seems clear that you would be acting differently if you weren't depressed. I don't think you're ready to deal with the reality of the situation yet." If she had been less severely depressed, he might have explored her failure to act in her own best interests, uncovering her defensive inhibition of assertion.

A third principle, after stimulating the patient's hope and protecting him from self-injury, involves reducing his guilt. Here, the physician addresses himself to the expiatory aspects of the patient's behavior. The suffering of depressive illness is associated with the unconscious hope that forgiveness will follow. If the doctor comments, "You have suffered enough," or, "You deserve a better life," he can alleviate some of the patient's guilt.

Conscious guilt is more often related to the secondary effects of depression. The patient may say, "I am such a bother to everyone. They'd be so much better off without me." He is guilty because he is unable to perform his work or provide for his loved ones. The doctor can reply, "You're sick. You've done so much for them, now it's their turn to take care of you." The patient may not respond, and occasionally it is necessary for the doctor to invoke the patient's guilt about the anger that he unconsciously discharges through his symptomatology. This manipulation utilizes guilt about expressing aggressive impulses to help suppress depressive withdrawal, and allows the patient to function more adequately with his friends and family. For example, the physician can say, "You aren't being very considerate of their feelings. They want you to get help and feel better."

Although the depressed patient needs considerable support, he becomes uncomfortable if the interviewer is overly warm or friendly. He feels unworthy, and is unable to reciprocate. Beginning psychotherapists, particularly those without a medical background, are sometimes overeager in their expression of positive feelings. When their depressed patients withdraw, they become even nicer, with the result that the patient becomes anxious rather than comfortable. He may experience the therapist's positive feelings as an attempt to reassure him because he really *is* bad.

The use of humor is a problem in the interview with the depressive. If the patient demonstrates any remaining sense of humor, it is better to encourage and respond to this than for the doctor to initiate humorous interchanges himself. The depressed person is likely to respond to the doctor's spontaneous attempts at humor as evidence that he is misunderstood, or even that he is being ridiculed.

The doctor may use the term "depressed" when he summarizes the patient's description of his problem, or he may offer it in his own formulation, saying, "It sounds as if you have been quite depressed for some months." This is in sharp contrast to the usual avoidance of diagnostic terms. The same doctor would not say, "You are suffering from hysterical symptoms." There are several reasons for this difference. One, which has been discussed earlier, is the dual meaning of the term "depressed," which refers both to a clinical syndrome and a related affective state. While it may be unusual for the doctor to employ diagnostic labels in the interview, he frequently identifies the patient's emotions, and "You seem depressed" may be seen as being analogous to "You seem angry." However, this does not tell the whole story, as it is common for the doctor to say, "You are suffering from a depression," clearly referring to the clinical entity. The reason for this can be understood if we consider the principle behind the usual avoidance of diagnostic labels. Patients often employ such labels in order to support their projective defenses. Thus they claim, "There's nothing I can do about it, it's my neurosis," as though a neurosis were a foreign agent, such as a virus, that is the cause of their problems. An important issue in treatment is to help that patient to experience neurotic behavior as being under his control as a preliminary step to exploring methods of changing it. Any phraseology that suggests that the patient has a disease will work counter to this goal and will therefore be antitherapeutic.

With the depressed patient, and occasionally with some others, this problem is reversed. The patient not only accepts responsibility for his difficulties, but he exaggerates his own role and tortures himself with guilt and self-condemnation. His self-accusations conceal a denial of his true role in his illness, but nevertheless the initial problem in treatment is often to dilute the patient's conviction that he is to blame. Phrases that suggest that he is suffering from an illness assist in this attempt. At the same time, the thought that the patient is sick suggests that he may get better, and challenges the depressed person's view of his situation as hopeless and eternal.

ORGANIC THERAPY. Pharmacological and organic treatbent are important therapeutic methods. They will only be considered here in terms of their impact on the interview. Regardless of their physiological mode of action, these treatments always have magical unconscious significance to the patient. The doctor may want to enhance this, or to interpret it, but he should keep it in mind. The placebo effect of medication is increased if the doctor suggests that his pharmacological regimen is potent and will alleviate the patient's symptoms. It is preferable to encourage the patient to associate his placebo reaction to the treatment as a whole rather than to any specific drug, since it may be necessary to change medication during the course of therapy. The doctor can say, "We have several powerful drugs, and we may want to switch from one to another." Comments such as, "We'll see if this does any good, and if not we'll try something else," have a negative effect. If there is a latent period before the drug has a therapeutic effect, it is well to warn the patient in advance, or he will feel that the treatment isn't working. Minor side effects, such as dryness of the mouth, can be interpreted as evidence that the drug is beginning to take effect.

The patient may introduce the discussion of organic treatment by questions such as, "Is there any medication that could help me?" or, "Do I need shock treatment?" These questions reflect the anticipation of intervention from an omnipotent external force, in the form of either magical assistance or punishment. The doctor can learn more if he delays his reply and instead asks, "What did you have in mind?" One patient said, "I understand there are some new pills that will make this all go away." Another replied, "You can do anything you want to me if only it will help. I don't care if it takes shock treatments, or even a lobotomy." The first person was hoping for the intervention of a good parent, whereas the second had to atone for his sins before he could feel better. The doctor rarely interprets these wishes early in the treatment, but they are important nevertheless. The first patient may well respond to psychological suggestions that the treatment will be potent and effective. The second needs to see treatment as punishment, and excessive reassurance about its safety or comfort might actually have a negative effect.

Electric shock therapy is widely used as a treatment for depression, and it is frequently discussed in interviews with depressed patients, either because the doctor suggests it or because the patient has heard of it previously and raises the subject. Shock treatment is explained and discussed like any other form of therapy, but the doctor should recognize that the phrase "electric shock" implies magical power and danger. Patients often indicate fears of what this treatment will do to them, and they often unconsciously equate it with early traumatic experiences and physical punishment. In contrast, they usually have early life experiences with pills and medicines, which lead to feelings of trust and security. The doctor can ask about the patient's fears. Pain, loss of control, death, change of personality, and infantile regression are all common ones, and his reassurances should be as specific as possible. The patient will feel more comfortable if he is prepared for what he will experience, such as the pretreatment injections. It is not helpful to discuss the technical details of the treatment. The patient will require some preparation for the organic mental syndrome which follows, and the more matter-of-factly this is discussed the more easily he will accept it.

When the doctor describes any organic treatment, he should provide as clear and specific a statement as possible. He should discuss not only the practical aspects of the regimen, but also the anticipated therapeutic effects. For example, it is preferable to say, "These pills will help your spirits to improve," rather than, "This should help the problem." There are aspects of depression that cannot be helped by organic therapy, and it may be helpful to spell these out. The doctor can say, "Of course the medicine won't help you get your husband back," or, "The pills will let you feel better, and then you may be able to deal with the financial problem more effectively." The patient will feel more self-confidence and self-esteem if he sees the physician as helping him to solve his own problems rather than resolving them for him.

INTERPRETATION OF PSYCHODYNAMIC PATTERNS

Supportive treatment is the only possibility if the patient is severely depressed or so despondent that he is unable to talk to the interviewer or to participate in the routine of everyday life. The doctor may use psychotherapy, antidepressant drugs, or electric shock, but his intent is to alleviate the patient's suffering, irrespective of its etiology. In the interview, he will listen to the patient's concerns and will try to reassure him about his fears. He will search for islands of adaptive functioning that are relatively intact and try to focus on them, expressing less interest in the developmental roots of the patient's character if the patient himself is not preoccupied with them. For many patients, this type of therapy is often adequate to eradicate depressive symptomatology, and there may be no motivation or indication for further treatment.

However, for those patients who are to be treated in analytic psychotherapy, the doctor shifts his basic clinical strategy after the immediate crisis is under control, acknowledging the risk of transiently aggravating the symptoms. This second approach in the treatment of depressed patients requires more active participation on the patient's part. Unlike the first mode of treatment, which is aimed at alleviating symptoms, it offers the possibility of influencing the course of the patient's life, decreasing the likelihood of future depressions, and diminishing his depressive character pathology. Clarifications and interpretations are designed to expose the unconscious psychodynamic factors that underlie the symptoms. The doctor interprets the defenses in order to uncover the thoughts and feeling which the patient is trying to avoid.

These two methods of treatment, suppressive and exploratory, are inherent in the nature of psychotherapy, and they are combined in varying proportions in the treatment of all neurotic conditions. However, there is more conflict between them and more difficulty combining and integrating them in the treatment of depression than in other disorders. Depression is the most painful of neurotic symptoms, and therefore the patient is concerned with rapid symptom relief. Also, denial is an important defense against depressive feelings, and if the doctor enhances this defense to increase the patient's comfort, he is working directly counter to uncovering therapy.

In the initial interview with the mildly depressed patient, the doctor may offer interpretive comments that are designed to test his ability to deal with insight. For example, a middle-aged man became depressed after moving to a new city. He told the doctor of his wife's unhappiness about the move, and her constant complaint that everything had been fine until he uprooted their home because of his professional ambition. She had refused to help furnish or decorate their new home. He finally cried and said, "If there were only some way to escape, to get away from it all. I just can't take any more." The doctor listened and then said, "You must get pretty angry at her." The patient immediately began to berate himself, saying, "I've been an awful husband. My whole family is upset and it is all my fault." The doctor's interpretation was accurate, but the patient's response revealed that, at this point, his reaction to such knowledge was to become even more depressed. The doctor decided that even this tentative exploration of the patient's repressed rage would be more effective later in treatment.

At times, what the doctor thinks has been uncovering exploratory therapy is experienced by the patient as supportive. One common pattern for the interview with the depressed patient is for the patient to start slowly, have difficulty talking, and seem somewhat retarded. As the doctor reaches out, inquires about symptoms, and explores the origins of the patient's difficulties, the patient grows livelier and more animated, participates well, and seems to search actively for the meaning of his behavior and to explore it in the interview. The doctor feels pleased and reassured, and then tells the patient that the interview is drawing to a close. The patient lapses back into hopeless gloom; the insight of a moment earlier has become irrelevant. He was responding to the supportive relationship implicit in the interview process, and the content of the uncovered material was of little therapeutic significance.

The psychodynamic origins of depression are often apparent to the interviewer long before awareness of them can be of any conceivable value to the patient. Beginning psychiatrists are often eager to practice interpreting, and when something is clear to them they want to share it with the patient. The depressed person provides a willing audience. He is glad to listen, and rarely challenges what the doctor says. However, the therapist must remember that insight is a means, not an end in treatment. If the patient uses the doctor's comments to verify that he is worthless, the doctor is interpreting prematurely, no matter how accurate and insightful his observations.

The tendency of depressed and masochistic patients to take the doctor's interpretation and use it as a weapon against themselves has been termed a "negative therapeutic reaction." When it becomes a problem in the interview, the doctor either alters his interpretative approach or tries to deal with the patient's response as a form of resistance. For example, he might say, "You seem to search for evidence that you're bad."

Direct interpretations of the patient's anger are more likely to be disturbing than supportive. However, euphemistic phrases, such as, "You are very disappointed in him," may be acceptable. The doctor takes care not to challenge the patient's right to feel the way he does. Usually this neutrality will be interpreted as active support for the patient's feeling. Some therapists, upon learning that depression results from anger directed against the self, openly encourage the patient to direct his anger at key figures in his life. Although this is occasionally effective, the results are more often disastrous, as the patient becomes frightened that his controls may not be effective and that all of the dangers that he fears from expressing his rage will occur. The result is commonly a loss of confidence in the doctor and a flight from treatment.

Patients have frequently heard of biological theories and biological treatments of their illness, and they may use them as a defense against its psychological meaning. This is also true of schizophrenic patients, but their theories are more bizarre and the defensive role that they serve is more obvious, so the interviewer has less difficulty dealing with them.

The patient who raises the question of a chemical or hormonal basis of his depression is usually challenging the doctor's discussion of psychological factors. The patient feels that it is bad to be depressed, that somehow it is his fault, and that he is less culpable if he can find a physical cause. His desire to defend himself from feeling that he is to blame for his troubles is a positive sign, and should not be challenged by the doctor. The patient utilizes the biological explanation in the service of psychological denial, and the overall strategy of therapy will determine whether this is to be interpreted or supported. Usually, rather than interpreting this as a defense, the doctor simply indicates that there is no contradiction between the psychological meaning of the patient's depression and any physical basis that it might have. This explanation must be adjusted to the patient's level of sophistication. For example, a relatively uneducated person who has asked if he might just be run down physically could be told, "There is no question that you feel run down, and that is part of your problem. At the same time, I think you are worried and upset about what has happened, and feel disappointed in yourself. I suspect that makes things worse."

The preceding discussion of psychotherapy has been relatively superficial, but as mentioned above, this is intended to counteract the tendency of beginning psychiatrists to go too deep, too fast in treating depressed patients. Major clinical improvement and extensive diagnostic information are often obtained by a simple supportive approach.

INTERVIEWING THE FAMILY

The family of the depressed patient is often seen by the doctor, whether they accompany the patient to the initial interview or come later in treatment. They may be sympathetic and concerned about the patient or angry with him. Usually these two feelings are both present, although one may be concealed. The doctor is interested in obtaining information from the family, in modifying their behavior as part of the treatment for the patient, and in exploring the interaction between patient and family.

A few clinical illustrations may highlight some characteristic problems. An adolescent girl sought help because she was despondent and contemplating suicide following the disruption of a relationship with a boyfriend. The psychiatrist advised treatment, but she was sure that her parents, who lived in another city, would refuse to support such a plan. The doctor offered to see them, and the patient called a few days later, saying that her mother was coming to the city, and arranged an appointment. When the mother arrived, she was obviously angry at both the patient and the doctor. She started the interview by speaking of the over-indulgence of contemporary adolescents, and the need for will power and self-discipline in emotional disturbances. The doctor asked, "What has your daughter told you about our talk?" The mother replied that the girl had described the disruption of her relationship with her boyfriend, her subsequent visit to the psychiatrist, and their extensive discussion about suicide. "Furthermore," she added, "I think it's terrible that you talked to her so much about suicide. You're likely to put ideas into her head." The doctor half turned toward the girl while asking her mother, "Did she tell you why we talked so much about suicide?" At this point the girl interrupted, sobbing loudly, and telling her mother for the first time of a suicide attempt she had made some months earlier. The effect was dramatic; the mother was insistent that the doctor arrange for immediate treatment and questioned him about the advisability of the girl remaining in school. This concern had been concealed by the mother's need to deny her daughter's difficulty, but the doctor had enlisted the girl's aid in a confrontation that had broken through her mother's denial. At the same time, the doctor had challenged the girl's distorted image of her parent's attitude toward her welfare, and had laid the groundwork for later interpretations concerning the patient's role in their apparent indifference to her difficulties.

Another situation is illustrated by the middle-aged, depressed woman who was accompanied to the initial interview by her husband, a successful attorney. He spoke of his concern about her condition and bewilderment about what to do. He said that she had been worried so much that he felt she needed a rest, a vacation, and urged the doctor to prescribe one. He made it clear that money was no object where his wife's health was concerned. At the same time, he indicated that business pressures made it impossible for him to go away with her. His wife sat through this discussion silently, staring at the floor. The doctor responded by turning to her and asking, "Do you feel he's trying to get rid of you?" The husband protested vehemently; his wife looked up with a flicker of interest. Later, when speaking to the husband alone, the doctor was able to explore his conscious irritations and dissatisfactions with his wife, which he had concealed lest he aggravate her problems. When the doctor again pointed out the hostility that had emerged in the husband's therapeutic suggestion, he became quite distraught. He then revealed that he was having an affair with another woman, and that much of his anger at his wife covered feelings of guilt that he was the cause of her problem. When these were discussed, his attitude shifted to a more realistic acceptance of her illness. He was still dissatisfied and angry with her, but no longer angry because she was sick.

It is not unusual for the family to provide crucial information concerning the precipitants or stresses in the patient's life that he has denied so completely that they do not emerge in the early interviews. One middle-aged man said that there were no problems at home, but later, when his wife came with him, she revealed that their son was flunking out of high school. The patient interrupted, saying that he felt his wife was exaggerating the problem, but when it was discussed more fully, it became apparent that he had refused to accept it.

In each of these episodes, the doctor's interview with the family served to facilitate treatment. Members of the patient's family had developed fixed attitudes that contributed to the patient's difficulties and that were perpetuated in part because the patient was unable to question or confront them. The doctor assumed the role that would otherwise be played by the patient's healthy ego, and thus reversed a vicious cycle that had contributed to the depression and the increasing rigidity of the family conflict.

The family of the depressed person may prefer that he remain depressed. This is often related to the patient's inhibition of aggression and his masochistic willingness to tolerate his family's exploitation. If this is the case, they will be opposed to any treatment that threatens to lead to change, and the doctor will find that they are more accepting of a poor prognosis and a stable hopeless situation. This may provide an indication for family therapy. It is not unusual for this family to interfere with treatment just as the patient shows signs of improvement.

Depressed people feel deprived and rejected, even without realistic provocation. It is usually an error for the doctor who is treating a depressed person to treat another member of the patient's family himself, as it will usually contribute to the patient's feeling of rejection and deprivation. Of course, this does not apply to family sessions that include the patient, which may be helpful in treatment.

THE MANIC PATIENT

The interview with the manic patient is a dramatic and unforgettable experience. The patient is usually talking before the doctor comes on the scene, and he talks continuously throughout their contact. His initial response is likely to be a provocative comment about the doctor's age or appearance. An attempted introduction provides an opportunity for clang associations to the doctor's name and a series of jokes, made so rapidly that it is difficult to keep up, let alone respond. For example, a manic young man was talking to a nurse when the doctor came onto the ward. When he caught sight of the new arrival, he said, "Here comes the sawbones; I guess we're going to have some surgery now. Hey, are you Dr. Kildare or Ben Casey? Are you a real doctor or a television doctor? You must be a real doctor, because a television doctor wouldn't be so ugly." At this point the doctor interrupted, saying, "My name is Dr. Williams." The patient immediately started singing, "Wee Willie Williams—wanted to make billions—so he became a shrink and look at him now."

In a situation like this, the doctor is tempted to listen silently, make his observations, and retreat. However, this reduces the patient to an object of study, and although he may seem to invite this kind of treatment, it will soon become apparent that he is just as disturbed by it as the manifestly depressed patient would be.

At times it is possible to join the patient's mood and respond to it with a smile and a comment such as, "You seem to feel quite playful today." The doctor can attempt to introduce himself and ask the patient a few simple questions. Even if these aren't productive in the sense of direct answers, they do help orient the patient to the doctor's interest, and this may be useful later in treatment. In addition, they allow the doctor to make the first crucial interpretation with a truly manic patient: "I get the feeling that you don't want to talk with me." Manic behavior is complex and overdetermined, but in the interview situation it must first be handled as a defense against emotional contact with the interviewer.

Interviews with manic patients are, of necessity, rather brief. Often the patient gets to know the doctor from seeing him on a hospital ward rather than in the formal interview situation. However, once the patient develops some familiarity with the doctor, a new type of behavior emerges. The patient's clever sarcastic quips become bitter, and are sometimes directed inward. At the same time, his mood shifts from elation or euphoria to isolated moments of despair. The doctor must sense and respond to these quickly, although often the patient will deny them and take off on a new manic flight. However, it is the interchange that, repeated often enough, provides the basis for the therapeutic relationship. For example, a manic college professor was entertaining a staff conference by telling them, "I can read your souls from your ties. Wide ties, narrow ties, red ties, blue ties. Your ties are better than your eyes. They're even better than my lies." With this last comment, his eyes suddenly filled with tears. The psychiatrist who was interviewing him leaned forward in his chair and softly said, "You're upset." The patient looked at him seriously for a few seconds, and then angrily shouted, "Get away from me, you damned mindreader!" For a moment he had dropped his defenses, and he now took up the fight anew. However, as he improved, he developed his closest relationship with the doctor who had interviewed him.

The patients described above represent full-blown manic psychoses, a relatively rare condition that almost always requires hospitalization and pharmacological or other organic treatments. More common are those with hypomanic syndromes, the patients who use manic defenses but do not lose their contact with reality. The hypomanic patient seems easy to interview; he is garrulous and talks freely about almost any subject. He tends to be irritable and provocative, but is usually more able to control these traits with the doctor than in the outside world. He rarely has any insight into his difficulty, and as a result hypomanic character traits are more often an incidental finding than a chief complaint. The major problem in the interview is to get the patient to talk about his problems rather than the myriad other subjects that are of greater interest to him.

TRANSFERENCE

In response to his feeling of helplessness, the depressed patient develops a clinging, dependent relationship, with the expectation that his therapist has the magical omnipotent power to effect a cure. He tries to extract nurturant care through his suffering, cajoling or coercing the doctor into helping him. He may become openly angry or more depressed if he fails at this attempt. This mixture of dependency and anger characterizes the transference. On the surface he is hopeless, but his unconscious hope is revealed by his feeling that the doctor has the capacity to help him.

The patient's dependent feelings emerge as he reveals his inability to make even simple decisions. Usually he does not directly ask for the doctor's help, but his obvious helplessness elicits the doctor's pity and concern. Without realizing it, the doctor may find that he is guiding not only the interview, but also the patient's life, and that he is, implicitly or explicitly, offering advice about his practical problems, his family relationships, or almost anything else. These silent requests for the doctor's aid are often combined with tributes to his wisdom and experience. For example, the patient may say, "I just can't decide whether to take the job. I wish I could be decisive, like you." The doctor is placed in the position of either taking responsibility for the patient's decision or depriving him of valuable advice and guidance. If he declines to give advice, saying, "I think that you should make that decision yourself, but we can certainly discuss it," or, "I don't have any special knowledge about your job, but let's talk about the questions you have about it in your own mind," the patient reacts as though he were deprived and rejected. He feels that the doctor could provide direct help but, for some reason, has decided not to. On the other hand, if the doctor supplies the advice, it is common for new information to emerge that makes it clear that the advice is wrong. For example, if the doctor had said, "Well, it seems like a great job to me," the patient might reply, "Good, I'm glad you said that. I wasn't sure, because it would mean an extra two hours of commuting each day." The doctor is now on the spot; does he withdraw his first statement, inquire why the patient withheld this critical data, or simply keep quiet? None of these alternatives is satisfactory; the first leaves the patient wondering whether the doctor feels he isn't able to handle the challenge, the second is taken as criticism, and the third creates the danger that the patient will act on the doctor's suggestions and escalate the problem one step further.

This pattern reveals the close relation between the patient's dependency feelings and his anger. He wants something, but he assumes in advance that he will not get it, and is angry as a result. When the frustration actually occurs, it only confirms his feelings. If, on the other hand, his wishes are gratified, he still has difficulty. He feels even more dependent, and is ashamed of his childishness. To receive what he craves is to relinquish any view of himself as an independent, competent person. Furthermore, he resents any suggestion that he is in some way an extension of the therapist, a relationship that is felt as similar to that he had with his family.

The patient often finds frustration and rejection more comfortable than gratification, since, when his wishes are gratified, his anger is exposed as inappropriate and guilt follows. One depressed woman called the doctor at home on a Sunday afternoon, saying that she was upset and asking if he would see her right away. To her surprise, he agreed. By the time she came to his office, she was contrite and apologetic, fearing that she had disturbed him for something that wasn't truly an emergency. Her guilt about assuming that he would not help was more prominent than her original concern.

In time, the therapist must interpret this entire pattern, pointing out the inevitability of frustration and disappointment in the patient's mode of relating to potential sources of dependency gratification. However, before such an interpretation is possible, the doctor has usually gone through this sequence many times, and has erred on both sides of the dilemma. Perhaps one of the most critical aspects of treating the depressed patient is to respond to such experiences with understanding rather than irritation. This will be discussed further under countertransference.

The discussion of suicide can become a vehicle for the patient's transference feelings. Allusions to suicide are sure to elicit the doctor's concern, and at times may be primarily motivated by this goal. As the patient becomes involved in therapy, suicide may also become a vehicle for angry or competitive transference feelings. The patient may learn that the most effective way to challenge the doctor's self-esteem is to demonstrate how impotent he is in stopping the patient's self-destructive behavior. One young girl who had been hospitalized after a suicide attempt became angry when the therapist wouldn't permit her boyfriend to visit her. She would appear for each appointment with a razor blade or some sleeping pills, repeatedly exposing the hospital's inability to really protect her adequately. The patient who informs the therapist that he has a cache of sleeping pills at home "just in case" is demonstrating similar feelings. The inexperienced therapist feels that his grandiosity has been challenged, and tries to get the patient to give up the supply or to promise not to use them. The patient experiences this as the doctor's attempt to disarm him and render him helpless. Any outpatient who wants to kill himself, can, and the therapist who accepts the patient's power in this situation has taken a step toward analyzing the underlying transference feelings.

Discussions of suicidal behavior that are motivated by transference feelings may become an important resistance. However, talking about suicidal feelings is a much preferable form of resistance to acting them out, and premature interpretations may force the patient to prove that he really meant it. The suicidal patient usually acts out in other ways as well, and the interpretation can often be attempted in less dangerous areas of behavior before it is applied to suicide.

In addition to the patient's dependent, angry, and guilty transference feelings, the patient often evokes anger or guilt in the interviewer. His suffering itself tends to make others feel guilty, and this may be accentuated by comments such as, "I hope you had a nice weekend; it's nice that some people can enjoy life." Early in treatment, it is best not to interpret the aggression in such remarks. Later, when the envy and anger are closer to the surface, the interviewer may comment on them. The therapist's vacations are particularly important in the handling of the depressed patient's transference feelings. The patient's dependency needs and his anger at the doctor's refusal to gratify them are accentuated, and his powerlessness to control the doctor's behavior is underlined. Suicidal behavior may appear as a means of either holding onto the doctor or punishing him for going. Often this whole constellation is denied until the doctor has actually left, and forceful and repeated interpretations are necessary in the weeks preceding the vacation. With the seriously depressed patient, it is always a good idea to let the patient know where the doctor is going, how to get in contact with him, and who will be available for emergencies.

The patient's masochistic trends sometimes invite sarcastic or frankly hostile comments by the doctor. These are rarely helpful, although it may be useful to interpret the way in which the patient attempts to provoke them.

COUNTERTRANSFERENCE

The depressed person elicits strong feelings in those who have close contact with him. Most prominent is the empathic depression that can be such an important diagnostic tool in the interview with a patient who denies his own depression. Whenever the doctor feels his own mood lowering during an interview, he should consider whether he is responding to the patient's depression. This response is not countertransference, but simply the identification that the skillful interviewer always experiences with his patient.

In addition to this normal empathic reaction, the doctor may respond in a less realistic way. For example, the dependent transference, which was discussed above, may elicit a complementary omnipotent countertransference. The patient acts as if to say, "I'm sure you have the answer," and the doctor responds with agreement. A paternalistic or overprotective style is the most common manifestation of this problem. One doctor suggested that his patient, a middle-aged depressed man, read certain books, and encouraged him to learn tennis for recreation. The patient at first responded positively, but then began to complain that he didn't have the energy to pursue these activities, and he felt that the doctor was disappointed in him. The depressed patient is initially pleased by active interest and encouragement, but his dependent craving is always greater than the doctor can possibly gratify, and he often comes to feel frustrated and rejected. The doctor who has actually played the role of the omnipotent parent finds it difficult to interpret the transference origins of these feelings. This common pattern of countertransference is related to the universal desire to be omnipotent, if only in the eyes of others. Many physicians have an unusually strong wish for power to control the lives of others.

One of the most dramatic manifestations of omnipotent

countertransference is the doctor who assures the suicidal patient, "Don't worry, we won't let you kill yourself." This statement can never be made with absolute certainty, and the patient realizes that the doctor is promising more than he can deliver. At the same time, any responsibility that the patient may have felt for his own life is diminished. One patient later reported that his inner response to this assurance was, "We'll see!"

A second pattern of countertransference with depressed patients involves the doctor's feelings of guilt and anger. The patient conceals his angry feelings, and often expresses them by using his suffering to make others guilty. The doctor who does not understand this process may respond to it nevertheless. A depressed man did not appear for an appointment during a heavy snowstorm, but did not cancel it. When the doctor called, the patient answered the phone and said, "Oh, I thought you'd realize I wouldn't be in, but don't worry, I'll put your check in the mail today." The implication was that the doctor was calling because he was concerned about payment, not because of his interest in the patient. The doctor started to defend himself, protesting, "No that's not it," but the patient interrupted, saying, "I shouldn't have said that. Anyway, I'll see you next week." The doctor felt that he had been misunderstood, and at first worried that he shouldn't have called. This type of guilty response to the patient's covert aggression is common. When the pattern has been repeated a few times, the doctor is more likely to become angry. Doctors sometimes express their anger at depressed patients openly, often rationalizing their reaction as an attempt to mobilize the patient or to get him to express his feelings. The doctor's guilt or anger may also be a response to his feeling of helplessness in the face of the patient's overwhelming demands. It is difficult to tell a hopeless, crying patient that the session is over, and it is an annoying imposition to extend the time into the next patient's hour.

A third manifestation of countertransference is the boredom and impatience commonly felt while treating depressed patients. This serves as a defense against the doctor's concealed feelings of depression, guilt, or anger. It usually occurs after several sessions; the first interview with a depressed patient typically causes less anxiety than usual in the doctor. The decrease in normal anxiety results from the patient's preoccupation with himself, which prevents him from taking an active interest in the doctor.

However, the doctor's initial comfort rapidly shifts to boredom as the patient's constricted interests and painful feelings become apparent. The doctor who wants to be entertained by his patients will have little success treating depressed patients. Disinterest and indifference are far more destructive to the treatment than more obviously negative feelings of anger or guilt, since the latter are usually closer to consciousness and easier to work through. The doctor who feels bored with a depressed patient may subtly try to drive that patient out of treatment without being aware of it, and the patient's feelings of rejection will reinforce his depression, and may even precipitate a suicidal crisis.

It is easy to exploit the depressed person. He submits masochistically, and his slowness to respond and inhibition of aggression make him a ready victim. If the doctor finds that there is a patient upon whose time he is likely to intrude, or whose appointments he often changes, it is usually someone who is depressed.

Medication is important in the treatment of depressed patients, and it plays a role in the countertransference. The doctor may initiate pharmacotherapy or switch to a new drug, not because of clinical indications, but because he is tired of the patient's symptoms. The patient may correctly feel the physician's impatience and react by feeling rejected and more depressed. The doctor is more comfortable if he thinks that it is the patient rather than his treatment that has failed.

Depressed people want to be cared for, but a central aspect of their pathology is that they drive away the very thing they crave. If the doctor recognizes the inevitability of this pattern, he is less likely to overreact to the patient's needs and also less likely to reject the patient for having them. This intermediate position allows him to respond appropriately, interpret effectively, and play a truly therapeutic role.

Interviewing the depressed patient requires sensitivity and a capacity for empathic understanding of severe psychological pain. The psychiatrist will find few clinical situations that so test his basic humanity as well as his professional skill. However, the stakes are high. Depression often affects productive and potentially healthy individuals who have an excellent prognosis for recovery, but it is the only common functional psychiatric syndrome with a significant mortality. Treatment may strongly influence the outcome, and here, as nowhere else, the psychiatrist is in the traditional medical role of healer and saver of lives.

REFERENCES

Bieber, I.: The meaning of masochism. Amer. J. Psychother., 7:433, 1953.

Brenner, C.: The masochistic character. J. Amer. Psychoanaly. Assoc., 7:197, 1959.

Cohen, M., et al.: An intensive study of 12 cases of manic depressive psychosis. Psychiatry, 17:103, 1954.

Freud, S.: Mourning and melancholia. Standard Edition of Complete Psychological Works of Sigmund Freud, Vol. XIV. London, Hogarth Press, 1957, pp. 237–258.

Freud, S.: The economic problem of masochism. Standard Edition of Complete Psychological Works of Sigmund Freud, Vol. XIX. London, Hogarth Press, 1961, pp. 157–170.

Gaylin, W. (ed.): The Meaning of Despair. New York, Science House, 1968.

Havens, L.: Recognition of suicidal risks through the psychologic examination. New Eng. J. Med., 276:210, 1967.

7
THE SCHIZOPHRENIC PATIENT

Psychopathology and Psychodynamics

The syndrome of schizophrenia is varied in its psychopathology, psychodynamics, etiology, and clinical course. Two patients, both diagnosed as being schizophrenic, may appear to be totally different. This variability has led to the understanding of schizophrenia as not one, but a group of clinical entities.

The schizophrenic patient suffers from disturbances in several areas of psychological functioning. The most prominent difficulty can involve overt behavior patterns and interpersonal relationships, subjective mental processes, or even physiological regulation. For example, one patient may present with extreme social withdrawal, retreating to bed for weeks at a time, another with episodes of depersonalization and feelings of being controlled by external forces, and still a third has marked anorexia with severe weight loss. This is in contrast to other major psychiatric entities, in which, although several areas of functioning may be affected, one is seen as central to the disorder.

A patient may show great variation in symptomatology, both at a given time and over the course of his life. The illness may be so circumscribed as to resemble an acute organic psychosis, or it may be as inseparable from the basic personality as a character disorder. It may recur with such regularity as to be designated "periodic." At any given time, there can be striking inconsistency in various areas of the patient's functioning. Thus, a scientist may conduct superior research while his personal habits isolate him from even casual social acquaintances, or a woman capable of tender sympathy for a stranger may feel no fondness for, and willfully neglect, her own child. Inconsistent fragments of behavior may coexist in a single person. For example, a young man may pay meticulous attention to grooming his hair, but refuse to wash or bathe for many days, or a woman may alternate between gorging herself on compulsive eating binges and rigorous dieting to the point of malnutrition.

THE DISTURBANCE OF AFFECT

The schizophrenic patient has a disturbance in the regulation and expression of his affect or emotions. The interviewer relies upon the patient's affective responses as a guide to how the patient is relating to him, and therefore he must adjust to the patient's mode of affective communication.

The patient's subjective emotional experience may be diminished, flattened, or blunted. In addition, he has difficulty expressing and communicating the emotional responses of which he is aware. More subtle gradations of feeling tone are lost, and the emotionality that does emerge often seems exaggerated. Warm and positive feelings are sporadic and unreliable. The patient somehow fears them, as though his continued independent existence would be threatened if he felt tender toward another person. When affection does appear, it is often directed toward an unusual object. Commonly, a schizophrenic patient will most comfortably feel love for someone with whom he has little real contact, or whom others might consider far beneath him in social status, such as a servant. One adolescent girl who was hospitalized for several years claimed to have no concern for her family, but was intensely involved with her pet cat.

This affective deficit not only leads to estrangement from others, but also to an inability to enjoy the solitude that results. The patient is a lonely, unhappy person. Anhedonia, or the absence of pleasure, characterizes his entire life, although it is rarely the presenting complaint. One man, recovering from a prolonged psychotic episode, said that he never remembered feeling really happy in his whole life. The schizophrenic feels inner conflict about his very existence, and even minor pleasures seem out of reach. In contrast, the neurotic patient maintains areas of pleasure in life, and can enjoy himself thoroughly in activities that remain free from conflict.

Some schizophrenic patients say that they feel as if they are only playing a role, or that other people seem to be actors. The sensation of play acting results from the patient's defense of emotionally isolating himself in response to a disturbing situation. In this way he remains distant from both his own feelings and those of others. Hysterical and sociopathic patients may also seem to be playing a role, but this is rarely described by the patient himself; rather, it is an observation of the interviewer.

The physical and bodily components of affect may rise to central importance. These, of course, are present in everyone, although they frequently escape conscious recognition. The schizophrenic patient will often be fully aware of them, but will deny their emotional significance and explain them as responses to physical stimuli. Thus, an anxious patient will attribute the beads of sweat on his forehead to the warmth of the room, or a grieving patient will wipe away his tears as he explains that something got into his eye.

The interviewer may find it difficult to empathize, or may not trust his own empathic responses to the patient. Affects that he expects to find in the patient do not appear, and the signs that normally help him to understand the patient's feelings are unreliable or denied. A successful psychiatric interview always involves emotionally significant communication, and if the patient appears to have minimal affect, the problem is to evoke and reach this affect by whatever means are available. Some therapists use dramatic or unusual methods to develop an affective interchange with relatively affectless patients. They realize that they must use their own feelings as stimuli before the patient will permit an emotional interaction to develop. In spite of the possible pitfalls, this is preferable to a passive technique of scrupulous neutrality, which allows the interview to unfold without emotion.

The beginning psychiatrist is reluctant to use his own feelings in so active a manner. He fears that he will create problems or disturb the patient, and is concerned lest he inadvertently reveal too much about himself. He may indeed make mistakes, but if these help to generate an affective interchange where none was present, they may be preferable to a safer but emotionally bland approach.

The patient's feelings may seem inappropriate to the apparent content of his thought, or to the interview situation, or to both. However, emotional responses are always appropriate to the patient's inner experience, although these may be hidden from the interviewer. After identifying the patient's emotions, the interviewer's task is to elicit and identify the thoughts that evoke them. Often the patient has responded to something that seems trivial or unusual to the interviewer. The physician will better understand the patient if he attempts to unravel the meaning of the patient's reactions as the patient experiences them. The interviewer should not expect customary emotional responses in schizophrenic patients; the patient may sense this expectation and react by concealing his true emotions. For example, if a social acquaintance spoke of his mother's recent death, the spontaneous response would be sympathy and an indication of willingness to share the experience of grief. The interviewer's response to most patients would be similar. However, this might disturb a schizophrenic, because it would indicate that the physician expected a response that differed from the patient's actual feelings. The patient would then react with evasion and withdrawal, unable to correct the interviewer's error. His true feelings would not emerge. An open-ended inquiry concerning his feelings allows the patient greater freedom in his response.

The Disturbance of Thought

The schizophrenic patient has difficulty organizing his thoughts by the usual rules of logic and reality. His ideas emerge in a confused and bewildering sequence. Every conceivable aspect of organization is potentially defective, as exemplified by loosening of associations, tangentiality, circumstantiality, irrelevance, incoherence, and so forth.

The disorganization of thought and communication is not random. Although the capacity to develop such difficulties may ultimately be explained biologically, the process of disorganization can best be understood in a dynamic framework. Disorganization blurs and confuses, and appears when the patient experiences emerging anxiety. In a sense, the patient's confusion serves as an unconscious mechanism of defense by obscuring the uncomfortable topic.

These cognitive defects have secondary effects as well. Circumstantiality and tangentiality are likely to annoy the listener, and therefore may become a vehicle for expressing hostility. Gross incoherence and loosening of associations evoke sympathy, although at the cost of emphasizing the patient's difference from other people and promoting his social isolation. These effects may be exploited by the patient, usually unconsciously. In general, they should not be interpreted early in the treatment, as they represent a minimal gain that helps to compensate for a large loss. Later, they may become an important source of resistance that must be worked through.

The attention span of the schizophrenic patient may be diminished, and he may have difficulty shifting the focus of his thoughts. Frequently the patient seems preoccupied with minor details, and at times this emerges as an unusual capacity for mastering irrelevancies. For example, one young schizophrenic boy was preoccupied with the detailed schedule for every subway station in New York City.

The schizophrenic may also have difficulty with the symbolic aspect of language, manifested by his tendency toward inappropriately concrete or abstract thinking. Not only are the connections between words disturbed, but the words themselves have a different range of meanings than is generally accepted by others. He will frequently interpret the interviewer's words in a strangely literal way, as when a patient who was asked what had brought him to the hospital replied that he had taken the bus. At times the opposite will occur, as when a college student who was acutely psychotic complained of a fear that "My behavior has violated the categorical imperative." It was several hours before he revealed that he was worried about masturbatory impulses. He had transformed his guilty feelings into ruminations about abstract philosophical systems that deal with right and wrong. By the time that he came to see the psychiatrist, it was these philosophical systems, and not sexual thoughts, that consciously preoccupied him.

Language functions that are normally autonomous become involved with sexual or aggressive feelings. Seemingly every-day words are assigned special meaning. One young hebephrenic girl became embarrassed when the word "leg" was used in her presence, because she felt that it had sexual significance.

In addition to his difficulty in organizing his thinking and in maintaining an appropriate level of abstractness, the schizophrenic patient may accent obscure features while ignoring central issues. For example, a hospitalized man with paranoid delusions who had formerly worked as an attorney became involved in a major campaign to get the United States off of the gold standard, writing letters to the President and members of Congress. At the same time, he was uninterested in resuming his regular employment, or even in more traditional political activities. Another paranoid patient, a post office employee who developed tuberculosis, spent several years collecting affidavits attesting to the unsanitary conditions to which he had been exposed during his employment. His realistic problems with his health, his family, and his occupation were ignored while he pursued a relatively small disability compensation. When his persistence was finally rewarded, he became even more disorganized.

The schizophrenic patient spends much of his time preoccupied with fantasies that have little meaning to the outside world. They may be bizarre or autistic, but they do have meaning to the patient, and if the patient trusts the interviewer enough to reveal his thoughts, they can provide valuable insights concerning his emotional life. However, the patient is afraid to expose his fantasies to others. For the schizophrenic, as for any other person, fantasies represent a retreat from reality and an attempt to solve problems by constructing a private world. However, this universal function of fantasy may be less apparent because of the patient's personalized use of symbols and his peculiar style of thinking. Furthermore, he is not sure where fantasy stops, and at times his overt behavior can be understood only in terms of his inner reality. The interviewer may respond to the bizarre or idiosyncratic nature of the fantasy, rather than to its dynamic significance. In general, the psychotherapeutic exploration of the dynamic origins of fantasies is best deferred until later in treatment, since premature focusing on his fantasy life may further impair his contact with reality.

The psychological function of the patient's fantasy life is illustrated by the young man who spent many hours planning trips to other planets and developing methods for communication with extra-terrestrial beings. His life on Earth was lonely, and he had never mastered the more mundane art of communicating with friends and family.

The schizophrenic patient may develop more complex systems of ideas, entire worlds of his own, if his fantasies are elaborated. When reality testing is intact, these are confined to his mental life, but if the patient is unable to differentiate fantasy from reality, the fantasy becomes the basis of a delusion. Often these ideas are religious or philosophical in nature, as the patient's struggles with the nature of his own existence are generalized into questions about the meaning of the universe. Religiosity is a common symptom, and schizophrenic patients have often turned to studies of Eastern religions or existential philosophy before seeking therapy more directly. Less sophisticated individuals may become deeply involved in their church, usually with the accent on fundamental questions of theology rather than the daily activities of the parish. A preoccupation with the existence of God is a typical example. The more delusional patient feels that he receives messages from God or has a special relationship with Him. Other related disturbances involve magical thinking in the form of extrasensory perception, mind-reading, or mysticism. This is discussed further in Chapter 8.

BEHAVIORAL DISTURBANCES

The chronic schizophrenic patient typically lacks initiative and motivation; he is bored, listless, and apathetic. He does not care what happens and is not interested in doing anything, fearing that any activity may reveal him as inadequate and ridiculous. His obvious problems seem to distress his family or the interviewer far more than they do the patient himself.

Like the apparent absence of affect, the apparent absence of purpose or motivation can serve as a means of avoiding discomfort. It often leads to frustration and hopelessness in others, further increasing the patient's isolation. The interviewer can overcome this defense by searching for those areas in which the patient remains capable of admitting involvement and, at the same time, exploring the fears that inhibit his interest in the remainder of his life.

Negativism is another characteristic abnormality of behavior. This patient relates to the interviewer, but at the same time asserts his own independence and control by doing the opposite of what is requested. The interviewer can facilitate a more flexible relationship by indicating that he accepts and agrees with the importance of the patient's independence. He can also point out that automatically to say "No" is to relinquish self-control as much as it is to say "Yes." The interviewer's temptation to suggest that the patient do the opposite of what is desired would only lead to difficulties. The patient would soon learn that he is being treated dishonestly and with condescension, and this reinforces his desire to act like a defiant child.

The schizophrenic may insist on the lack of awareness of inner drives in even the most elementary areas of behavior. A young man with anorexia nervosa stopped eating for several weeks but claimed to feel no hunger. Later, as he improved, he asked how often he was supposed to be thirsty, and how many times he should swallow at the water cooler. Through this mechanism, the patient denied responsibility for his desires, but at the same time he was able to sustain his minimum needs. In extreme cases, he may blindly follow the doctor's advice without regard to what is best for himself, at the same time denying his genuine involvement with the doctor as a separate person.

The behavior of the schizophrenic patient is often disorganized and inappropriate. He pursues goals that are unrelated, inconsistent, or obviously maladaptive. This chaotic behavior can offer valuable clues to his conflicting motives and feelings. For example, a hospitalized patient pleads for an opportunity to obtain a ward pass, but then provokes a fight with another patient and becomes agitated just before he is to leave, revealing a conflict between his desire for independence and his fear of the outside world.

The Disturbance in Interpersonal Relations

The schizophrenic has difficulty relating to others. He has few friends and does not trust people. Although he is sometimes capable of unusual empathy and sensitivity to others, he may be indifferent to the most compelling emotions. His acquaintances tend to respond by avoiding him, thereby increasing his loneliness and isolation. When he does develop a friendship, it is often with someone who is also an outcast, or who exploits the patient in return for companionship.

This disturbed pattern of social interaction was first experienced in the patient's relationship with his family. Trust, warmth, and the capacity to relate to others develop in a child's early years. Studies of the families of schizophrenic patients reveal a high incidence of parental psychopathology and subtle disorders of communication. The child growing up in this environment does not develop the skills that are necessary for successful social adaptation. He does not feel that he can rely on his understanding of how others think or feel, and even mistrusts his perception of his own mental processes. Instead, he learns to protect himself by maintaining emotional distance, preferring his own autistic world to shared experiences in the world of others. At times, his feeling of always being on the outside looking in is represented quite concretely through such phenomena as derealization and depersonalization. Other people appear to be relating to each other with warmth and intimacy while he, alone, is excluded. This patient may be so starved for affection and emotional contact that, rather than withdraw from personal relationships, he will ignore the most obvious dangers and suspend his critical judgment in the pursuit of these experiences. For example, a young girl who was withdrawn and hallucinating became pregnant after a fleeting contact with a stranger.

The schizophrenic patient has emotional reactions to other people that are simultaneous and contradictory. Ambivalence is found in all important human relationships, but most people manage to keep the less acceptable side of their feelings out of consciousness. The early family experiences of the schizophrenic stimulate such intense rage, and provide such inadequate controls, that repression is impossible. The conscious ambivalence of the schizophrenic extends to all of his relationships and contributes to his erratic and inconsistent behavior in his contacts with others.

The mistrust, fear of closeness, ambivalence, and clinging dependency of the schizophrenic patient influence all of his human contacts, and thus determine the general quality of his transference behavior toward the interviewer. Dynamic psychotherapy utilizes the exploration of transference as a major tool in helping the neurotic patient to understand his conflicts and to modify his patterns of behavior. This assumes that the patient has a simultaneous non-neurotic relationship with the doctor that allows him to look at his transference feelings objectively. It was once thought that the schizophrenic did not establish a transference relationship, and therefore could not be treated by analytically oriented psychotherapy. In fact, he often establishes a transference quickly, but the intensity of the resulting feelings may threaten the basic alliance between patient and therapist. The greatest problem is to maintain the relationship through the violence of his transference reactions, and, in view of this, interpretations of the neurotic origins of the transference must be deferred until a therapeutic alliance has been established.

The schizophrenic patient employs behavior patterns based upon techniques that have protected him in his family setting. One example is his skill in eliciting guilt in others. The patient may subtly imply that the interview is either causing or intensifying his suffering. If the physician responds with guilt, the patient reacts as though his accusation were confirmed, with a resultant increase in his dramatization of suffering. In time, the interviewer becomes angry, and thereby further convinces the patient that he is being treated unfairly through no fault of his own. It is difficult to respond spontaneously, avoiding both guilt and anger, and at the same time help the patient to see his pattern of behavior.

SECONDARY SYMPTOMS AND SECONDARY GAINS

Secondary symptoms such as hallucinations, illusions, delusions, and bizarre behavior are the dramatic derivatives of primary disturbances in thinking and feeling. The anticipated responses of other individuals would inhibit normal persons from exhibiting such bizarre behavior. The schizophrenic patient is not affected in this way, even though he is aware of the reactions of others. His primary pathology not only provides the material for the development of secondary symptoms, but also destroys the mechanism that would normally control and inhibit them.

Such symptoms have dynamic significance, and must be explored and understood like any others. They represent attempts to adapt to the patient's primary deficit, defend him against anxiety, repair the psychological damage that his illness has caused, and help him to regain contact with the real world. For example, hallucinations offer an opportunity to externalize inner conflicts while providing the individual with a sense of importance and narcissistic gratification and protecting him from loneliness.

Special problems occur in the interview because the interviewer tends to respond negatively to the social deviance and craziness of these symptoms. The patient may sense this response and retreat further into isolation. The interviewer may deny his true reaction in an attempt to avoid this, suggesting that the symptom is an acceptable way to deal with the problem. This will usually cause the patient to push the matter until the interviewer's real feelings are revealed. The patient then rightfully objects to this hypocritical treatment. For example, a young schizophrenic man was constantly embroiled in struggles with his parents over his bizarre dress and grooming. His clothes were a mixture of Edwardian elegance and cowboy rustic, and he shaved each half of his face on alternate days. The therapist suppressed his spontaneous reactions in order to support what he interpreted as beginning steps toward separating from the patient's family, never discussing the general social response to the patient's appearance. One day the patient accidentally met his doctor while walking to their appointment, and the physician's obvious discomfort when they entered his building together made the patient feel rejected and betrayed. Inevitably, he overreacted to the doctor's response, and was mistrustful for many months afterwards. A bizarre symptom, like any other, is a maladaptive attempt to resolve a conflict over the expression of a drive while providing partial gratification, with a resulting inhibition of healthy functioning. The symptom can be used as a measure of the patient's psychopathology, but, more importantly, it is meaningful, communicative behavior that offers potential insight into his thoughts and feelings. When the interviewer understands this, he can comfortably indicate his interest without encouraging the patient's deviance.

Secondary gain, or the utilization of pathological mechanisms for goals that are unrelated to the dynamic origins of the behavior, may complicate any of the symptoms of schizophrenia. The modern psychiatric hospital, with its physical convenience and therapeutic milieu, may provide so much secondary gain for a schizophrenic patient that it becomes a major obstacle in his treatment. To get better means to leave the comfort and support of the hospital for the stress and sometimes the relative squalor of the outside world. Secondary gain appears directly in the interview, if the patient perceives that the doctor is more interested in some aspect of his psychopathology than in his feelings and problems. He may unconsciously exaggerate or conceal his pathology as a means of controlling the interviewer's responses, thereby explaining the well-known phenomenon that psychotherapists of any theoretical persuasion always find ample confirmatory evidence for their beliefs in the material that their patients present to them.

Some schizophrenic patients claim to have conscious control of their psychotic symptoms and to exploit them for personal gain. However, this claim usually represents an attempt to maintain some sense of omnipotence and self-control. For example, one man explained that his catatonic posturing allowed him to purchase theatre tickets without waiting in line, and a woman insisted that she would start hallucinating in order to resolve arguments with her husband. One example of the possible conscious use of psychotic behavior for secondary gain in the interview situation occurred in the waiting room of one of the authors. Two women arrived at the same time, one an older, well-integrated neurotic who had come an hour early by mistake, the other a young schizophrenic. The neurotic patient looked at her watch as if she were in a great hurry, and suggested that perhaps she could have the appointment, since she had a busy afternoon and didn't know if she could make a later time. The psychotic woman was unable to defend her rights openly, but walked into the corner of the room, turned her face to the wall, and proceeded to sob convulsively. The older woman quickly altered her attitude and fled the waiting room, saying she would return later. The psychotic patient entered the office and sat down for what promised to be a difficult session. She then uncovered her face and proceeded with the session as though nothing had happened. It is difficult to determine whether psychotic behavior is ever under the patient's control or whether the occasional patient's claim that he is able to use it consciously is only a rationalization.

CENTRAL CONFLICTS

The psychopathology of the schizophrenic syndrome has been described, but there are, in addition, certain psychodynamic issues that usually provide the content for the patient's psychological conflicts. Some of these are related to the developmental experiences of the child growing up in a family with disturbed patterns of communication. Others are universal human problems that assume a characteristic style when integrated into a schizophrenic mode of thinking and feeling.

THE PROBLEM OF PERSONAL IDENTITY

The schizophrenic patient has both a wish for and a fear of merging in a symbiotic union with other people. Originally this stemmed from his attempt to maintain a relationship with his mother, but it extends to other individuals in his life and to the interviewer. As a child he was confused and frightened by the experience of alternate rejection and smothering overprotection in his relationship with his mother. He reacted as if the only resolution was a magical union with her. At the same time, he was terrified by the consequences of this merger, and disturbed by his difficulty in accurately perceiving the boundaries that separate him from the rest of the world and, particularly, from other people. He wants to be distinct and separate, to have an existence and identity of his own, but fears the isolation, abandonment, and loss of security that might result.

Some writers describe the schizophrenic's fears of being eaten or incorporated by another person. One young catatonic girl said that she was afraid that her mother was going to chew her up and swallow her. These images are metaphors, but they have been created by the patient's thinking and feeling, not by the author of a textbook.

The interviewer's active attempts to establish and maintain emotional contact with the patient will arouse fears of symbiotic merger. On the other hand, if he allows the patient to structure the interview, or provides less feedback, the patient will fear abandonment. The interviewer feels as if he were walking a tightrope, and the patient may complain about the inconsistency as the interviewer changes his style in response to this dilemma. The interviewer is left with the feeling that whatever he does is wrong.

The schizophrenic patient's difficulties in differentiating himself from others contribute to a defective sense of self. This is frequently complicated by distortions of body image based on the perception of his parents' unusual attitude toward his body. For example, an adolescent girl described her earliest memory as her mother berating her for having hair all over her body, just like a boy. The normal individual constructs a sense of personal identity by integrating his body percept and concept, his awareness of thoughts and feelings, and the values and goals that he has absorbed from his family and society. If any of these components are defective or inconsistent with the others, the synthetic ability of his ego allows him to resolve this discrepancy and create a workable self-image. However, the schizophrenic has defects in each of these components and, in addition, lacks the integrative capacity required for the task of synthesis. As a consequence, he fails to achieve a normal sense of personal identity. Frequently, he will borrow an identity from someone else. This contributes to the role playing quality of schizophrenics, which we mentioned above, and also to the well-known social contagion and suggestibility of symptoms among schizophrenic patients. It provides a mechanism for dramatic psychotherapeutic effect in acute crises, but is also a major pitfall in the interview and in therapy. Apparent recovery may be only the transient acceptance of a more desirable role.

Dependency

The schizophrenic individual has increased dependency needs and a decreased ability to gratify them. His psychopathology impairs his adaptive skills; he is realistically less able to care for himself and more dependent on the help of others. His self-confidence and his own estimate of his ability to get along in the world are also impaired; he sees himself as even less able to cope than is actually the case. This actual and fantasied helplessness leads to regression to a dependent mode of adaptation, in which he relies upon others for what he feels he cannot do himself.

As the patient expresses his dependent feelings, his self-esteem is diminished, and he feels threatened by passivity and submissiveness. For the schizophrenic, these threats are particularly severe, and are further associated with threats to his sense of personal identity. He has difficulty establishing any interpersonal contact and is frightened by even the normal dependent aspects of intimate or loving relationships.

The result is either pseudo-dependence or pseudo-independence. The patient attempts to act out the roles, but if he tries to be dependent, he is unable to enjoy the sense of safety and security that accompanies true dependency, and if he tries to be independent, he fails to achieve the experience of mastery and enhanced self-esteem that accompanies true independence. This dilemma is illustrated by the catatonic adolescent boy who decided to move away from home, but was unable to care for himself, so that his mother visited him weekly with food and clean clothing. When he finally moved back, his intense ambivalence to his parents led him to avoid all social contact with them, and he would spend days without speaking to another human being.

ASSERTION, AGGRESSION, AND THE STRUGGLE FOR POWER AND CONTROL

The schizophrenic patient harbors hostile and angry feelings that he perceives as overwhelming. These are related to his conflict over symbiosis and individuation, as described above. The child who is uncertain about his boundaries and his freedom to separate from others will be terrified at even slightly angry feelings, because they may destroy both the outer world and himself. Repression is not an adequate defense, as it presupposes a degree of psychological maturation that may not exist.

The schizophrenic is anxious, lest these hostile feelings emerge and he be allowed to destroy others. He usually suppresses his healthy assertive capacity along with his violent rage, and this can be a major source of the apathy previously mentioned. His judgment is poor in evaluating both his destructive potential and his ability to control it. Although excessive inhibition is the usual result, there are times when his fear seems well-founded, and he may be capable of violence. Therapy attempts to develop his awareness of his inner hostility and of his controls, without forcing him into premature and frightening assertive behavior. One patient was unable to obtain a driver's license because he could not tolerate the frustration and resulting rage at having to wait in line, and he was fearful of his inability to control his responses.

The schizophrenic individual feels himself inadequate and impotent. He compensates by demonstrating his control over others and attempting to exaggerate his power. The struggle for power and control is also a dominant theme in the psychodynamics of the obsessive individual. However, whereas the obsessive perceives others as dangerous antagonists or threatening rivals, the schizophrenic struggles to maintain a sense of identity and independent being, rather than be submerged into nothingness.

The desire for power and control, together with his feeling

of inadequacy and tendency to withdrawal and fantasy, leads to an interest in magic. By ignoring the rules of logic, he hopes to gain what he otherwise cannot have. The magic of the schizophrenic may resemble the wishful magic of the hysteric or the coercive magic of the obsessive, but it is characterized by a more complete withdrawal from reality, and by a tendency to the bizarre or autistic that does not appear even in the fantasies of the neurotic.

Although schizophrenic patients do have special characteristics, their problems and conflicts are the same as those of neurotic or normal individuals—hopes and fears about family, work, sex, aging, illness, and so on. The schizophrenic is an individual with an unusual way of thinking, feeling, and talking about the same subjects that all of us think, feel, and talk about. The interviewer can often serve his most valuable function by relating to the patient as a separate and important person.

Management of the Interview

It is difficult to establish emotional rapport with a schizophrenic patient. His intense sensitivity to rejection leads him to protect himself through the use of isolation and withdrawal. In most psychiatric interviews the patient reveals his conflicts and problems with as little intervention as possible from the interviewer. The psychiatrist is a neutral figure who avoids becoming a real object, recognizing the patient's needs but not gratifying them directly. The interview with a schizophrenic patient requires modification. The patient feels rejected if the interviewer merely recognizes his needs. It is necessary for the doctor to convey his understanding more actively by revealing his own emotional response or by providing symbolic or token gratification for the patient's needs. Should this patient ask the interviewer to recommend a coffee shop near the office, the therapist would answer directly and provide the information, whereas with a neurotic patient he might interpret the patient's wish for dependency gratification or his evasion of more meaningful material. The schizophrenic patient has had much emotional deprivation during his life, and additional deprivation during the early stages of treatment is destructive. In the early phase of work the psychiatrist accepts whatever limited emotional contact is possible. The patient will accept gratification from the therapist only on his own terms. The therapist should accept these terms as the basis for the initial relationship, as long as they are within the realm of reality.

THE DEVELOPMENT OF
THE THERAPEUTIC RELATIONSHIP

DISORGANIZATION AS A DEFENSE

The most common defense encountered in the interview with the schizophrenic patient involves his unconscious use of disorganization.

This is not to say that the schizophrenic patient's difficulty in organizing his thinking is always defensive in origin, but his unusual style of thinking frequently assumes defensive significance. For example, a schizophrenic patient may speak freely from the beginning of the interview, manifesting little anxiety or hesitation; however, the interviewer soon encounters difficulty in following the trend of the conversation. The patient starts to answer a question but then leaves the topic. The interviewer may respond with confusion, boredom, or anger. Often he does not realize that the patient has changed the subject until the patient is in the middle of a new topic. On other occasions, the patient may seem to adhere to the topic under discussion; his words and even his sentences make sense, but somehow they do not fit together. This disorganization tests the interviewer's interest and serves to block effective communication. The interviewer must reveal his difficulty in understanding the patient, rather than responding, as in most social situations, with feigned understanding and concealed boredom, eagerly anticipating the termination of the contact. He can support the patient by avoiding statements that tend to berate him or that suggest that he is responsible for the interviewer's lack of understanding. Rather than saying, "You're not making yourself clear," the interviewer can say, "I'm having difficulty following what you are saying." Similarly, "I don't understand how we got on this subject," is preferable to, "Why do you keep changing the subject?"

Although it may be possible to understand the content of the disorganized patient's communication, it is important to deal with the process of disorganization and its effect upon the developing relationship between the interviewer and patient. The long-term goals of treatment include helping the patient to communicate more effectively with other figures in his life, as well as with the therapist.

Disorganization is sometimes apparent within the first few moments of the interview. The schizophrenic patient seems unable to describe a chief complaint. He might say, "I haven't been feeling too well lately," or indicate that one of his close relatives thought that he should come to see the doctor. One young man came to a hospital emergency room late at night, asking to see a psychiatrist, but unable to formulate any specific problem; he simply stated that he was upset. His waxlike face and vacant stare suggested a psychotic illness. When the psychiatrist directly inquired about his current life, he revealed that he had just come back from a business trip, and had discovered that his wife had taken their small child and left him. He felt panicky and helpless, but in his own mind he did not connect these feelings with the traumatic events that he had just experienced.

When a patient answers the interviewer's opening inquiry with a vague reply, it is helpful to inquire whether the patient himself decided to consult a psychiatrist. If the patient indicates that it was not his own idea, the interviewer can explore why another person felt that such a consultation was indicated. Furthermore, the interviewer might inquire whether the patient felt he was "dragged against his will" or pressured to come. Sympathizing with the patient's resentment concerning such a process facilitates early rapport.

The interviewer might then inquire if this is the first time that the patient has consulted a psychiatrist. If not, prior contacts are carefully explored. In discussing previous psychiatric contacts, explicit inquiry about past psychiatric hospitalization is important. A schizophrenic patient often indicates that there have been prior hospitalizations, but seems unable to describe the symptoms involved. The interviewer could ask about the circumstances of the hospitalization and whether there were any secondary symptoms. It is appropriate to inquire about a previous history of secondary symptoms with every grossly psychotic patient. While making these inquiries, the interviewer communicates his interest in understanding the patient rather than his interest in establishing a diagnosis. For example, instead of merely asking the patient if he heard voices, the interviewer would go on to ask what they said, how the patient interpreted them, and what he felt had caused these experiences. If the patient does describe the symptoms of previous psychotic episodes, the interviewer can inquire about their recurrence in the present.

The psychiatrist actively assists the schizophrenic patient in defining problems and focusing on issues. This is true even of the patient who does not have a serious disorganization of thought processes. Despite such efforts, some patients remain unable to identify the problem that is the theme for the interview. The interviewer can help by pursuing specific precipitants of the request for consultation. Questions such as, "What was the final straw?" or, "Why did you come today, rather than last week?" may be helpful. It is also valuable to inquire about the patient's expectations of the interview. For example, if he communicates that he has difficulty in finding a job, the interviewer attempts to pinpoint the specific difficulty encountered. The physician can gradually shift the focus from the external environmental problem to the intra-psychic issues. Often this will involve interpretive comments concerning precipitating stresses in the patient's current life. As an illustration, the interviewer might say, "Your trouble at work seems to have started at the time that your wife became ill; perhaps this upset you in some way?"

It is easy to overlook the adaptive skills of a psychotic patient. In focusing the interview, the physician can direct attention to the patient's assets and areas of healthy functioning as well as his pathology. The emphasis of the interview thereby shifts from exposing the patient's deficiencies to supporting his attempts to cope with the stresses in his life and the conflicts within himself.

The interview may seem to be rambling or aimless despite the interviewer's attempt to provide structure. In this situation, the interviewer looks for topics and themes that recur repeatedly, even though they may not occur sequentially in the interview. Thus, the interviewer might say, "You keep coming back to the trouble with your boss. I guess that is what is on your mind." Even if the interpretation is inaccurate, this comment indicates an interest in searching for the meaning of the patient's thoughts, rather than treating them as incoherent productions. Accuracy is only one determinant of the effect of any interpretation—timing, tact, and the transference meaning of the interpretive activity are all important factors that influence its impact on the patient. In addition, the therapist tries to demonstrate that he is interested in understanding rather than judging or condemning. Accuracy becomes increasingly important as a patient learns to trust the therapist and to use the insight that he gains in therapy. This process is particularly slow with schizophrenic patients, and therefore it is an error for the therapist to refrain from interpretive activity early in the treatment because he is not sure what is happening. If he is open about his uncertainty and invites the patient to join him in a search for meaning, the development of a therapeutic alliance will be fostered even if he is wrong in his interpretation. Phrases such as, "I'm not sure I fully understand what has been happening here, but it seemed to me . . . ," or, "I'm sure that this is only part of it, but could it be . . ." are helpful.

As the patient becomes better acquainted with the physician, he may reveal a surprising degree of insight into the social significance of his disorganized thought processes. For example, a young girl told one of the authors that if another person nodded agreement although they did not really understand her, her communication would become more diffuse and incoherent.

Some patients express acute emotional turmoil in association with the disorganization of their thought processes. The interviewer first works with this patient's feelings. He utilizes any communication that seems related to the patient's overall feeling tone and links it to the emotion the patient displays. For example, an agitated, disturbed young woman appeared in the emergency room of the hospital muttering incoherently. The interviewer noticed that although her medical chart was labeled "Mrs.," she was not wearing a wedding ring. He inquired about her marital status and learned that her husband had just abandoned her. She calmed considerably after this topic was discussed.

THE PROBLEM OF PRIVACY

The schizophrenic person has a great need for privacy and secrecy. This stems from his difficulty in establishing an individual identity and in separating his image of himself from his images of other members of his family. The interviewer may help the patient by indicating his awareness of the patient's conflict in this area and accepting the patient's need to proceed in his own way. If the patient expresses reluctance to discuss a personal issue, the doctor might say, "You're not comfortable talking about this yet; maybe we can come back to it later." The interviewer's acceptance of the patient's difficulty alleviates his anxiety and increases his trust in the physician. The patient's need to have a secret is often more important than the content of the secret. The schizophrenic has frequently been taught to feel guilty about his need for privacy. For example, a patient may attempt to answer the interviewer's question, but may speak as though the information were being extracted under torture. The interviewer could stop the patient and comment upon this phenomenon, thereby allowing the patient to discuss his fear rather than to submit passively to the interviewer's coercion.

The patient's concern about privacy and his fear that he may be damaged if the interviewer knows him too well lend a feeling of slowness or heaviness to the interview. Although it may take years for the patient to trust the interviewer and feel comfortable with him, the patient's time schedule must be respected. For example, a woman mentioned having had a nervous breakdown in the past that had required psychiatric hospitalization, but was unable to describe it. Some months later, on the anniversary of her original hospitalization, she again referred to this episode, but was now able to relate her symptoms and her experiences during the acute psychosis.

In his pursuit of privacy, the schizophrenic tends to withdraw from normal socialization. The interviewer may comment on the withdrawal and utilize it as a means of engaging the patient, if it is an important means of avoiding contact with the interviewer. In general, the interviewer accepts the emotional distance at which the patient feels most comfortable, while repeatedly interpreting it and gradually trying to promote greater intimacy without excessive anxiety.

THE PHYSICAL EXAMINATION

Since the grossly psychotic patient is frequently interviewed in a hospital setting, the physical examination provides an important opportunity for the facilitation of emotional engagement. The schizophrenic patient characteristically has distorted or devalued images of his own body that he is reluctant to discuss with the physician. If the interviewer is also going to be the patient's medical physician, the physical examination with its touching and direct contact may be for the patient the most meaningful part of the initial interview, but it is often misperceived as an addendum to the interview by the doctor.

The physical examination may also become pertinent after the initial relationship has developed. A patient may experience somatic symptoms or reveal thoughts about his body that have not previously been discussed. The psychiatrist's interest in these matters may help the schizophrenic patient feel that his doctor cares for him as a total person. Although the psychiatrist may not be qualified to treat the physical problem that troubles the patient, he nevertheless indicates an interest in the patient's body and his feelings about it. The interviewer will then refer the patient to an appropriate physician for further consultation.

MODIFICATIONS OF THE INTERVIEW

THE ROLE OF THE THERAPIST

The patient's disturbance of affect leads to an extension of the psychiatrist's traditional role. The patient may be better able to express his emotions in response to some similar expression on the part of the interviewer. Therefore, the interviewer follows the patient's emotional cues and utilizes them to intensify the affective tone of the interview. These cues are often difficult to detect, and the interviewer may have to be active in helping the patient both experience and express his own feelings. He may directly inquire if the patient is experiencing some particular feelings, asking, for example, "Are you angry right now?" The patient will often respond to such interventions with a total denial of any feeling similar to that suggested by the interviewer. After acknowledging that he may have been wrong, the interviewer can then discuss his difficulty in determining the patient's feelings. This will lead to an examination of the motivational aspects of the patient's defenses against feeling rather than an argument about who knows more about the patient's inner mental state. If such an exploration is premature, the interviewer can let the subject rest. It is common for a schizophrenic patient to vigorously deny a response suggested by the interviewer and then, weeks or months later, refer to the episodes as though he had been in complete agreement. For example, a catatonic girl burned a hole in the office chair with her cigarette. When the interviewer asked if she were annoyed, she denied that the behavior had any significance at all, insisting that it was only an accident. Several months later she referred to the episode as "the time I was so mad that I burned a hole in your chair."

There are occasions when the interviewer has no idea what the patient is feeling and the interview seems dull and flat. Flatness and the lack of interaction reinforce the patient's sense of loneliness, isolation, and alienation. The interviewer might utilize his own emotional response in such situations as a guide to the further conduct of the interview. To illustrate, the interviewer could say, "As I listen to your description of your life, a sense of boredom and loneliness comes through. Perhaps you have similar feelings?" or, "It sounds as if your life feels purposeless and filled with meaningless detail. Was there ever a time when it was different?"

When the treatment has progressed sufficiently, the physician may modify his role in other ways. For example, a patient might come into the office and comment, "It's a beautiful day outside." The physician who has developed a stable positive relationship with the patient might agree and add, "Shall we go out for a walk?" The spontaneous suggestion of a change in routine may open up areas of rigidity in the patient, expose fears about obtaining forbidden pleasure, or initiate a discussion about his perception of the doctor as a real person. If the patient is able to accept such contact with the psychiatrist, an opportunity is provided for sharing a new experience. The doctor must feel comfortable before making such a suggestion, or the patient will perceive and interpret his discomfort as indicating that the doctor is ashamed to be seen with the patient in public.

INTERPRETATIONS OF THE DEFENSIVE PATTERN

With the ego's weakened capacity for repression, the schizophrenic patient may reveal unconscious material in the initial interview that would take months to uncover in a neurotic patient. The beginning interviewer is often intrigued by hearing the patient discuss conflicts that are normally unconscious in the same terms that appear in the textbook. This intellectual insight into the unconscious is not to be encouraged, as it is a manifestation of the patient's basic psychopathology. The schizophrenic patient is quick to sense that the doctor has become intrigued, and might continue to produce such data in order to maintain his interest. The interviewer can best respond to such productions by asking the patient if he was helped by his attempt to understand his Oedipus complex, or whatever other term the patient may have used. If the patient indicates that he was not, the interviewer can ask why the patient wishes to discuss the topic or suggest that they direct their attention to some other area that might be more useful.

The schizophrenic patient retreats from reality and the external world of goal-directed behavior to an inner world of fantasy. Although it may be a long time before the psychiatrist gains entrance to this inner world, he may nevertheless acknowledge its existence to the patient and thereby underline its importance. He may further comment on the consequences of the patient's retreat from the external world in terms of the pain associated with isolation and loneliness.

Rather than participate in the fantasy material, the interviewer will often deal with it as an avoidance of the anxieties associated with the every-day life experiences of the patient. It is valuable to explore the minute details of day-to-day living with the schizophrenic patient, as it is his difficulty with these aspects of life that drives him to a defensive retreat into an autistic world of his own. For example, a young schizophrenic girl came to the doctor after a shopping expedition that left her quite depressed. She was silent for the first 10 minutes, but with the doctor's encouragement, she related her conversation with the saleswoman, and it became apparent that she had been coerced into buying something that she did not want because of her guilt about wasting the lady's time. She had been quite unaware of her response, or of her anger and withdrawal that followed it, and had felt only a sense of gloom. However, she was able to report the events in detail, and with the therapist's help, she reconstructed and re-experienced her emotional responses as well.

On some occasions, the psychiatrist's successful understanding of some aspect of the patient's private fantasy life may intensify the patient's fear of having his mind read and of losing his identity. The patient may retreat to a defensive posture and his communication may become more obscure. It is important that the psychiatrist then acknowledge his inability to understand, as this will assure the patient that he is able to re-establish a separate identity and that he will not fuse into oneness with the interviewer. For example, a seriously disturbed young girl had developed a strong positive tie to her therapist after several years of work. One day she presented a dream, an unusual event in the treatment, that concerned her anger at a grade school teacher who had paid less attention to her than to her classmates. As was characteristic, she had no associations. The therapist intuitively understood the dream as soon as he heard it, recognizing its transference implications and relating them to a very attractive woman who had been in his waiting room the preceding day. He told the patient his associations, and she was silent for some minutes. She then said that she thought that dreams were meaningless anyway, and that was why she rarely discussed them. Over the next few months she became increasingly guarded and evasive, until she finally quit treatment. Certainly this single episode was not the only cause, but it came to symbolize her fear that therapy represented a threat to her personal integrity, and that as long as she was a patient she could not be a private individual.

The interviewer will be more successful if he attempts to see the world as it appears through the patient's eyes. In order to accomplish this he must be prepared to share the patient's loneliness, isolation, and despair. The schizophrenic patient may evoke feelings of confusion and intense frustration in the psychiatrist. It is often helpful if the physician admits to the patient that he is experiencing such emotions and inquires whether the patient is experiencing similar feelings.

THE MUTE PATIENT

The interviewer introduces himself to the mute patient and asks an initial question but receives no reply. The patient may not even look at the interviewer or acknowledge his presence. After a pause, the interviewer rephrases his question or asks another. The patient still does not reply, and the physician begins to feel helpless. Silence is not an absence of communication in the interview, but rather, a specific type of communication that can be understood in the context of the relationship between the participants. The ambiguity of silence may be reassuring for the patient who fears giving a specific communciation. Silence also avoids responsibility for the meaning of a communication, and therefore is comforting for the patient who is fearful of such responsibility. A patient may utilize silence to coerce the physician into increased activity, or to indicate his disinterest and contempt for the physician. In this manner he rejects the physician before he can be rejected himself.

Rage is the most common emotion underlying the mute schizophrenic patient's inhibition. Angry, passive defiance characterizes his reaction to the doctor's expectation that he communicate. He withdraws from contact with the world since, if he were to express himself at all, he might totally lose control of his aggressive, destructive impulses. Silence and withdrawal are defenses against the expression of such emotion.

Confronted with a wide range of possible meanings of any period of silence, the interviewer relies on the non-verbal behavior of the patient and his own empathic responses in order to interpret its significance. A mute patient speaks by his posture, movements, facial expressions, and demeanor. Frequently, however, the interviewer is aware of his own empathic response before he can identify what in the patient has produced it. The interviewer will then attempt to translate his understanding of the silence into words, and thereby help the patient express his own feelings more directly. The interviewer can offer some general comment about the silence, such as, "You don't seem to feel like talking today," or, "What does the silence mean?" If the patient does not reply, the interviewer may sit quietly for several minutes before saying anything else. On the other hand, if the patient transmits a feeling of anger, the interviewer might remark, "What would happen if you really got angry? Are you afraid that you will lose control of your feelings if you speak?" Many hours may pass before the mute patient responds to the physician's attempts to establish a relationship. In spite of his unwillingness to communicate, the patient is cognizant of everything that transpires in the session. Patients have commented after recovery that the persistent relationship with their therapist was a key factor in maintaining a glimmer of hope throughout their most withdrawn phase.

Although the catatonic patient may steadfastly refuse to communicate with the interviewer at a verbal level, it may be possible to establish other kinds of communication. For example, a patient who remained mute in response to the interviewer's attempts to converse was quite cooperative when the interviewer proceeded with a physical examination. As the physical examination drew to a close, the patient took the interviewer's hand and held it. The interviewer then sat by the patient's side and continued to hold his hand, and the patient began to speak.

Inexperienced interviewers frequently do not allow enough time for the silent patient to respond to a question. If the patient has not replied after a few seconds, they immediately offer another question, perhaps fearing that their first one was offensive to the patient. This communicates an attitude of impatience and increases the likelihood that the patient will not respond. The interviewer should give the patient adequate opportunity to reply before introducing another question.

THE REGRESSED PATIENT

The bizarre behavior of a regressed patient has a disconcerting effect on most interviewers. The patient may sit on the floor in the corner of the room, holding his coat over his head, or constantly interrupt the interview to converse with a third, but non-existent, person. The interviewer can help this patient to control such behavior and promote rapport by indicating that he expects something different. If the behavior does not annoy the doctor, he might say, "Are you telling me that someone considers you to be crazy?" Another interviewer might sit on the floor in the corner with the patient. This indicates that the interviewer is neither impressed nor intimidated by the patient's crazy behavior. If the doctor is annoyed, it is best to first explore the hostile or provocative aspect of the patient's behavior. The impact of the doctor communicating his expectations is illustrated by the physician who was called to the emergency room to see an acutely psychotic patient who was standing in a corner and shouting at the staff, "Repent your sins. . . . Jesus saves!" The doctor interrupted the patient and said, "You'll have to sit down here and stop screaming for a few minutes if we are going to talk." The patient responded promptly to the interviewer's expectation of normal social behavior.

The patient's bizarre behavior may include inappropriate demands upon the interviewer. A patient may enter the office and, without removing his overcoat and two sweaters, ask that the interviewer turn off the heat and open the window because he may become overheated and then catch a cold when going out of doors. The interviewer is well advised not to comply with such unrealistic demands.

In exploring the content of a bizarre delusional system, the interviewer may ask questions concerning the details of the delusion as though the delusion were reality. In doing this, it is important that the interviewer not imply that he believes the patient's delusions. For further discussion of the interview with a delusional patient, the reader is referred to Chapter 8.

If the patient exhibits destructive behavior, the interviewer should stop the patient from doing damage to the interviewer's or the hospital's property, as it is not helpful to allow a patient to infringe on the rights of others. The patient who is permitted to continue such behavior will often become ashamed and guilty when he is less psychotic, and will justifiably be angry with the doctor who did not supply the needed controls.

THE CLOSING PHASE

With the schizophrenic patient, the most meaningful emotional contact may be at the close of the interview, as the patient is about to leave. It is crucial that the interviewer maintain the customary tact of the professional relationship with this patient —the greeting and farewell, the attention to promptness, and the reliability in keeping appointments—that mark his relationship with other patients. Toward the end of the session, he advises the patient concerning the time of the next appointment. The patient may look forward to this contact in spite of his apparent lack of interest in the interviewer. The withdrawn, catatonic, or bizarre regressed patient may seemingly ignore the content of the formal interview but nevertheless may say, "Goodbye," at the end of the session. A patient who has otherwise been unresponsive throughout the interview might be willing to shake hands with the therapist at the termination of an appointment. These acts ultimately provide a bridge to more traditional communication. If the patient elects these means to initiate emotional contact, the interviewer will exercise caution in interpreting such behavior. Rather than pouncing on the patient with an interpretation, he can reply in kind by merely saying, "Good-bye."

Conducting an interview with a seriously schizophrenic person can be frustrating and trying, even for the most experienced psychiatrist. This patient demands not only an enormous degree of patience, but a capacity for empathizing with the most profound human suffering as well. The schizophrenic person taxes the resources of the interviewer as a psychiatrist, as a physician, and as a human being. The slightest progress in developing a relationship based on trust and understanding furthers the treatment. Although the patient will often deny such progress, it is essential that the physician recognize and acknowledge each small step.

REFERENCES

Arlow, J. S., and Brenner, C.: The psychopathology of the psychoses: A proposed revision. Int. J. Psycho-Anal., *51*:159, 1970.

Bleuler, E.: Dementia praecox or the group of schizophrenias. New York, International Universities Press, 1950.

Bowers, M. D., Jr.: Pathogenesis of acute schizophrenic psychosis. Arch. Gen. Psychiat., *19*:348, 1968.

Brody, E. G., and Redlich, F. C.: Psychotherapy with schizophrenics. New York, International Universities Press, 1952.

Fromm-Reichmann, F.: Principles of Intensive Psychotherapy. Chicago, University of Chicago Press, 1950.

Fromm-Reichmann, F.: Psychotherapy of schizophrenia. Amer. J. Psychiat., *11*:410, 1954.

Frosch, J.: The psychotic character. Psychiat. Quart., *38*:81, 1964.

Hoch, P., and Polatin, P.: Pseudoneurotic forms of schizophrenia. Psychiat. Quart., *23*:248, 1949.

Jackson, D. D. (ed.): Etiology of Schizophrenia. New York, Basic Books, Inc., 1960.

Knight, R. P.: Borderline states. Bull. Menninger Clinic, *17*:1, 1953.

Kolb, L. W., Kallman, F., and Polatin, P. (eds.): Schizophrenia. International Psychiatry Clinics, Vol. 1, No. 4. Boston, Little Brown and Co., 1964.

Lidz, T., Fleck, S., and Cornelison, A.: Schizophrenia and the Family. New York, International Universities Press, 1965.

Mishler, E., and Scotch, N.: Sociocultural factors in the epidemiology of schizophrenia. Psychiatry, *26*:315, 1963.

Will, O. A.: Human relatedness and the schizophrenic reaction. Psychiatry, *22*:205, 1959.

8 THE PARANOID PATIENT

Psychopathology and Psychodynamics

Paranoid mechanisms are found in everyone and can be clinically prominent in a wide variety of schizophrenic, psychopathic, organic, and neurotic disorders. Although the range of psychopathology is great, there are psychodynamic patterns and mechanisms of defense that are common to all of these patients. The greater the degree of paranoia, the more difficult the interview, since the paranoid patient resists the establishment of a therapeutic working relationship. The patient typically comes to complain about something other than his own psychological difficulties, or he may be brought to the psychiatrist against his will. The paranoid patient is not readily liked and accepted by other people, and the psychiatrist also responds negatively to him.

PARANOID CHARACTER TRAITS

SUSPICIOUSNESS

The paranoid person is tense, anxious, and basically unsure of himself. He is mistrustful of others and suspicious of their intentions, and looks for hidden meanings and motives in their

259

behavior. He has few close relationships, and although he may have contact with many others, he feels himself to be a loner. He may be impressive and even charming at first meeting; however, as people know him better, they like him less.

The paranoid person sees himself as the center of the universe and views events in terms of their bearing upon himself. All actions, attitudes, and feelings of others are understood and reacted to in terms of their reference to him. The paranoid patient lacks awareness of his own aggressive impulses but instead fears that he will be attacked or treated unfairly by others, whom he views as unreliable and untrustworthy, thereby justifying his own secretive and seclusive behavior.

CHRONIC RESENTMENT

His inability to relate to others realistically causes him to feel awkward and ill-at-ease in social situations. Every slight is interpreted as a personal rejection. He collects injustices, and his vivid memories of these experiences are never forgotten. He is argumentative and quarrelsome, manifesting impatience and angry emotional outbursts in situations in which others are able to contain themselves. Inappropriate reactions of anger occur in heavy automobile traffic, while waiting in line, or in response to being pushed and bumped in a crowd. The paranoid person, like the narcissistic character, expresses resentment over his feeling of being unloved and unappreciated by the world. The paranoid, however, goes further, as he attributes malevolent motives to those who do not appreciate him. He frequently fixates these feelings on a specific individual or group who he feels do not like him. The narcissistic patient says, "That is just the way people are," with an attitude of arrogant contempt. The paranoid person, however, says, "He has been out to get me," with angry resentment.

JUSTICE AND RULES

Justice and fairness are a major preoccupation for the paranoid person. In his concern about safeguarding his rights, he often obtains instruction in the arts of self-defense, such as boxing or karate, and he may possess firearms, knives, or other weapons. A compulsive concern with honesty and dedication is a thin disguise for his concealed rage. The mistrust of the paranoid patient underlies his concern with the literal interpretation and rigid enforcement of rules and regulations. At the same time, he is unable to appreciate the spirit of rules, and he tends to interpret them without considering people's feelings.

He also uses the rules to control the direct expression of his own aggression. For example, one patient described how he had spent many hours scrutinizing the laws in anticipation of preparing his income tax return. He reported triumphantly that he could deduct the cost of the postage for mailing the forms. He was determined to get everything that was due him without breaking the law. He was not psychotic, but had paranoid character traits. The patient's own minor violations lead to exaggerated fear of detection, but at the same time he searches out loopholes that permit him to express some of his aggression, although denying the significance of his behavior.

A similar rigidity concerning rules is found in obsessives, but the obsessive person is more likely to bend the regulations for his friends. The obsessive patient is concerned with the authority and status issues represented by rules—who has the power to make them and who has the power to violate them? Rules stimulate his obedience-defiance conflict. Since paranoid and obsessive traits frequently co-exist, it is common to find both mechanisms in the same patient.

GRANDIOSITY

Paranoid patients create an impression of capability and independence, neither needing nor accepting assistance from others. They are opinionated and insist that they are right. Their tactlessness and attitudes of superiority, arrogance, and grandiosity antagonize other people. These traits also make them an easy target for insincere flattery and praise and such recognition quickly re-establishes childhood feelings of grandiose omnipotence. Paranoids are resentful of others when appreciation is not immediately forthcoming. That person is then viewed as stupid, contemptible, and incompetent. These patients frequently report receiving recognition from some authority before they have earned it through adequate achievement. They describe such experiences with a feeling of having been rescued, and may relate that their performance actually improved following this unearned and unconditional acceptance.

Because the paranoid person is confident that his goals and ambitions are for the betterment of mankind, he sincerely believes that his ends justify his means. He frequently develops missionary zeal and expects to convert the world to a more perfect place, but loses sight of how he treats other human beings while accomplishing his purpose. The paranoid personality is attracted to extremist groups, both political and religious; he is more concerned with the rigid application of a system of ideas than the principles contained in them. He is a revolutionary, but is always disenchanted, even if his revolution succeeds.

SHAME

It is common for the paranoid patient to report that he was treated sadistically in early childhood, with repeated experiences of shame and humiliation. Many of the patient's problems stem from his constant sense of humiliation over his failure to control and regulate himself and his environment properly. When he becomes aware of some deficiency, he reacts as though he had soiled himself publicly and everyone were ridiculing him.

He finds it difficult to apologize for a transgression and equally difficult to accept the apologies of others. The paranoid confuses forgiveness with the admission of having erred. One patient who had experienced a realistic slight from her therapist delineated this problem by saying, "If I forgive you, that means that I was wrong."

ENVY AND JEALOUSY

Envy is a prominent paranoid character trait. Paranoid persons are more concerned with the privileges and gratification that others receive than with their own deprived and emotionally barren existence.

The paranoid person is extremely jealous because of his inability to love and his strong narcissistic needs. He has an intense longing to be loved and an equally intense fear of betrayal. This is discussed in greater detail under the classical theory of paranoia.

DEPRESSION AND MASOCHISM

Paranoid patients have an underlying depressive trend. Paranoid illnesses may be seen as defenses against depression, in the same way that manic states are traditionally viewed. Clinically, when a paranoid defense is no longer effective, depressive feelings overwhelm the patient. Suicide is not uncommon in acutely paranoid patients. The paranoid person believes that he is not loved, has not been loved, and never will be loved. Feeling persecuted, he considers himself a loser, and his life is spent in suffering (according to his view) at the hands of others. Even the patient with grandiose delusions loses, as he is inevitably confronted by reality when these delusions do not come true. The paranoid person is an eternal pessimist, always expecting the worst. He interprets his misfortunes, disappointments, and frustrations not as chance, but as the result of personal malevolence from someone else. He is unable to ask for love directly and can only obtain it through pain, self-sacrifice, and humiliation. The intensity of his demands is exorbitant and insures disappointment. Unable to accept real gratification of his need to be loved, he substitutes fantasies of revenge. His chief enjoyment comes from observing the misfortunes and failures of others rather than from his own success.

Success also creates difficulty for the paranoid person. He expects that others will react to his success with intense jealousy and that he will soon become the victim of their retaliatory rage. Therefore, his acceptance of success leads to fear and anticipation of punishment. He cannot enjoy being a winner any more than he can enjoy the role of loser. He disbelieves or depreciates his success to avoid feeling that he has outdone his competitors.

Grandiose paranoids are better able to accept success, particularly when it is associated with some idealistic cause. This would include certain religious leaders and men like Hitler. Their success is always for the enhancement of "the cause" rather than for personal gains. In their private lives, the masochistic aspect becomes more apparent, with asceticism a prominent feature.

Obsessive-phobic characters also have fears of success, but the psychodynamic conflict is more clearly related to the patient's competitive relationship with the parent of the same sex for the love of the parent of the opposite sex. The conflict in the paranoid is at an earlier level.

THEORIES OF PARANOIA

CLASSIC PSYCHOANALYTIC THEORY

THE BASIC CONFLICT.   Freud felt that the basic drives that are projected by the paranoid patient relate to unconscious homosexuality. In the Schreber case, Freud showed how unconscious homosexual tendencies were warded off by denial, reaction formation, and projection. The feeling, "I love him," is denied, and through reaction formation becomes, "I do not love him; I hate him," and then through projection it is transformed into, "It is not I who hate him, it is he who hates me." The patient once again experiences the feeling of hate, but now he rationalizes, "I hate him because he hates me." This series of defensive maneuvers is involved in delusions of persecution. In the formation of grandiose delusions, the denial of homosexual impulses occurs through the process, "I do not love him; I do not love anyone, I love only myself." The same basic sequence occurs in the production of erotomanic delusions, in which the patient asserts, "I do not love him; I love her," and then this feeling is projected to become, "She loves me; therefore I love her." The original emotion has now returned as part of the projection. Fear and mistrust of the opposite sex prevent this patient from establishing a love relationship except in fantasy. The person upon whom the fantasy is projected symbolically represents both someone from the patient's past and a part of himself.

Freud felt that unconscious homosexuality is the foundation for delusions of jealousy. The patient's preoccupation with jealous thoughts is the residue of his ego's attempt to ward off threatening impulses. Through the mechanism of projection, unconscious wishes of the patient are attributed to others. The patient asserts, "I do not love him, she loves him." The "other man" whom the paranoid patient suspects his wife of loving is actually a man to whom the patient feels attracted. This is often borne out clinically when the wife of the patient confides to the physician, "I actually have been interested in other men, but it has never been anyone whom he suspects." The paranoid man often wishes to possess a beautiful female in order to attract the attention of other males. His self-esteem is elevated by other men's attraction to his "showpiece woman," just as though it were his penis that was being admired. Heterosexual impulses to be unfaithful also may be projected to the spouse, leading to jealousy. In the classic psychoanalytic view, the dynamics of unconscious homosexuality described for the male patient are the same in the female.

Narcissistic regression has contributed to the unconscious homosexual wishes in that the paranoid patient has withdrawn his interest from others and concentrated it upon himself. His ambivalent feelings of self-love and self-hate are expressed when he becomes enamored of another person, who unconsciously represents himself. He inevitably turns against these love objects, attacking them for the same qualities that he hates in himself. This process is the same whether the love object is a real person or a delusional figure. The intense interest in persons of the same sex arouses erotic feelings and fears of homosexuality. The patient's narcissistic wish to meet his own body and parts thereof in the external world is reflected by certain clinical material. Patients may reveal that some parts of the body of persons in their delusional world remind them of parts of themselves. Often the buttocks are involved in such thoughts. The frequency of anal preoccupation in paranoid patients reflects the person's obsessive conflicts and his passive submissive longing for intimacy with his father. This will be explained in greater detail under developmental psychodynamics.

Although conflicts referring to homosexuality are clinically common in paranoid illness, Freud's view of the etiological significance of unconscious homosexuality is not universally accepted. Some writers claim that a significant number of paranoid patients have no concern with this problem. It is difficult to test his theory, since paranoid patients are typically secretive and often withhold material from the interviewer that pertains to homosexual conflicts. For example, one patient initially denied homosexual concerns in association with his delusions of being poisoned. Finally he admitted that the "poison" was "hormones," and then he acknowledged that it was "sex hormones," and ultimately he revealed his belief that he was receiving female sex hormones. Some paranoid patients are treated for years before disclosing such material.

MECHANISMS OF DEFENSE.   Primitive denial is a significant defense in all paranoid persons. It is most prominent in the overtly delusional patient; the less paranoid patient utilizes reaction formation and projection to a greater degree. These defenses are first encountered early in the interview, when the patient indicates that he has no problem and does not need to be a patient or does not require hospitalization. The paranoid person utilizes reaction formation to defend himself from awareness of his aggression, his needs for dependency, and his warm or affectionate feelings. In this way he is protected from betrayal and rejection by others. One patient reported, "If I say I don't care about you, then you can't deflate me."

The paranoid person utilizes denial to avoid awareness of the many painful aspects of reality. Fantasy serves to bolster his denial. This mechanism underlies delusions of grandeur as well as other feelings of omnipotence. Although the paranoid patient sometimes reports his own experiences in great detail, he often completely disclaims any emotional response to a given event. Despite the fact that the paranoid patient is hypersensitive to those traits in someone else that he denies in himself, he is an inaccurate observer of the feelings of others.

The paranoid person first attempts to cope with painful feelings and unacceptable impulses by repression. However, when repression fails, denial, reaction formation, and projection are utilized to cope with the feelings that are not adequately repressed.

The paranoid person is consumed with anger and hostility. Unable to face or accept responsibility for this rage, he projects his resentment and anger on to others. He then relies upon rules to protect himself from fantasied acts of attack or discrimination, which represent his own projected impulses. The patient denies the aggressive significance of his own behavior and is therefore insensitive to the impact of his behavior on others. If the patient with persecutory delusions is able to recognize some of his anger, he feels that it is an appropriate response to the persecution he receives in his delusional world. The patient with grandiose delusions is more apt to feel that others resent him because he is so great. He, of course, considers himself to be above feelings of anger. The mechanism of projection enables the patient to imagine that he is loved by someone to whom he is attracted, or he may use projection as a defense against unconscious impulses that he finds unacceptable in himself. The latter case is exemplified by the spinster who imagines that men are breaking into her apartment with some sexual designs. Her delusion reveals not only her sexual frustration, but also her projected hostility to men.

A third aspect of projection is exemplified by the patient's own super-ego criticisms that are projected when denial and reaction formation fail to handle his guilt feelings. This is illustrated by the patient who believes that his persecutors are accusing him of dishonesty. Most delusions are critical or frightening, thereby implying a projection of super-ego processes. Furthermore, paranoid mechanisms are often triggered by intense feelings of guilt.

The defense of externalization as used by the paranoid person is similar to projection in its genesis. The patient accepts no responsibility in interpersonal situations because of extreme inner feelings of shame and worthlessness. Everything that goes wrong must be seen as someone else's fault. Obviously, the paranoid person alienates himself from others by constantly blaming them for his own misdeeds or failures.

Paranoid symptoms involve regression to earlier levels of functioning. This regression affects the entire personality, including ego and super-ego functions. Super-ego regression is revealed by a return to the early stages of conscience formation, when the patient was fearful of being watched by his parents.

MODIFICATIONS OF THE CLASSIC THEORY

Following Freud's initial work, others have suggested that paranoid defenses are not only pre-Oedipal, but that they even precede autoerotic stages of object choice. Some have objected to the theory of a latent homosexual basis of paranoia because of the coexistence of paranoid schizophrenia and overt homosexuality in the same patient and because of the absence of latent homosexual conflicts in certain cases. Some clinicians have argued that the coexistence of paranoia and overt homosexuality does not contradict Freud's hypothesis. They cite cases in which the patient accepts oral homosexual impulses but defends himself from passive anal homosexual desires through paranoid mechanisms. In fact, unconscious homosexual feelings are found in every patient and often are associated with intense psychological conflict. The lack of specificity in the paranoid suggests that this patient deals with unconscious homosexual feelings as he does with all conflicts, i.e., by the use of denial, projection, reaction formation, and regression. The presence of homosexual conflicts in paranoid patients is not convincing proof of an etiological connection.

The fundamental feeling that is projected by every paranoid patient is his self-image of inadequacy and worthlessness. In the male patient, this is symbolized by the self-accusation of homosexuality, which our culture depicts as the maximal state of masculine degradation. The projected accusations in the delusions of female paranoid patients often involve prostitution or fears of heterosexual attack and exploitation rather than homosexuality. This difference can be traced to the girl's early relationship with her parents. When she turns to her father for the maternal love that she is unable to receive from her mother, she begins to develop heterosexual desires rather than homosexual wishes. These are later repudiated and projected in the fears of heterosexual attack or hallucinated accusations of prostitution. In renouncing her Oedipal desires, the female paranoid has become unable to accept a passive feminine role and develops an intense fear of competition with other women. The common theme in both male and female patients is that of being a degraded and worthless sexual object.

The paranoid patient's childhood power struggle with figures of authority also contributes to his fear of homosexuality. The homosexual thoughts and feelings reflect the incomplete resolution of this power conflict, with the resulting development of inappropriate attitudes of submission and regression to dependent modes of adaptation, which are symbolically represented by homosexuality. Phrases such as "getting screwed" or "getting the shaft" illustrate the symbolic homosexual significance that our culture attributes to a situation in which one is forced to submit to unfair treatment. Because of intense ambivalence over such wishes, both male and female paranoids may resist normal cooperation on one occasion only to submit voluntarily to some totally unreasonable demand on another.

PARANOID SYNDROMES

HYPOCHONDRIASIS

Hypochondriasis is not a disease entity, but a symptom complex found in paranoid illnesses, schizophrenia, depression, obsessive and phobic neuroses, organic psychosis, and some personality disorders. Paranoid patients complain of insomnia, irritability, weakness, or fatigue, as well as strange sensations in their eyes, ears, nose, mouth, skin, genitals, and ano-rectal area. These areas represent the chief routes through which the patient's body can be penetrated or invaded by others.

Paranoid hypochondriasis is a manifestation of regression to an infantile narcissistic state. This regression occurs as a result of withdrawal from emotional involvement with other people. The ego develops as the infant differentiates his own body from the external world. Direct observation of infants reveals that the initial discovery of one's own body is a pleasurable process. However, in hypochondriasis the rediscovery of the body is intensely painful. As the patient's interest fixates on his physical self, he experiences fears of damage and death. This may symbolize castration anxiety or it may directly reflect an awareness of impending psychological disorganization. The threat of psychosis is defended against as the patient attempts to localize or wall off the disintegrative process in one part of his body.

The negative or painful feelings associated with hypochondriasis reflect the patient's hostile, antagonistic feelings that have been withdrawn from others and turned against himself. Although these patients have always experienced some social isolation, the further withdrawal of interest from others is now accelerated. The patient reports that since the onset of his physical preoccupation he has quit his job and stopped seeing his few friends, and now devotes all of his time to matters related to his illness.

The specific symptom choice may symbolically represent the patient's ambivalent identification with a parent or parent surrogate. To illustrate, a patient who was preoccupied with his bowels revealed that his father had died of a carcinoma of the rectum. Exploration of the symptom revealed both the positive aspect of the identification and the hostile competitive feelings toward the father that were now turned inward. The interviewer can learn much about the patient's psychodynamics through a careful study of his hypochondriacal symptoms.

Beginning interviewers are sometimes tempted to make early interpretations of the psychological meaning of physical symptoms. However, in the patient's view, his social withdrawal is caused by his physical suffering. He is therefore pleased to find an organic basis for his suffering that further fixates his attention.

If no organic basis for his complaint is found, he is likely to seek medical help elsewhere. In more severe cases, the interviewer will respond to the hypochondriacal symptoms as he would to a delusion, as is discussed below. A discussion of the interview with a patient who has less severe hypochondriacal symptoms is found in Chapter 11. Another variant of hypochondriacal reactions occurs in depressed patients and a discussion may be found in Chapter 6.

PARANOID PSYCHOSES

The majority of paranoid psychoses are schizophrenic, but the reaction also occurs in organic mental syndromes. Although the etiology of these conditions is different, the problems in interviewing are essentially the same. Paranoid states are functional psychotic syndromes in which the paranoid features dominate and schizophrenic symptomatology is absent. The authors feel that these states represent one end of the spectrum of paranoid schizophrenia.

The paranoid schizophrenic psychosis usually has a gradual onset. The patient withdraws from emotional contact with the people in his life and regresses to a state of narcissistic preoccupation with himself. Hypochondriasis often precedes the appearance of secondary symptoms. Although there is some controversy over the significance of delusions, the classic psychoanalytic view is that they serve a reparative function. The patient who has been preoccupied with himself shifts his interest from his own body and attempts to re-establish contact with those persons from whom he has withdrawn. He is unable to accomplish this, and the world appears to be chaotic and disturbing. In his regressed narcissistic state, he cannot make sense out of the behavior of others, and he desperately searches for the clue that will explain their actions. The delusional concepts that emerge represent the patient's effort to organize himself and to re-establish contact with the real world. Norman Cameron coined the term "pseudo-community" to describe the group of real and imagined persons who are united (in the patient's mind) for the purpose of carrying out some action against him. As the patient becomes a more active participant in his pseudo-community, he behaves in a more grossly psychotic manner. The fantasy world of the delusion is also designed to protect the ego from the pain of reality.

A delusion is a fixed misinterpretation of reality based upon denial, reaction formation, and projection. It reflects a degree of confusion between the ego and non-ego. The essence of delusional thinking is not the lack of correspondence with external reality but the fixity of the patient's conviction and his inability to alter his ideas in response to evidence of their irrationality. The capacity for delusion formation rather than the specific type of delusion is the patient's basic pathology.

Closely related to delusional thought is the paranoid person's fascination with extra-sensory perception, mental telepathy, and similar phenomena. The patient's affinity for these strange modes of communication is consistent with his regression to the magical thinking of childhood. The process is defensive in that it validates the patient's reparative distortions and convinces him that he is right. It also reflects his basic social ataxia and lack of understanding of interpersonal relations. Since he has withdrawn his emotional investment from others and has narcissistically fixated on himself, his ability to relate to others is impaired. These unusual means of communicating represent his attempt to restore contact with other humans by those primitive techniques that are still available.

The content of the patient's delusions is determined by his psychodynamic conflicts, by the general cultural values of the society in which he lives, and by the specific characteristics of the family in which he was raised. The physician can learn the patient's psychodynamic conflicts most quickly through a careful study of the patient's delusions. The defense mechanisms and psychodynamics of delusions have already been discussed. The different types of delusions are delineated below.

DELUSIONS OF PERSECUTION.   These are the most common delusions found in paranoid patients. The persecutor represents not only the ambivalently loved object, but a projection of aspects of the patient as well. There usually is some realistic basis for paranoid projections, although it has been vastly exaggerated by the patient. The patient's tendency to distort reality is furthered by the patient's particular sensitivity to the unconscious motives and feelings of others. However, he cannot differentiate their unconscious feelings from his own.

Persecutory delusions usually reflect the social issues of concern to the culture in which the patient resides. Communist conspiracies, racism, and the Mafia are the most popular themes in

American patients today, whereas the Japanese and Germans were more prominent in delusions 30 years ago.

DELUSIONS OF GRANDEUR.   Feelings of great artistic or inventive talent or of being a messiah provide the most common content of delusions of grandeur. The patient may or may not be aware that his fantasied abilities are unappreciated by the rest of the world. Sometimes grandiose delusions have been preceded by delusions of persecution. The patient may seek to avoid the painful feeling of persecution by telling himself that he must be a very important person to merit such treatment. Compensatory grandiosity assists projection in defending the ego from the full significance of the entry of unacceptable impulses into consciousness as well as warding off feelings of inadequacy. Primary narcissism with accompanying feelings of infantile omnipotence also contributes to these delusions.

EROTOMANIA OR DELUSIONS OF BEING LOVED.   These delusions most often occur in female patients. The basically grandiose delusional system becomes centered and fixated upon one individual, usually an older male. The patient feels that this man has fallen in love with her and is communicating this love through various secret signs and signals.

Milder, non-psychotic forms of this problem are seen in the female student and the older male teacher—often an English or a French teacher. The student does extra academic work, stays after school to assist the teacher, and soon becomes his pet. The teacher is romanticized and endowed with magical omnipotence and omniscience. His attention and interest are misinterpreted by her as she attempts to compensate for feeling unattractive to boys her own age. This state blends imperceptibly into psychosis in the case of the girl who feels that her teacher's selections of poetry are chosen particularly with reference to her and that they contain covert messages of his devotion.

The erotomanic patient may develop intense rage toward the object of her delusion. Such reactions can occur independently of any real rejection on the part of this person or they may occur as reactions to a trivial slight.

SOMATIC DELUSIONS.   These patients have a more severe form of pathology than those previously discussed as hypochondriacal. Their preoccupations have fixed upon a particular part of their body and have reached delusional proportions. The parts of the body and the psychic mechanisms most commonly involved are the same as those discussed under paranoid hypochondriasis. The specific choice of symptoms always has psychodynamic significance.

DELUSIONS OF JEALOUSY.   Although all paranoid patients are extremely jealous, this can only be considered delusional when an organized system has been constructed by the patient. The patient's mate is the most frequent target for this delusional jealousy.

DEVELOPMENTAL PSYCHODYNAMICS

Although genetic, constitutional, and cultural factors are undoubtedly important in the development of paranoid disturbances, this section will focus on the role of psychological conflict. The statements that will be made in this section concerning typical family patterns stem from clinical observations. Their etiological significance is not clear. Nevertheless, it is hoped that these observations, although admittedly general, will provide the beginner with guidelines for investigation during the treatment of such patients.

The paranoid person experiences difficulty in establishing a warm and trusting relationship with his mother. His feeling of rejection leads to difficulty in developing a sense of identity in this early symbiotic relationship. Feelings of worthlessness alternate with contradictory feelings of grandiose omnipotence. Perceiving his mother as rejecting, the future paranoid turns to his father as a substitute. In the male, this leads to fears of passive homosexual wishes. These fears are accentuated by the parents' anxiety over their young son's turning primarily to his father for nurturing love and closeness. In the female, fears of sexual involvement arise as she turns to the father for the affection that she is unable to obtain from her mother, causing a regression to earlier homosexual attachments. These fears are later interpreted in Oedipal terms, with the result that the girl's fear of attack from her mother is intensified. She develops a secondary fear of attack by men as her incestuous desires are warded off through projection.

This patient learns early in life that his parents are motivated by feelings other than love and closeness. Their behavior is inconsistent with their words; consequently, he is forced to rely on his own observations and what he is able to read between the lines. Sadistic parental attacks are common from either or both parents. The father may be rigid, distant, and sadistic, or weak and ineffectual, or possibly totally absent. The obsessive patient typically receives parental love and approval as long as he is obedient. The paranoid patient, however, submits to authority only to escape attack and receives no nurturing love and warmth as a reward. The patient equates his parents' attacks as a form of rape and this is later apparent in his fears of penetration. This fear is also a defense against his passive, submissive feelings toward his father, which stem from a longing for his love, as well as a defense against the rage felt toward him. Intense feelings of anger and hate develop and are dealt with by denial, reaction formation, and projection. Identification with the aggressor becomes a prominent mechanism of defense in his actual life behavior as well as in the structure of his delusions.

The child's occasional intimate experiences with the mother typically lead to humiliation or rejection. The resultant fear of intimacy is prominent in the paranoid patient, and closeness is avoided at all cost. As a result, the future paranoid also learns to project his warm, tender, and sexual feelings.

The mother in such families is overly-controlling and frequently seductive, exposing the child to sexual stimulation either directly herself or indirectly through siblings, with total denial of the significance of such stimulation. If the mother is the sadistic parental figure, she is likely to have prominent paranoid features. Her grandiosity leads her to feel that she is always right and the child is always wrong. Under these circumstances, the child develops little sense of worth or individuality, but instead denies his ambivalence and attempts to ally himself with his all-knowing, all-powerful mother. The more the child is rebuffed in his attempt to identify with the aggressor, the more likely it is that persecutory attitudes will later develop. Since his self-esteem is achieved through identification with an omnipotent, aggressive parent, he feels that he should automatically and immediately be recognized, without demonstrating his worth. The patient's mother often attempts to dominate and control her offspring through the threat of frustration and withdrawal. Therefore, intimacy and closeness become dangerous. The child expects that all close relationships require the abandonment of independence and the adoption of a passive, submissive attitude.

The paranoid person frequently comes from a home in which success is measured by boastful claims rather than adaptive accomplishments. The child is treated as though he were exceptional and gifted. Any failure is viewed as the result of inadequate appreciation from others. Difficulties in school are blamed on incompetent teachers. Social problems are blamed on other children or their parents. The patient does not develop a realistic sense of his own worth, his strengths, and his weaknesses. His parents' attitudes towards his actual performance vary greatly. On some occasions they overevaluate his most trivial achievements, but on others, genuine accomplishments may go totally unrecognized. Both of these experiences contribute to the paranoid patient's feeling that he can achieve a sense of personal identity and recognition only through the most dramatic and awesome accomplishments. Not only must these be accomplished instantly and without effort, but the training and preparation required for such achievements are considered unnecessary.

As his parents have inadequate social skills, he too is unable to acquire the coping mechanisms necessary for acceptance by others in his environment. His parents' lack of consideration for his rights as a human being leads him to lack appreciation either of his own rights or of the rights of others. He compensates for his isolation and loneliness with an increase in his grandiosity. This offensive attitude in turn causes the patient renewed rejections from others and further entrenches the feelings of persecution.

It is difficult to differentiate the primary grandiosity that accompanies the fixation at a narcissistic level from the secondary grandiosity that is designed to repair the patient's damaged self-esteem. In general, the former is more related to grandiosity as a character trait and the latter is more prominent in the formation of delusions.

Although obsessive, phobic, depressive, and hysterical symptoms are common in childhood and pre-adolescence, paranoid symptoms are unusual before middle adolescence. Paranoid patients tend to show less severe regression or deterioration than other schizophrenics, an observation that seems in part to be explained by the later age of development. Although this is not well understood, it may be related to the fact that full-fledged paranoid syndromes require experience with a rejecting environment other than that of the patient's family. Another factor is the highly developed capacity for logical thinking associated with the production of delusions.

Paranoid behavior is, in part, learned behavior, and is based upon the attitudes of the parents. This patient may develop a close peer relationship during the preadolescent years; however, his parents warn him not to trust his friends and not to reveal confidences about himself or his family. Puberty, with its intensification of sexual impulses, creates problems for the paranoid person. He is unable to make the transition from preadolescence to adolescence with the consequent shift of emotional interest from members of the same sex to members of the opposite sex. His deflated sense of self-esteem and fear of sexual impulses cause him to remain distant and aloof from members of the opposite sex. The young boy is fearful of women and relates better to other males. His fears include both fear of domination and fear of rejection. His avoidance of women requires intensification of his defenses against homosexuality, as he is unable to shift his sexual feelings to persons of the opposite sex. Similar problems occur with a girl, as she fears either sadistic attack or rejection and disinterest such as she experienced from her father.

PRECIPITATING STRESS

There are two classes of psychodynamic stress that precipitate paranoid reactions. The first consists of situations similar to those that precipitate depressive episodes. These include the real, fantasied, or anticipated loss of love objects. Closely related are experiences of adaptive failure with loss of self-esteem. This loss of self-esteem, such as occurs after losing a job or failing in school, is contingent upon the expectation that significant other persons will reject the patient. Paradoxically, success as well as failure may precipitate paranoid episodes as a result of the patient's fantasy of retaliation from envious competitors. The second major category of situations that stimulate paranoid reactions includes those in which the patient has been forced to submit passively to real or fantasied assault. These range from injury incurred through an accident or an assault to situations in which the patient is forced into a passive submissive role in his occupation. In the latter case, the patient may project his wishes to submit passively, with the resulting fantasy of having been overpowered or assaulted. Competitive experiences may lead a paranoid person to feel that he must passively submit or they may stimulate intense feelings of aggression. Situations in which there is an intensified stimulation of homosexual feelings, such as confinement in a closed space with other males on a Navy ship, can lead to acute paranoid reactions. In all of these instances, the paranoid regression may be initiated by the intense guilt or feeling of shame that overwhelms the patient. He may experience this guilt over his failures, his successes, or his passive submissive wishes.

Management of the Interview

The paranoid patient's anger is a prominent feature in the initial interview. This may emerge as negativistic withdrawal, an angry filibuster, assaultiveness, or irrational demands. Once the interview is underway, the patient's profound mistrust presents additional problems. His hypersensitivity and fear of rejection make interpretation and confrontation extremely difficult. However, when psychotherapy progresses successfully, a trusting therapeutic relationship develops and the therapist becomes the most important person in the patient's life.

THE OPENING PHASE

ANGER AND SILENCE

The patient who has been brought for psychiatric care against his will frequently expresses his angry feelings by refusing to talk. However, unlike the catatonic or severely depressed patient, the angry paranoid person does not remain aloof from his human environment. His withdrawal is not only a defense against anger, but also a means of expressing such feelings. The patient welcomes any opportunity to give vent to his anger and hate. The interviewer can establish initial rapport with the patient by recognizing this and commenting, "You seem to have been brought here against your will," or, "I gather you feel you were railroaded into coming here." The doctor has not agreed with the patient's interpretation but has shown an interest in learning more about it. Usually such remarks will start the patient on a long, angry diatribe that allows the interviewer to engage the patient. If the patient is already hospitalized and this approach does not induce him to talk, it is helpful to say, "I assume that you were committed to the hospital for some reason, and until I have evidence that these reasons were not good, or are no longer valid, you will have to remain. Under the circumstances, talking with me can only improve your chances of being released." The interviewer must make it clear to the patient that although discussion may lead to his *eventual* release, it is not likely to be immediate. This honest approach will often enable the otherwise non-communicative paranoid patient to be interviewed.

The doctor can sympathize with the patient's feeling of being mistreated. For example, a hospitalized paranoid woman who had been interviewed by several different doctors earlier in the day began the interview by saying, "I have told my story to enough doctors and I am tired and fed up and I am not going to talk to you!" When the interviewer sympathized with the patient's feeling of injustice in being utilized in this way, the patient angrily continued, "Yes, and furthermore the male patients who have jobs are excused to go to work and do not have to be subjected to these interviews." This additional statement about the special treatment received by the male patients provided an opening for a sympathetic response, and in two or three minutes the patient was talking freely with the interviewer.

The more seriously ill paranoid patient, suffering from frightening hallucinations and delusions, is better motivated to communicate with the interviewer in order to obtain his protection; however, the pattern of the interview very quickly assumes the same characteristics as that with other paranoid persons.

THE PARANOID STARE

The paranoid patient observes every detail of the interviewer's behavior and of the surrounding environment. His "paranoid stare" makes many interviewers feel uncomfortable, and they may react by averting their gaze from the patient's eyes. This patient is reassured if the interviewer watches him closely throughout the interview. Experiencing this as evidence of interest rather than mistrust, he is reassured that the interviewer is paying close attention and is not afraid of him.

The Filibuster

The interview with a paranoid patient is better described as a filibuster rather than as interaction between two participants. This filibuster is usually most pronounced in the opening and the closing phase of the interview. Since the paranoid person, like the obsessive, experiences his greatest difficulty in establishing emotional contact and then in separating from another individual once contact has been made, it is easy to understand the adaptive value of this symptomatic behavior. By not allowing the other person to talk at the start of the interview, the patient controls the degree of his engagement in the relationship. Once he has developed emotional rapport, he must ward off the dangers of imminent rejection. He accomplishes this by rejecting the interviewer first, using words to keep him at a distance, but at the same time "hanging on" by continuing to speak.

A basic sense of worthlessness and inadequacy underlies the patient's attempt to dominate the therapist with his tirade of words. In order to permit engagement, the interviewer must allow the patient to tell his story. However, if this filibuster is permitted to continue throughout the interview, there will be no contact with the patient. Although one may occasionally confront this defense in the first interview with a comment like, "I have the feeling that I am being subjected to a filibuster," this technique will often alienate the patient. It is usually preferable to say, "I would like to hear the details of your story and over the course of our sessions together I certainly will. However, there are issues that we must discuss now in order that I may be able to help you." Another way to limit the patient's tirade, without provoking him, is to ask, "How can I be of help to you with these problems?" In this way the interviewer indicates that he will not be dominated by the patient and he takes some control away from him. It may be necessary to repeat similar statements on more than one occasion during the interview if the patient attempts to re-establish the filibuster.

Denial

The paranoid person often refuses to accept the role of patient. This is a form of denial. For him the acceptance of this role implies a humiliating loss of dignity. If the interviewer attempts to force this person to admit that he is a patient, it will further threaten an already tenuous balance of self-esteem. On the other hand, if he does not insist, the patient will often respond by demonstrating further psychopathology, once again inviting the interviewer to force him into the role of the patient. The interviewer, even though he recognizes and understands this cycle, should not interpret it to the patient during the early stages of treatment.

The patient who denies problems of his own and wants to discuss his delusional complaints of such things as being followed by detectives and wire-tapping, but who has come to the hospital voluntarily, offers an easy opportunity for engagement. After listening to the patient for 10 to 15 minutes, the doctor can say, "Since you have come to a hospital to consult a physician rather than the police, you must have had something in mind about how a doctor could be helpful to you." The patient's attention is thereby directed away from the content of his delusions. He may indicate that he had already consulted the police and that they laughed at him or told him that he was crazy. Emotional rapport is facilitated if the interviewer empathizes with the patient's predicament. For example, he might say to the patient, "It must have been terribly humiliating being treated in that way."

MISTRUST

The management of the patient's mistrust and hostility becomes the crucial issue in conducting the interview. Beneath the patient's hostility are deep wishes for, and also fears of, a close, trusting relationship. Any closeness with the paranoid patient leads to fear and mistrust with further hostility. This occurs because of the patient's fear of passivity and his conviction that only rejection can follow closeness, which is the reason that he wants to reject the doctor first. When the patient is not openly antagonistic and angry towards the physician, he will be distrustful and suspicious. The interviewer should refrain from assuring the patient that he is a friend, that he has come to help him, or that the patient can trust him as an ally. Instead, he can agree with the patient that he is a total stranger and that there is, indeed, no reason that the patient should immediately trust him or perceive him as an ally. The interviewer expresses his human compassion for the patient's pain without becoming his intimate friend. His relationship with the patient is real and authentic, but professional rather than personal.

The paranoid person has great difficulty in determining whom he can trust and whom he cannot trust. The interviewer's recognition of the patient's mistrust shows understanding of the problem. If the patient accuses the interviewer of having bugged the room, the patient could be given freedom to look about and check for himself. The interviewer might then pursue the patient's feeling that people are not trustworthy by asking him to relate experiences when he has been betrayed.

Non-psychotic patients with paranoid personality traits express their mistrust of the doctor in more subtle ways. The psychodynamic issues involved are the same as those found in the more seriously disturbed patients. Some patients show their suspicion at the start of the interview.

A patient may begin with a tone of firm conviction, "I was just curious, Doctor, did you leave that magazine on top of the pile so that I would see the cover story?" or, "I think you left that picture crooked as a test!" The interviewer is advised to pursue these ideas further before providing an answer. He could reply, "What might I hope to learn from such a test?" One patient answered, "Oh, you could see if I am an aggressive type of woman who goes around straightening other peoples' pictures." Since the patient resisted her impulse, she felt that she had passed the test and therefore had no such problem. The interviewer did not challenge this view, but mentally registered the incident as part of his evaluation of the patient.

Other patients evidence their suspicion and fear by attempting to keep "one up" on the interviewer. An example is the patient who says, "I'll bet I know why you asked me that question," or, "I know what you're trying to do; you want to get me angry." If the interviewer explores the motives that the patient ascribes to him, he will uncover the power conflict and the patient's fear of being controlled. Persons with paranoid character traits tend to be secretive about revealing the names of former doctors or even friends whom they are discussing in the interview. The patient typically asks, "Why do you need to know that?" The interviewer can explore the patient's fear of damaging other persons as well as his fear of betrayal by the doctor. If the interviewer tries to pressure the patient into revealing such information, it only reinforces the patient's fear. It is more helpful if the physician interprets the patient's mistrust of him.

DEMANDS FOR ACTION

On occasion, a paranoid patient may begin the interview not only with denial of any emotional problems, but with some bizarre demand based upon his delusional thoughts. For example, a patient came to the emergency room complaining that he had been shot in the back. When the intern could find no evidence of a wound, he suggested psychiatric consultation. The patient, however, replied that he had been shot with an invisible bullet and demanded an x-ray. Attempts to establish rapport with such a patient by acceding to his outlandish demands are doomed to failure. Some part of the patient's ego maintains awareness of the irrational aspect of his request, and the doctor who humors the patient subjects him to later feelings of humiliation. Instead, the interviewer can indicate that the patient's perception is valid but that his interpretation is impossible. One might say, for example, "You feel that you have been wounded in the back, which is frightening, but your explanation for that feeling is impossible. I would not consider taking an x-ray picture; there are no invisible bullets." The inexperienced interviewer often expects that the patient will angrily leave the emergency room at this point; however, if the physician is able to express his genuine interest, with his tone of voice and attitude, the interview will then proceed.

A similar situation occurred with a patient who came to an emergency room demanding an x-ray of his skull, claiming, "There is a radio in my brain." The patient was hallucinating, and again the interview was initiated by the physician's indication that he was sincerely interested in aiding the patient but that he did not accept the patient's delusional interpretation of his experience.

The interviewer is advised to limit his early confrontations concerning delusions to situations in which a patient demands immediate unreasonable action on the part of the interviewer. These demands can also be managed by exploring how the patient would feel if the x-ray failed to confirm his belief. This will sometimes provide an opportunity for discussion of the problem that the patient attempts to deny with his delusions. The patient may then be able to express his fear that the voice may be a hallucination and therefore a reflection of mental illness.

It is sometimes necessary to accede to some unrealistic request on the part of a paranoid patient in order to establish an initial therapeutic relationship. For example, a paranoid patient entered the physician's office and at once complained that he could not discuss his problems unless the interviewer pulled the window shade because he was being watched from the next building. The interviewer granted his request, but it became readily apparent that, even though the shade was pulled, he still was not discussing his problem. When this was pointed out, the patient first became angry, but then proceeded to reveal his difficulties. In these situations, the patient's demand is not as bizarre as those described earlier and the interviewer set the stage for challenging the patient's rationalization by yielding to his request. One paranoid patient refused to be interviewed in a room where the partition did not go to the ceiling, even though he was assured that there was no one in the adjacent room. The patient's request for greater privacy was granted by moving to a different room.

A difficult problem is presented by the patient who refuses to be interviewed unless the physician will promise not to hospitalize him. Obviously, no such blanket promise can be given. The interviewer might reply, "I do not believe in forcing treatment on someone against his will, since it would be unlikely to help. On the other hand, people who have uncontrollable impulses to harm themselves, or others, are best treated in a hospital until they strengthen their own self-control." Often this will reassure the patient sufficiently that the interview can continue.

If the patient has come voluntarily but insists that the physician promise not to hospitalize him, the interviewer could say, "Unless I learn that you are in danger of hurting yourself or someone else, I will not force hospitalization." However, if further discussion convinces the physician that the patient would be best treated in a hospital, he should attempt to convince the patient to accept hospitalization, and if the patient still refuses, he can refuse to treat him unless he agrees. If the patient has been brought by someone else and the above techniques fail, with the patient insisting on the promise before speaking, the interviewer could say, "If I do not hear the problem from you, I will have to base my decision exclusively on what your relatives can tell me."

ESTABLISHING THE THERAPEUTIC ALLIANCE

CHALLENGING THE DELUSION

Every beginning psychiatrist is tempted to argue the patient out of his delusional system by the use of logic. The impossibility of this task soon becomes apparent. It is more helpful if the interviewer asks the patient what is responsible for this persecution—why people should be against him and what he could possibly have done that offended them. The interviewer neither agrees with the delusions nor challenges them. The patient, however, usually interprets the interviewer's interest as a sign of tacit agreement. It is essential for their later relationship that the interviewer make no deceptive statements in order to gain the patient's trust and confidence momentarily.

If the patient directly inquires whether the physician believes his story, the interviewer could reply, "I believe that you feel just as you say and that you are telling me the truth as you see it; however, the meaning that you attribute to your feelings is a matter of interpretation." The interviewer might address himself to the patient's anxiety about convincing the interviewer concerning the accuracy of his views so quickly and indicate that time is required to evaluate these problems. In general, the more bizarre the delusional material, the more open the interviewer must be in directly expressing his disbelief in the patient's interpretation of his experiences. In doing so, it is helpful for the interviewer to state the logical foundation behind his own position, but to avoid debating it with the patient. Frequently, this involves a challenge to the patient's grandiosity. For example, the physician might say, "I have no doubt that the green car you described actually drove around the block; however, I see no reason to believe that it contained Communists or that anyone in the car was interested in you more than anyone else. Nothing you have told me indicates why the Communists should consider you so important that they would bother to make your life difficult."

The interviewer can often point out that the patient's relatives disagree with his delusional system, and that they believe their view just as strongly as the patient believes in his. He can then ask, "Why should I believe that you are right and that your relatives are crazy?" Any doubt or fluctuation in the patient's feelings provides a foothold for establishing a therapeutic relationship. Later in treatment, increased or renewed delusional material should be related to specific precipitating stresses.

Differentiating Delusions from Reality

Every paranoid delusion contains some kernel of truth. When the delusion is somewhat plausible, beginning interviewers often attempt to determine how much of the patient's production is actually delusional and how much is real. This is an error, since it does not really matter exactly where reality begins and ends, and one can never actually make such a determination. It is far more important to establish rapport through the acknowledgement of the plausible elements of the delusion. The most important aspects of a delusion are the patient's preoccupation with it, his irrational certainty that it is true, and its use to explain his frustrations, dissappointments, and failures. The meaning of the delusion to the patient and the adaptive purpose it serves are the more crucial issues for discussion. One way to make contact with the patient is to indicate sympathetically that his preoccupation with the delusion interferes with a constructive and useful life. In this manner, the interviewer avoids arguments concerning the degree of truth in the delusion.

The interviewer inquires whether the patient has ever taken action or contemplated action based on his delusional system. It is important not to ask these questions in a tone that suggests that the patient should have taken action. The effects of any action that the patient did take will often enable the interviewer to evaluate the patient's judgement and impulse control.

The Treatment Plan

It is important that the patient function as an active participant in evolving the treatment plan. Otherwise, he is likely to feel passive and submissive and then express his resentment by not following the doctor's advice. To avoid this problem, the physician must stimulate the patient's motivation to receive help. The patient who is delusional may not feel that he requires treatment for his delusion, but willingly accepts help aimed at his irritability, insomnia, or inability to concentrate. He might acknowledge a problem in his social life or on his job that could be treated with psychotherapy. Once the patient has indicated that he recognizes problems for which he desires help, the doctor can offer a tentative recommendation for treatment. Statements such as, "These are problems we could work on together," or, "I believe I can help you to arrive at a solution to this difficulty," emphasize that the patient plays an active role in treatment and is not merely submitting to the doctor. If the therapist is overly enthusiastic in offering therapeutic recommendations, the patient is more likely to resist them.

When it is necessary to refer a paranoid patient to another therapist, the physician can anticipate trouble. The patient will often question the qualifications of the doctor to whom he is referred. The interviewer can review these qualifications and then ask, "Did you think I would send you to someone not adequately qualified?" The patient will usually hasten to reassure the interviewer that he had no such thought. The interviewer could then comment, "Perhaps you feel hurt or angry that I do not have time to work with you myself." If the patient acknowledges such feelings and the interviewer is not defensive, the referral is more likely to proceed smoothly. If the patient denies such feelings, the interviewer can expect a call from the patient saying that he did not like the new doctor for a variety of reasons. In general, the interviewer should advise the patient to go back to the other doctor and discuss these feelings with him, rather than send the patient to still another psychiatrist.

The paranoid is hypersensitive to restrictions of freedom or situations of enforced passivity. He does not readily accept medication or hospitalization. The interviewer should not bring up these subjects until he has established a trusting relationship with the patient. When hospital treatment is required, every attempt should be made to convince the patient to accept voluntary hospitalization, avoiding physical or social coercion (see Chapter 14). The paranoid patient's fear that others will exert influence over his behavior extends into the area of medication. The physician who hands a prescription to the patient and says, "Take this according to the directions," will have little success. Instead, the physician might advise the patient concerning the name of the medication as well as the therapeutic action and possible side effects to be expected. He can then ask the patient if there are any questions concerning the prescription. The patient is now a partner in planning the treatment and is more likely to work for its success.

OPENNESS AND CONSISTENCY

The therapist works to establish a relationship with the remaining healthy portion of the patient's ego. It is not the patient's delusional system that requires treatment, but the frightened, angry person who has created it. Firmness and steadiness characterize the secure therapist's attitude. The patient should be granted no special favors or privileges, and the doctor must maintain the most scrupulous honesty at all times. The punctuality, predictability, and consistency of the therapist's behavior are of great importance in enabling this patient to develop a trusting relationship. When a paranoid person is treated on an outpatient basis, a clear statement about the rules of treatment, the charges for missed sessions, and so on will help prevent misunderstandings that otherwise may threaten the therapy. For example, this patient can easily make the doctor angry by not respecting his personal rights or property.

The doctor does not help the patient by allowing him to intrude in the doctor's private life or to abuse the furniture in his office. The interviewer may sympathize directly with the patient's hate of hypocrisy, inconsistency, and unpredictability. Accurate perceptions should be reinforced, including perceptions about the interviewer, even though these may be negative. At all times, the interviewer must be forthright about areas of disagreement, making statements to the patient such as, "We can agree to disagree." Such statements underline that the patient and interviewer each have their own identity. Whenever possible, the therapist can emphasize and support the patient's right and ability to make his own decisions.

ANXIETY IN THE THERAPIST

Some therapists have such strong dislike or fear of paranoid patients that they should not treat them until these problems are resolved. If the therapist is frightened of the patient's assaultiveness, he should conduct the interview only in the presence of an attendant or other adequate safeguard.

The paranoid patient tends to disrupt his relationship with the therapist as he has done with significant persons in the past, first by making him anxious and then by perceiving his reaction as a rejection. The therapist must understand that there is some validity in the patient's complaints. The paranoid requires a secure therapist whose self-esteem is not challenged by angry, and at times accurate, criticisms.

When the patient expresses hostile, critical feelings, the therapist who needs to be liked and appreciated will feel hurt and will respond with anger or depression. When the patient expresses positive feelings, this therapist will accept the benevolent parental role that the patient ascribes to him, thereby inflating the doctor's ego and infantalizing the patient.

The interviewer may advise the paranoid patient that, in due time, he will grow suspicious of the therapist, but that this does not justify terminating the relationship. Instead, it is an indication for exploration, improved communication, and a better mutual understanding of the doctor's and the patient's feelings. Because of the patient's extreme sensitivity to rejection, he must be prepared long in advance for any vacation or absence from treatment on the part of the therapist.

Infinite patience is required in order to tolerate the continuing mistrust and suspiciousness that is directed at the therapist. The patient's extreme sensitivity to criticism and his alternation between clinging submissive ingratiation and defensive aggression often stimulate anger in the therapist.

Avoidance of Humor

The paranoid person thinks of himself as having a good sense of humor. In actuality, he lacks the ability to relax and to accept the subtlety and ambiguity required for true humor. His sardonic laugh reflects his pleasure in the sadism or aggression in a situation, but more complex types of humor are beyond his grasp. The interviewer, therefore, should avoid witty or humorous remarks, particularly if they are directed at the patient, as this person has no sense of humor about anything applied to himself. He reacts to such attempts, no matter how skillfully conducted, as though the interviewer were making fun of him. Irony and metaphor are also dangerous, as the patient's concreteness makes him likely to miss the desired meaning.

The most frequent joke attempted by the therapist is an exaggeration of the paranoid's tendency to be suspicious or mistrustful. If the "clever" sarcastic remarks of the paranoid are returned in kind, the patient feels hurt and misunderstood. For example, a paranoid patient made sarcastic, humorous remarks about her physician's scheduling her appointments during the lunch hour. The interviewer misperceived the meaning of the patient's "jokes" and quipped, "The next thing I know you'll be accusing me of trying to starve you." Not long thereafter, the patient developed a delusion that the therapist was plotting her starvation. The inexperienced physician displays his anxiety and unconscious hostility to the patient with such remarks.

INAPPROPRIATE REASSURANCE

The interviewer sometimes offers inappropriate reassurance prior to understanding the patient's specific fears. For example, an obviously paranoid patient began an interview by asking a resident psychiatrist, "Do I look 'crazy' to you, Doctor?" The resident replied that he did not, thereby hoping to foster a supportive therapeutic relationship. Although some initial rapport was established by this method, the doctor soon learned that the patient had many crazy thoughts and feelings. By allowing himself to be manipulated, the doctor appeared naive and foolish in the patient's eyes. It would have been better had he said, "What makes you ask if you are crazy?" or, "I can't really consider that until you tell me about yourself." The patient was testing the doctor to determine his willingness to admit uncertainty. The doctor's lack of hypocrisy despite the coercive pressure for an insincere reply would have been comforting.

THE USE OF INTERPRETATIONS

IMPORTANCE OF TIMING

Interpretations are intrusions in the patient's life, and paranoid persons are unable to tolerate intrusion. Clarification or explanations may be offered early in treatment, but interpretations must be delayed until a trusting relationship has developed.

Dynamic interpretations of grossly psychotic paranoid distortions must wait until the psychosis has improved. However, it is necessary to stimulate doubt and uncertainty in the patient's mind concerning his delusional systems. Teaching the patient to consider alternate explanations of his observations undermines his projective defenses. As an example, a patient reported that people in the apartment across the street were taking movies of him. The therapist agreed that there might indeed be people across the street taking movies, but suggested that there were other explanations of what was being photographed. When the patient argued that the purpose of the filming was to obtain evidence concerning his sexual practices, the doctor inquired whether the patient felt embarrassed and ashamed about his sex life. This was, in fact, the case, and it initiated a discussion of a major problem area.

Interpretations directed at the role the patient plays in bringing about his own misfortunes must be slow, gentle, and tentative. This topic can easily precipitate severe anxiety with total loss of self-esteem and overwhelming depression, a constant problem for the paranoid patient. When the patient does achieve some insight into this aspect of his behavior, he experiences a sense of acute panic and feels that the problem must be resolved magically, immediately, and permanently. For example, a therapist interpreted that the patient's fear of male figures of authority had caused him to behave provocatively with his boss. During the following session he reported, "Well, I have now solved that problem of being afraid of my father." Further exploration was thereby closed off. This makes any "uncovering" approach to psychotherapy difficult with a paranoid. He cannot afford to be intellectually curious about his deeper motives, as he fears that every discovery about himself will only lead to exposure of his badness, with resulting humiliation. The patient is unable to live up to his ego ideal and feels intense shame whenever the discrepancy is brought to his attention.

Early in treatment, the therapist can offer interpretive comments that are aimed at reducing the patient's guilt, even though the patient denies any feeling of guilt. The paranoid person is tortured by unconscious feelings of guilt, and such comments reduce his need to project his self-contempt on to others. Some early clarification of the patient's continuing search for closeness and his intense fear of it may be productive. Attempts to interpret unconscious homosexual conflicts must be extremely cautious, if they are made at all. Some exploration of the clinical material in this area is feasible provided the patient is able to deny its significance.

INTERPRETING THE TRANSFERENCE

When the patient produces fantasy material about the therapist in the early stages of treatment, it is helpful first to provide realistic data and then to explore how the patient came to his own conclusions. An analysis of the paranoid patient's transference fantasies while the therapist remains anonymous is doomed to failure.

As a positive relationship evolves, the paranoid patient typically develops an unrealistic overestimation of his doctor as omniscient and omnipotent. The interviewer can diminish this projection of the patient's grandiosity by occasionally dropping specific data about himself that challenge the patient's idealized distortion. For instance, a paranoid man indicated that the doctor was always fair and reasonable. The therapist reminded the patient that he had once overheard the physician speaking impatiently to the doorman. Another patient made a reference to a historical novel and the therapist indicated that he hadn't read that book. The patient immediately offered excuses for the doctor's ignorance, but the physician remarked, "You have uncovered an area in which I am not well informed and you seem reluctant to accept my deficiency." This technique can stimulate disturbing fantasies and must be utilized with caution and never early in treatment.

The interviewer can indicate to the paranoid patient that his recognition of slights from others may be quite accurate, but that his interpretation of their motives may be quite erroneous. The paranoid person views the world as though people had no unconscious motives and all acts were deliberate. The patient's accusations may pertain to the motivation of the interviewer. One of the author's patients, who was justifiably angry when he found the physician had forgotten to leave the waiting room door unlocked, suggested that this was evidence of the therapist's wish to get rid of him. The therapist responded by admitting that he had left the waiting room door locked, thereby supporting the patient's right to be angry, but then added, "You are certainly entitled to analyze me if you wish to do so; however, isn't it only fair that you find out what I think happened and how I feel about it before jumping to conclusions concerning my motives?" In this way, the interviewer not only addressed himself to the patient's feeling of righteous indignation, but also established a foundation for analyzing the patient's projective defenses. Every opportunity for the patient to expand his awareness of how he makes conclusions about the motives of others without adequate information has a therapeutic effect. It was later explained that the physician was unlocking his front door when the telephone rang. He rushed to answer the phone, leaving the door ajar but still locked. A passerby closed the door and soon thereafter the patient arrived. It is helpful to the paranoid for the physician to show the patient that other factors in the interviewer's life not related to the patient may at times affect the doctor's mood and his treatment of the patient.

The therapist must be tolerant of the patient's overreactions to the therapist's mistakes and shortcomings, an attitude that is the opposite of that expressed by the patient's parents. It is common for the patient to collect a series of minor grievances and withhold them from the therapist. He will often confront the doctor much later with something that the patient misinterpreted as a slight, quoting the physician's exact words. While he keeps his injuries secret, the patient may feel superior to the doctor. The patient's tendency to withhold his resentments makes examination and understanding impossible.

The paranoid patient attempts to maintain a one-up position on the doctor by anticipating his behavior and interpretations, and he defends himself from their impact by analyzing the motivation behind the therapist's comments. The patient's eventual awareness of his underlying grandiosity and its role as a defense against feelings of worthlessness and inadequacy is only the beginning. It allows exploration of the developmental problems that led to the utilization of such defenses. The constant introduction of reality into the treatment process provides an important therapeutic lever. However, in discussing the patient's delusional system in terms of reality, the therapist must protect the patient from feeling humiliated.

THE HOMICIDAL PATIENT

Homicide is most frequent in men in the age group of 20 to 40. The assessment of homicidal risk is in many ways quite similar to the assessment of suicidal risk. As with the suicidal patient, the interviewer inquires if the patient has formulated a specific plan as to how he would commit the murder and whether or not he has taken any action toward the implementation of this plan. The interviewer might ask if he has had similar feelings in the past and how he managed to overcome them on those occasions. A family history of murder or sadistic beating is of import. Inquiry into past episodes in which the patient had lost control of aggressive impulses and the outcome of these episodes provides important data. A past history of vengeful destructive behavior indicates that the patient may require external controls. In this regard, the interviewer could inquire if the patient has ever caused anyone's death. Precipitating stress is important in understanding the development of destructive impulses. When specific stresses can be uncovered, the physician has a greater opportunity to recommend helpful manipulations of the patient's environment. Persons accompanying the patient should always be interviewed, including police officers. Often the homicidal significance of the behavior is denied by the patient's relatives and professional personnel as well.

The interviewer should realize that it is possible to assassinate anyone. The patient who is unambivalent concerning his homicidal impulses is not likely to be interviewed by the physician, or at least he will not mention these feelings. If the patient brings the subject up for discussion, this is already evidence that he has not completely decided to commit murder and may therefore be influenced away from this course of action. The interviewer can interpret that the patient is undoubtedly frightened and upset at the prospect of becoming a murderer and comment on the predicament in which the patient finds himself. The therapist offers to help the patient understand the reasons behind his desire to commit murder and to help the patient obtain additional control in restraining his impulses if this is needed. The latter may be in the form of tranquilizing medication or temporary hospitalization until the patient feels more capable of controlling himself.

A 17-year-old boy was brought to the emergency room by his parents because he had become seclusive and refused to attend school. He had been seen cutting out advertisements for firearms and would sometimes lock himself in his room for hours. In the interview, he was sullen and withdrawn, responding evasively when asked about violent or aggressive impulses. A history of fire-setting and cruelty to animals was elicited from the parents. On one occasion he had almost choked another boy. He repeatedly denied any need for treatment and asked to be allowed to return home. The interviewer told the patient, "I have the uneasy feeling that you may be planning to kill someone." The patient did not reply, but looked away from the interviewer. The physician continued, "Under the circumstances, I feel that you belong in a hospital until I am convinced that you are well enough to return home." On other occasions, the interviewer's admission of discomfort with the patient would facilitate the interview. He might say to the patient, "If you are trying to scare me, you are succeeding. I can't help you if you put me in this position, so let's try and find out why you need to do this!"

It is worthwhile to remember that the patient who threatens the life of a doctor often behaves in this fashion because he is afraid. The interviewer who realizes that the patient is more anxious than himself has a distinct advantage. For example, a frightening incident occurred when one of the authors had started to deliver a baby at the mother's home when he was a fourth-year medical student. The expectant father suddenly burst into the room, intoxicated and waving a pistol. He shouted, "The baby better be o.k., Doc!" The student physician started to pack up his equipment and said, "If you don't put down that gun and leave immediately, I will leave your wife and not deliver the baby." The man put down the gun and left without further trouble.

It is not unusual for an interviewer to explore these issues and have all the data indicate that there is little danger. Nevertheless, the therapist continues to be uneasy. Such reactions may stem from unresolved neurotic problems in the therapist, often relating to anxiety about his own control of aggressive impulses. When a physician assesses that there is little risk of a patient's being homicidal, he should have confidence in his clinical judgement, just as he would with a suicidal patient.

Although a paranoid patient may be assaultive in initial interviews, it is rare for him to harbor specific homicidal impulses toward his therapist until treatment has progressed. It is easy to panic when a patient announces that he is formulating a plan to kill the therapist or some member of his family.

It can be devastating for the patient if the interviewer panics and calls the police behind the patient's back, arranging for him to be hospitalized under force. The arrangements for hospitalization must be openly discussed, *with the patient under constant observation,* until they can be implemented. If the patient indicates that he is carrying a weapon, the psychiatrist should ask him to relinquish it until the patient has re-established confidence in his ability to control himself. The therapist might well remember that the patient fears he will be rejected because of his intense homicidal impulses. The therapist's ability to accept the patient in spite of these feelings will often lead to their prompt amelioration.

THE CLOSING PHASE

Particular attention should be paid to offhand or casual comments made at the door, either by the patient or by the doctor. The beginner tends to consider such remarks as not part of the session, but for the paranoid patient this is often the most important part of the session.

Gradually, as the treatment progresses, the patient develops some understanding of how his attitudes and behavior affect others. As he learns to trust the support and affection of his therapist, he can then appreciate that life is not always black or white and that people are able to genuinely care about him without his becoming the center of their universe.

REFERENCES

Bullard, D.: Psychotherapy of paranoid patients. Arch. Gen. Psychiat., 2:27, 1960.
Cameron, N.: Paranoid conditions and paranoia. In Arieti, S. (ed.): American Handbook of Psychiatry, Vol. 1. New York, Basic Books, 1959, Chap. 25, pp. 508–539.
Dupont, R. L., Jr., and Grunebaum, H.: Willing victims: The husbands of paranoid women. Amer. J. Psychiat., 125:151, 1968.
Freud, S.: Psychoanalytic notes on an autobiographical account of a case of paranoia (dementia paranoides). Standard Edition of Complete Psychological Works of Sigmund Freud, Vol. XII. London, Hogarth Press, 1958, pp. 3–82.

Freud, S.: Some neurotic mechanisms in jealousy, paranoia, and homosexuality. Standard Edition of Complete Psychological Works of Sigmund Freud, Vol. XVIII. London, Hogarth Press, 1955, pp. 221–232.

Jackson, D.: A suggestion for the technical handling of paranoid patients. Psychiatry, 26:306, 1963.

Salzman, L.: Paranoid state, theory and therapy. Arch. Gen. Psychiat., 2:101, 1960.

Will, O., Jr.: Paranoid development and the concept of self: Psychotherapeutic intervention. Psychiatry, Chestnut Lodge Fiftieth Anniversary Symposium, Vol. 24, 1961.

9
THE SOCIOPATHIC
PATIENT

Psychopathology and Psychodynamics

NEUROSIS AND PSYCHOPATHY

Psychodynamic theory views behavior as a product of four interrelated factors: (1) basic motives; (2) those mental structures that control motives and regulate their expression; (3) the values, goals, and attitudes that the individual has incorporated from his family and society; and (4) external reality, including the significant other people in the individual's life. Within this framework, neuroses are seen as maladaptive patterns of control and regulation, in which the individual's basic motives are frustrated because of attitudes and feelings that stem from the past and that are not appropriate to current external reality. The gratification of impulses is sacrificed in order to protect the individual from anxiety related to unconscious fears of imagined dangers.

Sociopathy, or psychopathy, is seen in a somewhat different way. Behavior is psychopathic when the gratification of basic motives is of overriding importance. The controlling and regulating functions of the ego are defective, and the individual pursues immediate gratification with little regard for other aspects of psychic functioning or for the demands of external reality. The

297

primary goals of psychopathic behavior are to avoid the tension that results when impulses are not gratified, to avoid the anxiety that appears when frustration is imminent, and further, to protect the ego from feelings of inadequacy.

PSYCHOPATHIC TRAITS AND PSYCHOPATHIC CHARACTERS

Psychopathic mechanisms are found in everyone. There are times or situations when needs feel urgent, or inner controls have not been developed, and the executive functions of the ego are directly utilized to obtain gratification. The sexual behavior of a conventioner away from home, the heavy smoker deprived of tobacco, or the person who receives too much change from the cashier in a restaurant are familiar examples of psychopathic maneuvers. When these mechanisms become the major mode of adaptation, we speak of psychopathic personality types.

The sociopathic or psychopathic personality is less clearly delineated than the neurotic or psychotic reaction. The term is applied to a wide variety of clinical syndromes, and is used to refer to both psychopathological and psychodynamic features. When the impulses involved in psychopathic patterns are sharply defined, it can be disarmingly simple to employ them as specific diagnostic labels, ignoring other clinical features. Thus we customarily speak of alcoholism, drug addiction, sexual perversion or even specific perversions, pathologic gambling, anti-social criminality, kleptomania, pyromania, and so forth. If the specific impulses are less obvious, or other features are more salient, we may speak of "immature," "emotionally inadequate," or "acting out" personalities, and even of some borderline or pseudoneurotic states. When the problems in impulse control are only part of more general integrative pathology, we see certain schizophrenic and paranoid syndromes. The relationship of the patient's impulses to his psychopathology will be discussed below.

PSYCHOPATHIC CHARACTERS AND CHARACTER NEUROSIS

Although psychopathy refers to a characterological style, it is not synonymous with character neurosis. The neurotic character has developed ego syntonic modes of adaptation rather than neurotic symptoms as means of dealing with endopsychic conflict and anxiety. That is, he has acquired patterns of behavior that serve to partially gratify his impulses, bind his anxiety, and appease or satisfy super-ego demands without undue impairment of his autonomous ego functioning or his relations with others. Our discussion of the neurotic syndromes has focused on these characterological aspects of neurosis. The traits of the psychopathic character, on the other hand, are designed to ensure the gratification of impulses and to provide the security and tension relief that result. There is little regard for the demands of conscience, affectivity is shallow, and there is little capacity to tolerate anxiety. The psychopathic character's failure to develop adequate neurotic defenses makes it necessary for him to *escape* from frustration and anxiety, as compared to the neurotic, who has mental mechanisms that control anxiety while providing partial gratification of feared impulses. The psychopathic individual shuns responsibility and avoids situations that expose his affective deficit.

Frequently, both neurotic and psychopathic components are found in specific patterns of behavior. For example, the recent recognition of the neurotic component of perversions and addictions, which were previously seen as "pure" psychopathic syndromes, has led to modifications of therapeutic technique in these disorders. However, there are certain features that differentiate the psychopathic character's mode of pursuing gratification from that of the neurotic. The psychopathic individual is relatively indifferent to his objects apart from their relationship to him. He sees other people only as potential sources of danger or gratification, having little concern for their security, comfort, or pleasure. Inner drives are experienced as urgent and overwhelming—delay or substitution does not seem possible. Lastly, the feeling that results from gratifying his drives has a quality of tension, relief, or satiation, rather than the more complex happiness with tender feelings toward objects and with increased self-esteem that characterizes the neurotic. Those features that differentiate the psychopath from specific neurotic syndromes will be discussed below under "Clinical Features."

SOCIAL ATTITUDES

Both the term "psychopath" and the somewhat euphemistic and often preferred term "sociopath" have strongly negative implications. Many attempts have been made to minimize this unfavorable connotation. Nevertheless, the diagnosis retains its pejorative quality, and this accurately reflects the attitudes of most psychiatrists. Some of the problems in the interview with the psychopath are clarified by a study of the sources of the negative feelings that this patient so consistently elicits.

The young psychiatrist usually has great difficulty in understanding and accepting those patients who are least like himself. The feeling that the patient is different and somehow inferior is a common reaction to both psychopathic and schizophrenic patients. However, the contrast between responses to these two groups is enlightening. The doctor may feel pity or detached curiosity for the schizophrenic, but he is more likely to experience unconscious admiration or even envy of psychopathic patients. The patient is seen as getting away with behavior that is gratifying or pleasurable, but that is conflictual or forbidden for normal people. In reality, of course, it is the patient's primary deficit in the capacity for pleasure in human relationships that leads to psychopathic behavior as a striving for substitute forms of pleasure. The conflict and anxiety of neurosis are avoided, but the rewards of warm affectionate relations with other people are also missing. The doctor's unconscious envy is often accompanied by some degree of identification with the patient, and exaggerated negative responses to these patients may represent the doctor's rejection of similar unacceptable impulses in himself.

Although the formal diagnosis of psychopathy involves overt social behavior, psychodynamic issues are also an integral part of the syndrome. A psychopath does not conform to social standards, and participates in activities that are illegal or immoral, but "psychopathy" is not merely a technical term for social misbehavior. It implies that certain developmental experiences and psychodynamic patterns have led to fixed disturbances of behavior that are antithetic to the basic moral standards of the society in which a person was raised. However, there are times and situations in which apparently antisocial behavior may be psychodynamically normal. It is therefore important to take the patient's age and cultural background into account in evaluating his psychopathology. For example, normal adolescents will experiment with behavior that is superficially antisocial; in fact, the absence of such experimentation may be suggestive of psychopathology. Members of deprived and oppressed subcultures will exhibit similar tendencies, and the lack of opportunity to resolve their conflicts more adaptively is also associated with an increased utilization of seemingly psychopathic mechanisms. Persons raised in families that are committed to lives of crime and antisocial behavior may identify with familial goals and values, with resulting patterns of criminal behavior without psychological abnormality—a pattern that is called "dyssocial reaction." Such individuals are capable of loyalty and love, and can control their impulses so that they conform with the requirements of their own subculture. In each of these situations, overtly antisocial behavior does not signify psychopathy.

CLINICAL FEATURES

The psychopathic individual, failing to develop control over the expression of his basic needs, retains relatively primitive impulses as his primary motives. Thus, oral behavior is preponderant and symptomatic derivatives of orality such as addiction are common. Painful affects are poorly tolerated, and the capacity for mature pleasure and positive affectivity is impaired. Failure to develop mature ego functions is associated with inadequate or pathological object relations early in life, and adult object relations are severely disturbed. Therefore, the patient with a preponderance of psychopathic mechanisms is likely to show defects in (1) his basic impulses and his mode of handling them; (2) his affectivity, including anxiety, guilt and the capacity for pleasure; (3) his object relations; and (4) the resultant patterns of overt behavior.

IMPULSES

Impulses are the mental representations of needs and motives that form the driving force behind all behavior. Their central role in the integration of the psychopathic personality has been described. Some psychopathic patients experience their impulses as ego-syntonic—that is, they feel that they want to act on them— but others have a subjective sense of an urgent and compelling external force. Combinations of these attitudes are common. For example, an addict explains his desire for drugs by the pleasurable experiences that they offer, but he has neither the interest nor the capacity to defer the pleasure when he learns of the long-term dangers associated with it. If he is deprived of the drug, his need is experienced as more urgent. He is unable to postpone gratification because of the feeling that each opportunity may be his last, and that he must take advantage of it. This philosophy of immediacy is associated with a lack of concern about the consequences of his behavior.

The psychopathic individual is impatient and hedonistic, but the acts that are customarily associated with pleasure for others are more likely to bring him only a transient relief of tension. Those pleasures that he does experience have a primitive oral quality and are more related to physiological responses than to interpersonal relationships. The drink, the "fix," the opportunity for sexual gratification, or the acquisition of property, offer a temporary diminution of his inner pressure for gratification. There is no long-lasting shift in his psychic economy, no change in his perception of himself or his relationship to others. The neurotic patient who engages in a pleasurable sexual relationship develops a new attitude toward his partner, enhances his own self-esteem, and enriches his personal life in a way that lasts far longer than the effects of the physical sexual act. The psychopathic patient is more likely to experience the event as a relief of a bodily need.

The patient's inability to control or modulate his impulses leads to outbursts of aggression. These may be active or passive, and although they can be triggered by relatively minor slights, they usually involve a reaction to some frustration. The patient's deficit in empathy and concern for others may lead to extreme cruelty and sadism, although, characteristically, he will have little emotional reaction to his own behavior after it is over.

Psychotic patients also have a disturbance of impulse control. The schizophrenic patient who is concerned by his sensation of numbness or feeling of being dead will sometimes attempt to evoke intense affects or sensory experiences in himself. Self-mutilation, such as burning oneself, is one common method, but antisocial behavior can also be involved. One young man would kill small animals and make objects from their skin; a nurse would abandon her work for week-long binges of perverse promiscuity and drug abuse. The bizarre, primitive, and chaotic nature of the impulses suggests their basically psychotic origin. Furthermore, the psychopathic individual will claim that his impulsive behavior is pleasurable, whereas the schizophrenic is more likely to describe diminished or apathetic emotional responses.

Psychopathic patients must also be differentiated from paranoid individuals, who have difficulty controlling their anger and may have poor reality testing. This combination can result in episodes of explosive violence. When the paranoid patient's delusional view of the world is taken into account, however, his behavior is understandable. The paranoid patient may feel guilt and remorse after an episode of rage, he may attempt to defend his behavior, or he may disown responsibility for it, but it usually takes him a long time to simmer down. In contrast, the angry outbursts of the psychopathic person can disappear as suddenly as they began, and the patient may be tranquil, almost to the point of disinterest, following the episode. He cannot understand why others attribute such significance to his violence.

Affect

ANXIETY.   The psychopath is often described as having little or no anxiety. In fact, he has a very low tolerance for anxiety, and many psychopathic mechanisms are designed to forestall, defend against, or allay even minimal anxiety. The slightest threat that his needs will not be gratified leads to unbearable discomfort. He will go to great lengths to guarantee his security, but of course frequent frustrations are inevitable, and constant diffuse tension is the result. A common defense is denial, with the appearance of external composure leading to the erroneous claim that these patients do not experience anxiety. The patient is likely to deny not only his anxiety, but also the urgent, compelling nature of his inner needs. However, this denial can be maintained only if constant gratification is available. When gratification is not available and the denial fails, anxiety, depression, rage, and impulsive behavior are common.

GUILT.   The role of guilt is another controversial issue in the discussion of psychopathic patients. In one view, there is a diminished tolerance for guilt, but in the other there is a relative lack of guilt. In the authors' opinion, both of these features are present, and they are integrally related in the early development of the patient, as will be discussed below. The psychopathic patient experiences the more primitive precursors of guilt. He may feel shame and fear public disapproval for his unacceptable behavior, or he may become depressed if his behavior is exposed. However, he has not developed an autonomous internalized system of behavioral controls that function without the threat of discovery and that provide for regulation of impulses before they lead to overt behavior.

At times it is quite difficult to differentiate this patient from the obsessive character. Obsessive individuals are dominated by an overpowering super-ego and an unconscious sense of guilt. The obsessive may seek punishment in order to alleviate his guilt. He may commit minor violations of social mores or laws and flagrantly advertise these transgressions, all the while concealing others for which he feels unconsciously guilty. In effect, he appeases his conscience by substituting punishment for a lesser offense. The interviewer is easily fooled because of the obsessive patient's boastful tendency to exaggerate successful manipulations and transgressions. It is as though the patient reassures himself by saying he is not weak, passive, frightened, and guilty, but just the opposite; strong and defiant of the rules that everyone else must follow. The obsessive patient exaggerates his antisocial behavior to allay his castration anxiety; the psychopathic patient minimizes his defiant behavior in order to smooth the course of his social relationships.

SHALLOWNESS.   The affective responses of the psychopathic patient have a superficial quality. This may not be apparent at first contact, and even when it is, the inexperienced interviewer may think that it is himself, rather than the patient, who has failed to connect. The patient may go through all the motions, and even do so with a dramatic flair, but his feelings are unconvincing. When the patient's sham or façade affect is penetrated, one usually finds feelings that the patient may describe as depression, but that seem more like freefloating anxiety mixed with emptiness and a lack of relatedness to other people. These patients seek stimulation from the outside to fill this inner void, and any experience is better than the tense, isolated feeling that they are trying to escape.

Hysteric and schizophrenic patients have disturbances of affect that may present problems in differential diagnosis. The hysteric may seem insincere and shallow, with dramatic displays that do not represent inner feelings. However, as one gets to know the patient more, it becomes apparent that he has a genuine, varied, and deeply emotional life concealed behind his histrionic façade. The psychopathic patient's affective façade is often more convincing at first contact, but the feelings behind it are shallow and evoke little empathy. The scizophrenic patient has a flattened or inappropriate affect, and this is usually quite obvious. In cases in which the flattened affect of the schizophrenic is concealed behind a dramatic histrionic façade, the resulting clinical picture is often labeled borderline. This diagnostic group grades imperceptibly into the psychopathic syndromes.

Object Relations

The emotional investments of the psychopathic patient are narcissistically focused on himself. Other people are transient characters in his life; they come and go, or may be replaced by substitutes, with little feeling of loss. He is most concerned with how they supply his needs, so that his primary style in interpersonal relations is ingratiating, extractive, and exploitative.

A sado-masochistic relationship typically exists between the patient and one or both of his parents or their surrogates. When the patient marries, this attitude is displaced to the spouse, who becomes both the victim and the silent partner in the patient's anti-social behavior. As the victim, the parent or spouse is hurt directly or indirectly. An example is the wife of the compulsive gambler who suffers from economic hardships as a result of his delinquency. She retaliates and punishes the patient by her nagging and frigidity, thus maintaining the cycle. At the same time, she might get a job and give him her own salary, or borrow money from a friend and permit him to use it for further gambling. The psychopathic patient's need to punish his loved ones is universal, and often the patient has little awareness of the amount of rage that is discharged in this pattern.

The patient prefers to avoid controversial issues, and if he senses the interviewer's feelings on any point, he will declare a similar position first. He has little sense of self, and therefore no desire to take a stand that will leave him feeling isolated and alone.

Hysterical patients are also manipulative and extractive in personal relationships, and show great variations in values or behavior according to social cues. However, the hysteric establishes important relationships with other people, and is distressed when these do not go well. The psychopath views others more as vehicles for gratification, and is less concerned about the disruption of specific relationships. The hysteric patient also exhibits sham emotionality and role playing. However, the roles assumed by the hysteric are dramatizations of unconscious fantasies, and there are consistent themes that relate to the patient's inner conflicts. The role is a vehicle for expressing and resolving a conflict, not an end in itself. It may have manipulative or extractive functions within the immediate interpersonal context, but this is only a secondary issue. The hysteric tries to be someone else because he rejects certain facets of himself; the psychopath tries to be someone because he feels that otherwise he is no one at all. The hysteric will claim early in treatment that he doesn't know who he is or that he feels no sense of personal identity. The psychopathic patient may ultimately reveal similar feelings, but they will seldom emerge in the early stages of contact.

The psychopathic person fears passivity in his personal relationships. Much of his aggressive behavior is designed to avoid a feeling of submissiveness, and the episodes of criminal violence that occur in psychopathic individuals can be triggered by direct or symbolic threats that make the patient feel passive. Psychopathic prisoners are often more disturbed by the enforced passivity of prison life than by the disruption of social relations.

Because he is interested only in what he can get from other people, the psychopathic individual seeks out persons of power or status. He is not concerned with the weak or powerless unless he can earn favor from others by displaying this interest. He frequently becomes involved with members of the opposite sex, and his air of cool self-assurance may make him quite attractive sexually. His dashing and exciting exterior bears some resemblance to a romantic folk-hero, and he is appealing to those who seek exciting or glamorous romantic involvement. Here again, however, his primary interest is extractive, and his lovers are doomed to disappointment.

At times, the patient appears to be playing a game, and the phrase "as if" has been used to describe his role playing quality. This is exhibited in mild form by the man at a cocktail party who makes himself more attractive and interesting by assuming glamorous and exciting roles. One patient would pick up women in bars and relate elaborate descriptions of his job, social connections, and past life, varying the story to suit the interests of each new woman. The most extreme illustration occurs in the impostor syndromes, in which the patient consciously acts out a false identity. Frequently these involve prestigious or romantic roles as a scientist, explorer, or physician. One of the authors saw an English professor who lived a double life, traveling to Europe each summer and convincing his acquaintances there that he was an atomic scientist working on secret projects for the government.

The patient may sometimes simulate the role of psychological health. When an individual is interviewed in some depth and is seemingly without any emotional or psychological conflicts at all, not even the stresses and strains of normal life, one should suspect underlying psychopathy. Closer scrutiny may reveal deficits in affectivity and object relations. Another role that the patient may assume in the interview is that of the psychiatric patient. This usually involves claims of subjective distress. However, these are not communications of inner pain, but rather attempts to deflect the conversation from the more uncomfortable topic of the patient's interaction with his environment.

BEHAVIORAL PATTERNS

ANTISOCIAL BEHAVIOR.   Psychopathic antisocial behavior includes a wide variety of disturbances, such as pathological lying, cheating, stealing, and drug abuse. The motivational context of this behavior ranges from the apparently rational financial manipulations of the shady entrepreneur to the bizarre and highly sexualized fire-setting of the pyromaniac.

The psychopathic individual usually seeks to avoid punishment, but the threat of possible punishment does not serve as an effective deterrent to his behavior. The patient's inability to postpone gratification, poor impulse control, lack of guilt, and intolerance of anxiety contribute to an inability to consider the consequences of his actions. At the same time, the usual social restraints are less important to the psychopath; the shallowness of his object relations and his lack of tender or warm emotionality render him indifferent to the loss of social ties.

The patient often feels that he is *entitled* to do what he does, although he may recognize that others will not agree. He thinks that he has been unjustly treated in the past, and that his current behavior will help even the balance. For example, a narcotic addict who had been apprehended by the police for stealing explained that his early life was so marked by pain and deprivation that he felt he should suffer no further discomfort. He explained that he had a right to take things from others who were more privileged, and that the comfort he achieved by doing so was society's debt to him.

The specific choice of perverse or antisocial behavior has symbolic significance. For example, the exhibitionist is usually concerned about the adequacy of his sexual equipment, and seeks reassurance from the reactions of others. Some patterns of repetitive stealing reflect the feeling that the individual has been unjustly deprived of something which is rightfully his.

ASSETS. Psychopathic mechanisms lead to useful character traits. The absence of neurotic anxiety can be associated with a calm self-control and daring behavior that superficially resemble courage and bravery. The psychopathic individual may develop great skill at tasks that would cause considerable anxiety in most others. For example, psychopathic traits are common in persons who pursue careers in dangerous sports. These skills are most evident when a single episode of brilliance will suffice and sustained goal-directed efforts over a long period of time are not required. Lack of patience and susceptibility to impulsive distractions cause difficulty with long-term pursuits.

The psychopathic person's social skill and smooth charm make him successful in dealing with others, and he is a master at the art of manipulating people. To the uninitiated, he does not seem to be antisocial. He has often cultivated social manners and graces to an extent that ranges from "slick" to sincerely charming. Although the psychopathic individual might utilize antisocial behavior when he feels it is necessary to obtain personal gratification, ordinarily he uses his social skills in order to control the interviewer and to make the interview as friendly and comfortable as possible.

DEFENSIVE AND ADAPTIVE TECHNIQUES

In the psychopathic patient, anxiety leads directly to action, in contrast to the neurotic, whose mental processes are designed to control and bind anxiety or to substitute symbolic action. However, there are certain psychological defenses that the psychopathic individual does utilize. These involve attempts to deny anxiety and a variety of maneuvers, including isolation, displacement, projection, and rationalization, that minimize the guilt and social discomfort that he might experience.

DEFENSES AGAINST ANXIETY

The psychopathic patient attempts to transfer his own anxiety to others. If he is successful, his own fear is diminished. Phobic patients also try to elicit anxiety in others, but if they are successful, they become quite anxious themselves and usually search for calmer partners whom they cannot disturb as easily. The psychopathic patient, in contrast, prefers those who react most intensely, as he seems to gain some reassurance from the other person's discomfort. His provocation may begin with the opening words of the interview. One of the authors treated a psychopathic patient who started the first interview by mentioning that he was acquainted with one of the doctor's medical school classmates, and later dropped innuendoes regarding information he had concerning the doctor's earlier life. A favorite technique for evoking anxiety is to detect some weakness in the interviewer, and then to focus on it. One patient asked about the doctor's fidgeting in his chair and his habit of playing with paper clips, inquiring whether he was nervous about something. This behavior also occurs outside of the interview. A medical student would question his colleagues about obscure details before examinations, implying that he was familiar with this material, and that they were in serious trouble if they were not.

In addition to making the doctor anxious, the patient will deny his own anxiety, with the resulting picture of detachment described above. Psychopathic individuals are relatively skillful at concealing the overt expression of emotions, and the doctor may miss the clues to underlying anxiety that usually betray the neurotic patient.

THE PSYCHOLOGICAL CONTROL OF GUILT

The psychopathic individual copes with his discomfort about his impulsive behavior by a series of defensive maneuvers. The simplest is the patient who claims, "I didn't do it," denying his overt behavior. This is common, for example, in alcoholic patients, who frequently state that they drink very little and have no problem with alcohol.

Slightly more complex is the patient whose position is described by the statement, "I thought it was all right." He admits the behavior, but denies any awareness of its social significance. This attitude is common in adolescent delinquents.

A related defense is represented by the idea, "Everyone else does it." This involves a projection of the patient's impulses onto others. The individual with psychopathic trends often feels that everyone has a gimmick, and that other people are extractive and exploitative, looking out only for their own advantage. He quickly extends this view to the interviewer, and may more or less directly suggest that the doctor has a good deal going. This is done in a tone of grudging admiration, often coupled with an offer of conspiratorial assistance. The patient might suggest that he could pay the doctor in cash, with the implication that the doctor cheats on his taxes, or he may offer information about investments, legal advice, or whatever.

The next step in the sequence can be characterized by the feeling, "No one cares anyway." The patient feels that others are indifferent to his behavior. This patient may claim that others expect it. For example, a college student who wanted a medical excuse from an examination, although he was not ill, explained that his professor knew what was going on, but just wanted an official letter. Patients will frequently employ this mechanism in dealing with fees that are paid by or to third parties, such as clinics and insurance companies. They attempt to enlist the doctor's assistance in falsifying information in order to save money, insisting, "It's all part of the system."

The ultimate defense in this series can be represented by the claim, "I'm special." The patient may include the doctor in his "special" category, saying, "You and I aren't like the rest." Various explanations for this privileged position can be offered: that his needs are somehow different, that he is more sensitive than others, or that his earlier experiences entitle him to special consideration.

DEFENSES AGAINST FAILING SELF-ESTEEM

The psychopathic patient finds that others disapprove of his behavior. Although he may attach relatively little significance to specific other people, some general sense of respect from the world is important to him, if only in the form of an outer display of social approval. An example is the powerful mobster who is active in his church. If he is not able to gain this respect from others, he feels increased loneliness, and diminished self-esteem. These feelings lead to defensive and reparative operations.

One of the simplest defenses is to treat his vices as virtues. This patient presents his callousness, indifference, or ruthlessness as an admirable trait. Adolescent delinquents and individuals with deviant patterns of sexuality that cannot be concealed frequently demonstrate this mechanism. It appears in milder form in the individual who brags about his numerous brief sexual relationships. This behavior is related to obsessive patterns, but the obsessive individual often expects disapproval, whereas the psychopath wants the respect and admiration of others. The obsessive is more likely to emphasize his defiance of authority, denying his fear and submissiveness. The psychopath will speak of his skill or agility in getting what he wants.

Emotional isolation also serves to protect the patient from the pain of depression. It is common for the patient to become visibly more depressed as a relationship with the doctor develops and this defense diminishes.

ADDICTIONS

Environmental agents may become involved in psychopathic patterns of behavior, and their secondary effects may strongly influence the resulting clinical picture. The most common examples are alcoholism and drug addiction.

The addictive personality tries to recreate an early ego stage that is associated with security, freedom from anxiety and, at times, bliss. This is, of course, true for all mankind, but whereas most people seek this feeling through close human contact and love, the addict uses a pharmacological short-cut. The substitution of chemical substances for human beings protects the addict from the inevitable anxieties and frustrations of interpersonal relations, but at the price of social isolation, drug dependency, and undesirable side effects.

The patient's life becomes organized around obtaining a drug for the resulting elevation of his mood and self-esteem.

Since these effects are temporary, he experiences periodic cycles of need, consummation, satiation, and renewed need. He usually claims that the satiated state is the desirable one, and that his behavior is designed to regain this experience after it has been lost. Contact with these individuals suggests that the entire cycle is an integral part of their personality, and that it is as necessary for them to crave and to seek gratification as it is to experience the state of satiation and euphoria that results.

Society frowns on addicts, and legal and social institutions are often harsh to the point of cruelty. By finding a magic chemical route to pleasure, the addict acts out universal unconscious fantasies of magical gratification for oral dependent needs. Anyone who openly acts out the secret and forbidden wishes of others becomes an outcast. These societal attitudes become issues in the interview, and it is common for the patient to cast the doctor in the role of policeman or judge rather than therapist during the interview.

Specific drugs are associated with specific psychodynamic patterns, but these will not be discussed in detail in this book.

PERVERSIONS

Perversions are patterns of sexual behavior that society considers deviant, usually because the specific act, or the partner selected, does not conform to traditional standards. Many patterns that would be called perverse if they were dominant are considered normal or healthy if they are a prelude to traditional sexual contact.

There are important neurotic roots to perverse behavior. The fear associated with normal sexual functioning leads to inhibition so that sexual impulses are deflected to psychologically less dangerous, alternate patterns. However, the resulting impulses frequently acquire a peremptory and urgent quality far exceeding that associated with normal sexual behavior, and it is this that gives them their psychopathic flavor.

The patient who is able to maintain his perversion secretly avoids becoming a social outcast. For others, social reactions to perversion vary with the type of perversion and the segment of society. They may be intense and associated with disgust or primitive aggression. As in social response to addiction, these reactions are related to the universal nature of perverse fantasies and to the need to negate and punish one's own forbidden impulses when they emerge in others.

Perverse and addictive behavior also occurs in individuals who do not have psychopathic personalities. Psychotic patients frequently have poorly integrated sexual functioning, and primitive amorphous patterns of pregenital sexuality may reflect an underlying psychosis.

The most common perversion seen in clinical practice is male homosexuality. This patient's object relations are characterized by shallowness and transience, which leads to depression when the patient is unable to satisfy his intense craving for close human attachment. Homosexual relationships are less stable than heterosexual ones, and the depressive syndrome that results from termination of these relationships is a common chief complaint. In the interview, these patients may ask for help in changing their sexual behavior, but they usually explain their desire to change as secondary to their inability to find a suitable partner or their inability to have a family. They may be aware of anxiety in sexual situations with women, but have usually repressed their attraction to members of the opposite sex. Characteristically, these individuals talk of being homosexual, not of engaging in homosexual acts. That is, they see "homosexual" as a type of person rather than as a behavior pattern. This defends the patient from the need to consider his primary anxiety with heterosexual objects or his own responsibility for his actions.

PRECIPITATING STRESS

Psychopathic patients may seek help to relieve inner feelings of pain, such as depression in an alcoholic patient or anxiety in a homosexual. Some seek aid because of secondary complications of their behavior, e.g., reactions to alcohol or drugs or conflicts with the law. At times the patient will indicate no immediate problem with the secondary effects of his activity but will acknowledge the future risk. This may be offered as an explanation for seeking help because the patient thinks the doctor will approve of the motive.

These patients are frequently sent to a psychiatrist, rather than coming of their own accord. They may be pressured into coming by relatives or friends, be referred by courts or social agencies, or may become management problems in schools, hospitals, or other institutions. Some problems in interviewing the person who does not consider himself a psychiatric patient are discussed in Chapter 12.

It is important to deal openly with the patient's reason for coming to the doctor. One can interview, and even treat, a patient who is sent against his will if his feelings about coming are discussed objectively early in the treatment. The paranoid patient can also be sent to the doctor, but he quickly reveals his negative feelings, whereas the psychopathic patient is more likely to conceal this response. One man was sent to a psychiatric clinic by a court as a condition of parole, but it wasn't until several visits had taken place that this fact was disclosed by a letter from the court. When confronted with this, he explained that although he had been sent initially, he had subsequently decided that it was a good idea, and therefore now came of his own accord. He was seen for several more sessions, but stopped going as soon as the parole requirement ended.

PSYCHOPATHY AND THE FAMILY

Psychopathic mechanisms frequently involve interactions between several members of a family, and it is common for the family to be involved in the consultation or treatment. The child who develops psychopathic patterns of behavior has often learned from parental example, or at least has acquired his social attitudes and super-ego structure by identification with his parents. The family is not only involved in the origins of psychopathy, but also in its manifestations. In fact, a conflict between two psychopathic individuals in the same family may precipitate the consultation. A few examples will illustrate these points.

A young schoolteacher sought consultation when she learned that her husband, an attorney, was having an affair with another woman. During the interview, she revealed that she had been involved in repeated extramarital relationships for many years. She had concealed these from him because she wanted the financial security that she felt he offered. In a separate interview, he related that he had secretly arranged his financial assets so that she could not attach them, just in case he wanted a divorce. They both expressed concern over their only child, a 15-year-old son who had just been sent to military school after being expelled from a secondary school for chronic truancy and use of marijuana. Each partner felt that his own behavior was a reasonable response to the chronic rejection and misunderstanding suffered at the hands of the other. The complementary patterns of psychopathic behavior, each used as justification for the other, and the impact of the conflict on the child, are typical.

Another example is provided by a college freshman who was referred to the school psychiatrist after being arrested for driving a stolen car across a state line and then having an accident while intoxicated. The boy's father, a successful businessman, came to see the doctor. After the initial introduction, he turned to the doctor and said, "Well, boys will be boys, eh, Doc?" He was willing to dismiss all that had happened so that his son could return to school.

DEVELOPMENTAL PSYCHODYNAMICS

The psychopathic individual's mistrust of others begins very early in life. The normal child's feeling that his needs will be met is based on his early relationship with his mother, and his repeated experience that frustration and delay, however stressful, is inevitably followed by gratification and security. Although the child may respond to each frustration with anxiety and protest, this occurs within the context of repeated gratification. Furthermore, the child learns not only that his needs will be met, but that this will occur in spite of angry protests directed at the need-fulfilling objects, his parents. In fact, this protest behavior disappears if it is unsuccessful, and the child whose cries bring no aid eventually stops crying and lies quietly and passively.

There are several reasons that the psychopathic individual does not take this basic love for granted. Early experiences may lead to the feeling that no one can be trusted and that security must be derived from some source other than a close human relationship. There may be constitutional determinants that contribute to an increased pressure from basic drives or a decreased tolerance for frustration. Frequently these two sets of factors interact. For example, the infant whose tolerance for frustration and anxiety is low will find even the best of mothering relatively inadequate. Consequently, he will not respond with the pleasure and gratitude that are necessary to reward and reinforce maternal behavior. If, in addition, the mother is relatively indifferent or insensitive to his needs, or has little confidence in her mothering skills, she will perceive the child as rejecting. The result is a cycle in which each episode of infantile frustration leads to inadequate mothering, which in turn leads to further frustration.

When a child has been abandoned by his parents, or has drifted through a series of foster homes and child care institutions, syndromes that resemble adult psychopathy may appear very early in life. There is much overt display of affection, but little real feeling, and the shyness and inhibition that most children experience with strangers is absent. The child is skillful at extracting love and attention from adults, but the relationship that is so quickly established is of little importance, and it will quickly be severed if a more rewarding parental figure can be found. These children can be seen in orphanages or juvenile care agencies, where their immediate and appealing charm is quickly directed to every new adult who appears on the scene. It is clearly a highly adaptive pattern of behavior for such a life, both protecting the child from the pain of repeated separations and facilitating his immediate adaptation to new social situations.

The severe ego pathology arising in the earliest years of life is further complicated at the stage of the developing conscience or super-ego. The capacity of the ego to mature through identification with important objects fails to develop. Furthermore, the parental figures who were associated with the deprivations of the first years of life may offer pathological models for identification. The same mother whose care never led to a sense of basic trust may have social and moral attitudes that, when incorporated by the child, will lead to a distorted sense of right and wrong.

These defects in conscience formation can also occur in the absence of serious primary ego pathology. The concept of "super-ego lacunae" has been offered to describe individuals who have isolated specific disturbances in the functioning of their conscience that are relatively dystonic for the remainder of their personalities. For example, one of the authors knew a man who was a pillar of his community and an elder in his church, but whose business success depended upon selling overpriced merchandise to poor people who didn't understand time payment plans. His daughter was arrested for selling narcotics to her high school classmates. Although the overt behavior of her parents met the highest moral standards of society, the child perceived hidden or unconscious parental attitudes and translated them into action. If the family of a delinquent adolescent is available for a careful interview, one can frequently obtain a history of behavior patterns in the parents' earlier years that are similar to the child's current difficulties and that were carefully concealed from the child. For example, the mothers of promiscuous adolescent girls often describe similar episodes in their own lives, although these had been hidden from both their husbands and daughters. Parental attitudes are sometimes transmitted through reaction formation. The girl who is called a tramp or a slut when she comes home an hour late, and whose every contact with boys is interpreted as a sexual escapade, soon learns what is expected of her.

The peculiar attitude of the psychopathic individual toward tension and anxiety may also stem from early experiences with the mother. The child's needs are ignored on one occasion, but on another his protests are quickly silenced by overindulgence in an attempt to placate his anger and buy his affection. He grows frightened of the tension associated with his needs, since gratification is erratic and unreliable. At the same time, the process of getting what he wants becomes equivalent to extracting a bribe, and he is entitled to take everything he can possibly get, since he feels deprived of that which is most important: love and security. When this pattern continues to adult life, we see the ego syntonic and guiltless extractive qualities of the psychopath.

As the individual with prominent psychopathic tendencies enters puberty and adolescence, he frequently has less difficulty than his peers. Shifts in identity and allegiance present no problem to him, and he is not troubled by guilt in response to his defiance. His acquaintances look up to him and envy his social and personal ease. He has no close friends, but is an object of admiration for many. In later years, these same friends are surprised to learn that the former big man on campus ended up friendless and a failure.

Adult life, and particularly old age, present great problems. Marriage is seldom successful, and when it lasts it is usually in spite of a distant and impersonal relationship with the spouse. If there are children, they are seen as competitors or potential sources of gratification, attitudes that rarely lead to close family ties. Life is lonely and empty and solace may be sought in drugs or alcohol.

Management of the Interview

Although the interview behavior of the psychopathic patient is not as consistent as that of the obsessive or the hysteric, there are specific problems in interviewing that are associated with the patient's use of psychopathic mechanisms. These occur both in psychopathic characters and in others with psychopathic traits.

Several major themes can be described. The patient may be charming, ingratiating, and superficially cooperative, although simultaneously evasive and dishonest. This is a common initial presentation. Later, often in response to direct confrontation by the interviewer, he can become uncooperative or overtly angry. This attitude might appear initially if the patient has been coerced to see the doctor. As the patient attempts varying methods of pursuing his goals, these established patterns may alternate.

The psychopathic patient studies the interviewer from the very first moment of contact. He covertly searches for evidence that will help him to decide whether the doctor can be trusted and, at the same time, mentally registers any sign of weakness or uncertainty on the part of the physician. Although the doctor often feels on guard, he has difficulty identifying the source of the feeling. He may experience a negative reaction to the patient, or he may be overly enthusiastic and develop rescue fantasies, but he is uncertain about the reason for these responses.

Action is far more important than thought or communication for the psychopathic individual. A major problem in interview technique arises from the patient's tendency to act before, or instead of, talking. He does not see how talking to another person can be of any use, unless that person is a means to some concrete end.

THE OPENING PHASE

Pre-interview Behavior

The psychopathic patient seizes the initiative at the very first contact. When the physician greets him in the waiting room, he may inquire, "How are you today, Doctor?", and he will often chat while walking into the office.

He is sensitive to the doctor's interests and attitudes, but unlike the hysteric, he is more interested in establishing a general atmosphere of permission and receptivity than in eliciting a specific emotional response. He may comment appreciatively on a picture on the wall or the political views suggested by a book on the doctor's shelf, comments that are aimed at disclosing something about the doctor's status or position. "Nice setup you have here," or "Have you been in this office very long?" is a typical opening remark. One patient, noticing that a Harvard diploma was displayed on the wall, said, "I see you trained in Boston." The recognition of the doctor's status was slightly disguised, but nonetheless obvious.

THE FIRST MINUTES

As the interview continues, this behavior is mixed with his scrutiny of the doctor and his tendency to focus on any flaws that may appear. For example, one patient began his first interview by commenting, "I noticed an article in one of the old magazines in your waiting room." He went on to indicate that he agreed with the article's political views, and then added, "I guess you must be much too busy to really get involved in that sort of stuff." The message was clear; the doctor was not only successful, but perhaps preoccupied with his success and inconsiderate of the needs of others. These comments provide important information for the interviewer, but any attempt to reply to them early in the interview will leave the patient feeling angry, uncomfortable, and defensive.

The patient appears to be composed, pleasant, and engaging; at times he may be smooth and charming. He speaks freely, but at a level of generality that sometimes leaves the interviewer feeling that he is lost and must have missed some key material. In spite of this, every sentence is clear and relevant, and there is no suggestion of a thought disturbance. He compliments the doctor on the insightful comments he makes or the penetrating questions that he raises. The patient seems to say, "We'll get along just fine." The doctor may feel pleased and flattered, or he may sense that the praise is somewhat extreme and that something is not quite right. As a rule, however, any comment will be met with indignant denial, the patient insisting that he could not be more sincere. It is not wise to challenge or confront the patient at this point. He does not trust the interviewer anyway, and any indication that he is not trusted himself will only make things worse. The patient's false flattery is a product of his mistrust, and this mistrust will be a central theme in treatment. Mistrust can be interpreted most effectively after it has been brought into the open, and premature confrontation is likely to encourage the patient to conceal his negative feelings. It is preferable to ignore this attempt to con the doctor until the patient has more completely exposed his suspicions.

THE CHIEF COMPLAINT

The doctor must establish the psychopathic patient's reason for seeking treatment, a process that is not the same as eliciting the neurotic patient's chief complaint. The psychopathic patient's complaints sound quite similar to those of the neurotic, but they rarely explain why he has come for help now. He may describe conflict and anxiety, but seldom displays these feelings directly. If he complains of depression, he quickly shifts to expressing his frustration and irritation over a lost love object. The patient experiences more anxiety than is apparent to the doctor, and it is preferable initially to accept the patient's description of his feelings rather than to confront him with the superficial quality of his affective response.

The psychopathic patient often seeks some relatively concrete goal, and hopes to elicit the physician's assistance in achieving it. If he was referred by the courts, he hopes for an acquittal or a lighter sentence; if referred by a school, he hopes to be pardoned for delinquent behavior or excused from some responsibility. The patient may want a letter to a draft board, assistance in obtaining workman's compensation, or a psychiatric evaluation for a therapeutic abortion. Perhaps the most common situation is the patient who wants an ally in a battle with a spouse or other family member. In all of these situations, the patient also suffers from painful inner feelings, but he rarely comes to the doctor with any hope of help for his inner pain; he only seeks assistance in his struggle with the outside world. The therapist is perceived as a real person rather than a transference object.

EXPLORING THE PATIENT'S PROBLEMS
WITHHOLDING AND SECRECY

Since the psychopathic individual is frequently referred by another person or institution, the doctor often has some advance information about the patient. The patient frequently does not mention that he is in trouble, thereby presenting the interviewer with a problem. If the physician allows the interview to unfold in the usual manner, important material will not be discussed. On the other hand, if he introduces the information himself, he will have difficulty learning its emotional meaning to the patient. Also, such action is likely to be perceived by the patient as a judgment or criticism. The problem is further complicated if the patient knows that the doctor has the information. The doctor often learns that the "confidential" letter he received from the referring agency has already been seen by the patient, and that the question in the patient's mind is not what the doctor knows, but whether he will be open about it. As with any other patient, it is essential that the doctor not keep secrets. Therefore, he refers to the information in a general way, and asks the patient to discuss it. An example will best illustrate the problems that arise.

An adolescent male high school student was referred to a psychiatrist by his school because he had been caught stealing books from the school bookstore. He came to the interview and discussed a variety of academic problems, not mentioning the books. After listening for a while, the psychiatrist said, "I understand you've had some difficulties with the bookstore." The boy, quite characteristically, replied, "What do you know about that?" At this point the psychiatrist did not go into detail, but replied, "I guess you don't feel comfortable talking to me about it," thereby commenting on the boy's unwillingness to discuss the matter himself. The boy persisted in trying to find out what the doctor already knew, and the doctor then added, "I guess you don't want to tell me more than I already know because you don't fully trust me." This approach shifted the interview from an attempt to find out what happened in the bookstore—a fruitless and basically unimportant quest—to a discussion of the patient's mode of dealing with other people.

The psychopathic patient frequently invites inquisition rather than a psychiatric interview. He seems to be withholding or frankly lying; he may become openly resistant or uncooperative; and the material that does emerge may suggest antisocial or criminal behavior. The psychiatrist is tempted to try to piece together the truth by ingenious or coercive questioning. The psychiatric interview is not furthered by getting the goods on the patient, and it is far more important to earn his trust and respect than to pin down the facts. It may be helpful to interpret this dilemma to the patient, suggesting, "I'm interested in your problem, but I see no point in my conducting an interrogation. You seem to cast me in the role of district attorney." The patient is establishing a pattern of relationship based on his past experiences with authority figures. He tries to get the interviewer to play the role of the suspicious and mistrustful parent, unjustly accusing and exploiting him. If the patient is successful, he feels justified in concealing his behavior and trying to manipulate the doctor so that he can achieve his own goals. This is the way the patient deals with others, and he feels that it is the way they deal with him.

With most neurotic or psychotic patients, the physician will, in time, learn about the patient's inner mental life. This is not the case with the typical psychopath, who is unwilling or unable to share such material. In fact, he is not even likely to tell the physician the daily events of his external life, let alone his fantasies. This prevents the therapist from obtaining the essential psychological information that he utilizes with other patients in understanding the psychodynamics of the treatment process. Some of this missing data may be offered by ancillary informants, such as a telephone call from one of the patient's relatives. The therapist accepts this information, telling the patient about each call. It is mandatory that the physician not betray the patient's confidence in any way, but it is not necessary for the doctor to tell the patient everything that he has learned about him if this would alienate the relative. The doctor can utilize these events to discuss the difficulties created by the patient's withholding.

CLARIFICATION AND CONFRONTATION

As the interview progresses, the physician directs his attention to the patient's style of life and his mode of relating to people in general and to the interviewer in particular. The doctor must shift the discussion from those issues that the patient has volunteered to the painful feelings that he tries to avoid. This usually requires a more or less direct confrontation. Despite cautious phrasing and careful timing, a negative response frequently follows. A conflict of interest develops between the patient and the doctor. The patient wants to use the doctor to elicit an emotional reaction or to obtain some assistance in pursuing a concrete goal; the doctor wants to establish a relationship that will permit exploration of what the patient wants and how he goes about getting it.

The interviewer is often struck by the patient's callous indifference in personal relations or his apparent comfort in violating social and ethical norms. Such responses may be elicited by material that is peripheral to the explicit theme of the interview, but that reveals the patient's general attitude toward other people. Thus, one patient who was seen during the week following the assassination of John F. Kennedy commented that he couldn't understand "what everyone is making all of the fuss about." A female patient revealed a similar facet to her character when she was at first indifferent to and then annoyed by the friendly overtures of a small child who was in the waiting room of the doctor's office. The doctor's spontaneous reaction is to the lack of human feeling in the patient's behavior. For example, one psychiatrist asked a patient who was being evaluated after an arrest for sexually molesting children, "Have you ever had any normal sexual feelings?" Early in an interview with a narcotic addict, another physician asked, "Do you serve any useful role in society?" Such comments reveal the interviewer's hostile feelings and prevent the establishment of a relationship with the patient.

The interviewer attempts to explore this insensitivity by exposing some anxiety or other need about which the patient is concerned. For example, the doctor was at first repulsed by the patient's comment following President Kennedy's assassination. However, after a moment's reflection, he realized that the patient was suffering from loneliness and isolation, while observing the closely shared feelings of those around him. The doctor commented, "You must feel cut off from everyone," and allowed the patient to discuss these emotions while lessening his feeling that he was also estranged from the doctor. A similar example is the hospitalized narcotic addict who described great physical and emotional discomfort, which he attributed to drug withdrawal.

The doctor realized that the patient feared he was being given placebos, although in fact he was receiving a full maintenance dose. He commented to the patient, "But the drug on which you are being maintained would prevent any such symptoms. Perhaps you are worried that we will lower your dose." The interviewer's statement challenged the distress that the patient described, and at the same time it exposed the anticipated frustration that the patient concealed, but that was a source of considerable anxiety.

The initial confrontation should aim at exploring the patient's behavior or exposing his defenses, but not attacking them. For example, a young man sought consultation because of depression and somatic symptoms that were accentuated each time he was abandoned by a homosexual partner. He seemed somewhat depressed during the interview, but emphasized his incapacitating anxiety while discussing the reasons for his consultation. The patient seemed more interested in what he could learn about the interviewer than in relating his own problems, and started the conversation by commenting, "I understand that you're on the staff of the medical school. Do you spend a lot of time teaching up there?" These comments were made with considerable social charm, and it was easy to imagine the patient's success as a personnel manager, his chosen profession. After some minutes the interviewer interrupted, saying, "I guess you're more comfortable talking about me than discussing the difficulties you've been having in your personal life." This is a very gentle confrontation that is combined with considerable support. Any more direct statement this early in the interview will interfere with the patient's communication. For example, the question, "If you're so upset about your own problems, why do you spend so much time talking about me?" might provoke an angry or withdrawn response.

THE PATIENT'S ANGER

The psychopathic patient has his own program for the interview, and his own goals in mind. He presents an image of himself as he would like to appear, and he fears the humiliation that would result if this picture were challenged. He will go to great lengths, often lying, in order to prevent exposure, and does not welcome distraction or interruption. His response to early confrontation is unsually negative. This may take one of several forms, the simplest of which is angry denial. The patient insists that he does not know what the interviewer is talking about, that he is being misunderstood, and it is clear that he is quite hurt by the doctor's failure to understand him. The patient may be both insistent and convincing, and it is not uncommon for the beginning interviewer to retreat in confusion and guilt, apologizing for his comment and letting the patient continue to control the interview.

For example, a nurse was referred for consultation because of her extensive use of narcotics for vague abdominal pains. After she described her symptoms and her drug regimen, the doctor commented, "It sounds to me as if you have become an addict." The patient became enraged, and said that several previous doctors had sympathized with her pain and had prescribed the narcotics. His labeling of the patient as an addict had reflected a pejorative view, and he quickly became anxious and did not know how to respond when she detected this feeling and reacted to it. Now uncertain, he apologized and shifted to a more detailed discussion of her physical symptoms. Had he been more comfortable, he could have interrupted her attack and said, "You're responding as if I just accused you of a crime. Perhaps it sounded that way, but I'm sure you know of the addiction that can develop to narcotics, and I guess I was wondering how you have been handling that."

The example illustrates several points: first, the importance of carefully obtaining the data *before* making an interpretation; second, the value of searching for a phrase that will "save face" for the patient and allow a comfortable response (e.g., he could have said, "With that much use of narcotics, you must be worried that you will become addicted"), and third, the problems created by the interviewer's countertransference.

The patient's angry denial does not mean that the confrontation was not accurate or, for that matter, was not therapeutic. One of the authors interviewed a man who had been referred for evaluation by the court after being charged with exhibitionism. The man spent the entire interview denying the accusation and explaining that he was the victim of a terrible mistake. The interviewer responded, "Well, if it is really a mistake, I guess that you have no need for a psychiatrist. On the other hand, if you are saying this to help your case in court, and you do have a sexual problem, treatment could help you, and you can return when your legal situation is settled." Some months later, after the charges had been dropped, the man returned to the psychiatrist for treatment for his long-standing sexual problems and exhibitionism!

The patient's anger may be denied behind a façade of rationalization. He will offer elaborate explanations of why his behavior has a meaning other than the obvious one. This is intended to circumvent the meaning that the interviewer attaches to it, but to maintain the appearance of goodwill in the interview. A student who was referred to the college psychiatrist after he had been caught cheating in a major examination insisted that he had only been cleaning his pen on a scrap of paper, which the proctor thought was a "crib." He went on to elaborate on how the paper came from a book of lecture notes that contained material related to the course. The psychiatrist commented, "I guess the Dean didn't completely believe your explanation or he wouldn't have asked you to come here. What do you think he had in mind?" The student responded by further protesting his innocence, and explaining why he thought that the administration might be discriminating against him. The interviewer then said, "Obviously you are the only one who knows what happened at the examination, but I'm not sure that that is really so important. Whatever actually went on, you are now in a jam. Have you thought about what to do?" When the rationalization is both elaborate and transparent, the doctor is often tempted to reply by suggesting that so complex an explanation must be covering something. This is a fairly direct accusation of lying, and whether or not the patient is lying, it will seldom improve communication. When the doctor does want to confront the patient with an obvious lie, this can be done by comments such as, "I find it hard to believe that what you say is true." This allows the possibility of discussing why the patient's statement is unbelievable, even if he continues to insist that it is true.

The patient may respond to the doctor's confrontation by sullen withdrawal. He controls his angry feelings, playing the role of the injured party, thereby appealing to the guilt or sympathy of the interviewer. This was seen in a patient who frequented hospital emergency rooms, presenting multiple somatic complaints. She would collect prescriptions by lying about her previous medical contacts. When an intern who had seen her on a previous occasion recognized her and rather sharply questioned her about her story, she refused to speak and sat staring at the floor, at first pouting and then beginning to cry. The doctor, not certain of what was going on, immediately became warmer and more supportive, and the patient constructed still another story.

A different type of response to the interviewer's confrontation is acceptance, followed by renegotiation. The patient adopts a new tack as he learns more about the doctor, often openly admitting that what came before was a line, and suggesting that he is now serious and straightforward. The doctor may feel flattered as the patient praises his perspicacity and insight. It is this patient's manipulative style, his readiness to use and then to discard a line, rather than any specific tactic, that is the essential point.

For example, a physician learned that a recently hospitalized patient had become involved in an extensive net of gambling and bribery that involved several hospital employees. When confronted, the patient quickly sized up the situation and then said, "Okay—you're smart and you're right. I got hooked into this by the attendants, the whole staff situation is really pretty rotten, but I can help you find out who's behind it." The patient offered to make a deal to protect himself and to placate the doctor.

THE PATIENT'S RELATIVES

The psychopathic person's problems usually involve other people, and the doctor often has direct contact with the patient's family. This takes the form of letters, telephone calls, and interviews that may or may not include the patient. Psychopathic mechanisms that may be obvious in the patient are often mirrored, although in subtler form, in other members of the family.

A case treated by one of the authors will illustrate some of these points. The patient, an adolescent boy, entered treatment because of academic difficulties in school and conflicts with his family over his use of marijuana. His parents, whom he described as "middle class and materialistic," were divorced and lived in another city. Shortly after treatment began, the doctor received a letter from the patient's father expressing his support for the treatment program and enclosing some insurance forms. The items that the father had already completed suggested that he was capitalizing on the similarity of his own name to that of his son to collect on a policy that did not actually cover the boy. The problem became more complex when the boy started to miss sessions, insisting that whether or not he kept his appointments was privileged information that was not to be shared with his father. It was clear that the father would be enraged if he learned that he was paying for sessions that were not actually held. Thus the boy had enlisted the doctor in a conspiracy against the father by offering him a free hour with full payment, and the father had engaged the doctor's assistance in extracting money from the insurance company. Finally the doctor told the boy, "I'm not here to get paid to read a magazine." The boy replied, "You said what happens here is confidential; you can't tell him about my not coming." The doctor answered, "That's true, but if I decide you're not motivated for treatment, we will stop. If that happens, I'll have to tell your father that I felt further treatment was not indicated." At the same time, the doctor explored the boy's anger at what his father was doing with the insurance. Eventually the boy and his father were seen together, and the doctor demonstrated the family pattern that each member practiced himself while protesting similar behavior in the other.

It is particularly important to keep the patient informed of every contact that the doctor has with the patient's family, although the doctor may keep the details to himself. If the doctor receives a letter, he can show it to the patient; if he has a phone conversation, he should discuss it at the next session. If the relatives are to be seen by the doctor, it is usually advisable to have the patient present.

Relatives often use subtle devices to induce the physician to betray the patient's confidence. For instance, a boy's mother called the physician and said, "I guess Mike told you what happened with the car this weekend." Either "yes" or "no" betrays the patient. Instead, the doctor might reply, "Anything Mike does or does not tell me is confidential; what was it that you wanted to say?"

ACTING OUT

The psychopathic individual prefers action to words or thought. When he feels anxious, he is more likely to do something than to talk about it. If his relationship with another person gives rise to uncomfortable emotions, these will appear in his behavior rather than in his report of internal mental processes. For example, a young female patient with psychopathic tendencies would indulge in promiscuous sexuality shortly before her therapist's vacations, although she persistently denied any emotional response to his leaving. It is this tendency to action that makes the standard techniques of psychotherapy relatively ineffective with these patients.

The term "acting out," when used strictly, refers to behavior that is based upon feelings that arise in the transference relationship and are then displaced onto persons in the patient's every-day life. The purpose and result is to keep the expression of these feelings away from the therapist. Such behavior is a common resistance in all patients, but it can be particularly troublesome in those with psychopathic tendencies. Other neurotic patients also may displace their transference feelings, but they are more likely to inhibit the accompanying activity. The psychopathic patient has a lower threshold for action and less restraint on his impulses. The result is that feelings arising in the treatment situation may directly lead to inappropriate and maladaptive behavior in the outside world.

For example, a patient with a history of homosexual behavior would respond to all emotions by episodes of homosexual acting out. If he felt that the doctor was annoyed at him, he would become involved with anonymous men in transient episodes in which he felt demeaned. If he was grateful, or felt positive feelings for the therapist, he would quickly search for a partner toward whom he could feel close, thereby displacing his feelings for the doctor. In general, if either pattern were interpreted, he would shift to the other one, feeling thankful for the interpretation of his self-demeaning behavior and angry at the interpretation of his more gratifying sexual relationships.

The acting out of transference feelings can also occur within the treatment without displacement to other figures. It is this acting out in the transference that produces some of the most difficult technical problems in the interview. The psychopathic patient may not follow the rules of simply sitting in his chair and talking. He will frequently try to read the doctor's mail or go through the papers on his desk if the doctor is momentarily called from the room. These acts are usually concealed in the initial interview, unless the patient's defenses are inadequate or are too quickly challenged.

An example can be seen in the interview with the inebriated alcoholic patient. His usual social façade is impaired by the alcohol, and he may become aggressive and belligerent. More characteristically, his underlying dependent needs will become manifest, and he will attempt to cling physically to the interviewer, will hold his face closer than is customary, and will act "sticky." The task of the interviwer is to translate this behavior into a statement of the feelings underlying it, without giving the patient the feeling that he is being pushed away or rejected. The interviewer can comment that the patient seems sad, or lonely, or that he seems to want to be with someone. He can offer substitute gratification—a hand on the patient's shoulder or a cigarette. In effect, this amounts to an "acting-in interpretation" by the therapist, which may be the only kind the patient can utilize.

In general, the role of the interviewer is to link acting out behavior with the underlying feeling, and to point out the displacements that have occurred. It is rarely useful to interdict the behavior early in treatment, and almost never effective if these interpretations have not preceded the interdiction. The exception is when the behavior directly impinges on the rights or interest of the therapist. Here, as with the psychotic patient, it is not helpful to allow the patient to abuse his relationship with the doctor. The patient who cannot set his own limits requires others to assist him in this. For example, a hospitalized delinquent adolescent boy was angry, ostensibly because the therapist would not permit him to go home for the weekend. He picked up an ashtray from the doctor's desk and broke it on the floor, and was about to go further when the doctor obtained assistance from attendants on the ward and returned the boy to his room. In this situation, forcible restraint preceded the interpretation, but the doctor visited the boy later in the day and suggested that the outburst might have been connected with the doctor's impending vacation.

THE ROLE OF INTERPRETATION

The limited value of intellectual insight into the psychodynamic mechanisms underlying pathological behavior is nowhere so clear as in the psychopathic patient. These individuals may be quick to understand the therapist's interpretations, and they will frequently repeat and extend them at appropriate points in therapy. They are often misperceived as excellent teaching cases by beginning students. The diagnosis of psychopathy can be suspected when a young resident is defending his patient at rounds, explaining that he is really a highly motivated though unfortunate person who will profit from intensive uncovering therapy, although the more experienced clinicians present are both more pessimistic and less sympathetic.

Although the psychopathic individual may be skillful in manipulating abstractions, only concrete things have emotional significance to him. The simplest comment linked to an act or a thing is far more valuable than an insight into unconscious patterns that is not connected to an immediate object or behavior in the patient's life. The patient will make many concrete demands, asking for an aspirin, money for a parking meter, the use of the doctor's telephone, and so on. Initially, the therapist responds to these directly, either accepting or rejecting them. At some point, when the patient has at least partially accepted the mode of treatment, the therapist will suggest that these requests have an underlying psychological significance. The patient will either accept or deny this, but it will have little emotional impact. However, if the therapist links his interpretation to a change in his own behavior, no longer gratifying the demand that he has now interpreted, the patient will respond dramatically and at times violently. For example, a doctor frequently supplied aspirins to a patient who complained of headaches in his office. Then, at one point, he suggested that the patient's requests were an attempt to gain the doctor's implied agreement with the patient's view that the headaches were organic and had no psychological significance. The patient said that he thought that this was true, but seemed unimpressed. During the next session, he again asked for aspirin, and the doctor said, "I don't think that it would be helpful for me to continue supplying the aspirin, after what we said last time." The patient became furious —it was as though he never expected the doctor to change his behavior simply because of its *meaning*.

TRANSFERENCE

The patient's need for a sado-masochistic relationship soon appears in the transference. The most common manifestation is to stimulate the doctor's hopes that the therapy will succeed.

This is partially due to the fact that the patient's deep mistrust is not verbalized early in therapy, and instead, the patient will often feign trust by playing the role of a good patient. As treatment progresses, it becomes apparent that the problems do not magically disappear and the doctor is disappointed. Although the physician is fully aware that neurotic and psychotic symptoms do not vanish quickly, he seems to expect that they will in this patient. Such attitudes insure his disappointment. It must be remembered that deceit is a way of life for this person, and then it can be viewed as any other symptom.

It is the psychopathic patient, rather than the schizophrenic, who has a true narcissistic neurosis. Although the psychopathic patient's thought processes are coherent and relevant, his emotional life and the pattern of his important object relations is more similar to those of the schizophrenic than to those of the neurotic. Consequently, many of the interview techniques that have been discussed for schizophrenic patients will also be of value here. The importance of the concrete act rather than the abstract interpretation and the need for a real relationship with the therapist have already been mentioned. This patient cannot tolerate the frustrations of a classical psychoanalytic technique, and if therapy is to be helpful, the patient must perceive the doctor as a total individual. The psychopath has difficulty in relating to the doctor, and treats him as a source of supply or as an obstacle in the path toward some desired goal. Transference constitutes a repetition with the therapist of previous modes of dealing with significant persons, and this patient has treated important people in his past only as fragmentary objects, with little regard for them as total persons.

One result is that the personal identity of the therapist is relatively unimportant to the patient. He may forget the doctor's name, or have little concern about shifting to a new doctor. The psychopathic patient will show defensive interest in the doctor, and possibly curiosity about his status or his therapeutic technique, but he will be strangely devoid of curiosity about the doctor's more human attributes—his family and his personal life. When he does ask questions, they are designed to shift the spotlight to the doctor, either to charm him or to make him uncomfortable.

If, in spite of this, an important relationship with the therapist does develop, it is difficult if not impossible to replace him with a substitute. When the doctor finally does become a total object for this patient, he is a *real* object, not a transference object, and the patient may retain such a relationship, if only in fantasy, for the rest of his life. If the patient does begin to recognize the therapist as a person, his problems with trust will be manifested in a different fashion. For example, he might tell his friends some personal information that the physician has offered about himself. Here the doctor can comment, "You don't seem to consider things that go on between us as personal," or, "You have betrayed my confidence." This response shows the patient that the doctor really is different from his parents.

The patient's tendency to view the therapist as a non-person is illustrated by the adolescent boy who was seeing a psychiatrist because of chronic truancy. The boy perceived therapy as a route to increased privileges and the removal of restrictions on his freedom that his parents had imposed in an attempt to control his behavior. He came to the doctor, but involved himself only at a superficial level. His interest never deviated from the issue of when he would again be allowed to use the family car or to keep his own hours. He would talk about his feelings or discuss the day's events, but always with his mind's eye trained on his goal. When he regained the lost privileges, he abruptly stopped treatment.

It is valuable to make the patients' concerns as explicit as possible early in the treatment. For example, when the boy said, "I feel anxious about being tied down in the house all of the time," the doctor could have replied, "You must be annoyed about not being allowed to use the car." This directs the interview to the issue that is most prominent in the patient's mind. Later, the doctor could add, "I imagine you have some idea of what your parents want to happen before they'll let you use the car again. What do you think that is?" As the discussion shifts to parental demands, and the boy's response to these, the doctor can offer his services in helping the boy to understand the connection between his desires and his parents' behavior, and to work out a relationship with them that will accomodate both the boy and his parents. It is necessary to explore the parental encouragement of the boy's behavior. Why did the father buy a fancy sports car? What traits does the mother admire in a man and what avenues are available for the boy to emulate these? At the same time, the doctor must avoid taking sides. He must neither blame the parents, thereby relieving the boy of any sense of responsibility for his own behavior, nor scold the boy while ignoring the parents' implicit communications. If the doctor can resolve this dilemma, the relationship with the patient shifts from that of adversary or conspirator to a therapeutic framework.

COUNTERTRANSFERENCE

The psychopathic patient elicits major countertransference problems in the interviewer. The doctor is confronted with suspiciousness and distrust, coupled with evasion and, at times, outright deception. The patient shows little guilt or anxiety about this behavior, and angrily denies it if confronted directly. Furthermore, the doctor senses that the patient is trying to manipulate him. The most common patterns of countertransference are (1) the doctor who is oblivious to the patient's behavior; (2) the doctor who assumes the role of the angry parent, threatening and admonishing the patient for behavior that is often linked to unacceptable impulses of the physician himself; (3) the doctor who is more strongly motivated than the patient to continue treatment. His own therapeutic success makes the patient a feather in his cap, but this dream is short-lived, as the patient inevitably disappoints him. The doctor may then react to his disappointment much as the patient's parents have done; and (4) the doctor who consciously or unconsciously enjoys the patient's psychopathy, and encourages his acting out.

The inexperienced psychiatrist is particularly prone to accept the patient's self-presentation as valid, and to ignore more covert psychopathic dynamics. The young doctor expects to believe his patients, and he prefers to rely on the objective data that the patient provides rather than his own subjective, vague, and often contradictory responses. This is also the basis of much of the young doctor's resistance to unconscious material.

This countertransference response is illustrated by the resident who was evaluating a man referred by the courts after a fourth arrest for passing bad checks. The doctor was moved by the patient's description of his early life deprivation, his desire for another chance, and his plans for schooling and vocational training. However, the clinic administrator wouldn't support the doctor's recommendation that the court drop the charges, arrange a draft deferment, and refer the boy for vocational rehabilitation. Before the disagreement could be resolved, the patient had jumped bail and disappeared. The resident angrily explained the patient's behavior as a result of the clinic's failure to provide support and assistance. This view was modified when it was learned that the patient had continued his check writing habits throughout the initial evaluation, although claiming to the resident that he had gone straight. When the patient returned, he indicated a preference for the senior doctor, whom he had met briefly during a conference, and with whom the patient had developed a good rapport. The patient was aware of the disagreement among the staff, but felt more comfortable with a doctor who understood him than with one who was taken in by his subterfuges.

The physician who becomes inappropriately angry and judgmental, adopting a disciplinary rather than a therapeutic position, probably represents the most common countertransference response to these patients. This may follow the response just described, when the doctor feels that he has been duped and switches from blind acceptance to blind rejection. The patient is accustomed to similar responses in the outside world, and he will often work hard at provoking them in the therapist. If they occur, he knows where he stands, and his mistrust is justified. The patient who provokes countertransference rejection by placing the doctor in the role of inquisitor is a common example. An illustration is the adolescent boy who was institutionalized after becoming involved in several gang warfare espisodes. He would repeatedly violate minor hospital rules—curfew time, meal hours, playing his phonograph too loudly, and refusing to wear shoes in the public rooms. As a result, all of his time with the therapist was taken up by discussion of his infractions and the institution's response to them. The doctor repeatedly found himself in the role of disciplinary parent. Each time this occurred, he patiently explained that he felt he would be more useful to the boy if he were not forced to occupy himself with administrative issues, and that he disliked being placed in the role of disciplinarian. The boy would smile faintly, and make no reply. Finally, the boy came in one night many hours after curfew, obviously drunk, boisterously rousing the ward and breaking several items of furniture before he was taken to bed. The next day the therapist lost his control and berated the patient for his adamant refusal to cooperate with the treatment program. Only then did the boy reveal that he had learned of his grandfather's death on the previous day, and that his drinking was an attempt to handle his grief. The therapist's anger had already demonstrated what the patient had always assumed, that all of the protestations of wanting to help were just a façade for the doctor's desire to control his behavior.

The last form of countertransference, the encouragement of acting out, also repeats a pattern common among parents of psychopathic patients. The doctor vicariously enjoys the patient's behavior, although he may loudly condemn it. His pleasure is often revealed by the delight he has in recounting his patient's exploits in discussions with colleagues, or his fascination with the mechanical or operational details of the patient's behavior. One physician would entertain his professional friends with anecdotes of his patient's sexual conquests; another would explore his patient's technique of income tax evasion in great detail. The patient, sensing what was going on, would spend long periods of time tutoring the doctor in sophisticated methods of accounting. Psychopathic patients are quick to sense the conspiratorial potentialities of such a situation.

The doctor may be aware of his personal involvement with the patient's acting out, but convince himself that he can conceal this involvement and prevent it from influencing the treatment. This is not possible. For example, psychopathic individuals who are involved in the business world will frequently offer the doctor tips on the stock market. One broker, being treated for homosexuality, casually mentioned, "By the way, if you have any loose cash lying around, I know a company that's going to split next month, and the stock is sure to shoot up." The information was provided as an innocent piece of friendly advice, and the temptation is obvious. The doctor quickly interpreted, "I guess you feel that I'm only interested in you if there's something in it for me." The patient seemed moved by the doctor's interpretation, but a few minutes later he said, "Now, let me give you that stock tip." The physician replied, "No, I don't want to know about it." The patient insisted, but the doctor held his ground, explaining that such information changed the nature of their relationship. The patient finally acquiesced. In the next session he commented, "You know, Doctor, you are a real professional and I admire you for that." The easiest route—recording the patient's comment during the session and quickly calling a broker afterwards—creates a dual and essentially deceitful relationship with the patient. Further tips will be encouraged, but therapy becomes impossible. The ethical and highly motivated therapist, though, is still faced with a dilemma. Why not interpret the patient's behavior, but, since this first piece of information has already been acquired, take advantage of it? This always fails. The therapeutic transaction requires an honesty and openness in the doctor's interest in the patient, and this is impossible if a secret business relationship coexists. The situation would be parallel to the patient's relationship with parents who exploited him covertly while insisting that they were only interested in his welfare.

THE CLOSING PHASE

As the interview draws to a close, the psychopathic patient senses the doctor's intention of stopping. He may seize the opportunity to obtain some favor or permission, avoiding the necessity of full discussion. For example, a patient with addictive tendencies visited the emergency room of a general hospital during the course of his evaluation in the psychiatric clinic. He told the emergency room doctor of his anxiety since the last clinic visit, and discussed his family problems. The doctor reviewed the patient's difficulties, and confirmed that he had a follow-up appointment in the clinic. Just as he rose to terminate the interview, the patient said, "Oh, one more thing, Doc. I've just run out of my Seconal and I need a new prescription." The waiting room was crowded and the doctor was hurried. The patient was counting on this pressure to coerce the doctor to grant his request. There is obviously no time for exploration or interpretation in this situation, but the doctor could have replied, "Why don't you call your regular doctor in the morning and discuss a new prescription with him? I'll let him know about our talk tonight." The patient is forced to explore his behavior with his primary doctor.

The end of the interview provides an opportunity for the doctor to counteract the patient's tendency to relate to him impersonally. With this patient, as with the borderline, it is helpful for the doctor to foster and maintain a real relationship. Brief social amenities at the end of the interview—plans for the weekend or comments about the weather—are usually seen as a form of resistance in neurotic patients. The psychopathic patient has difficulty establishing interpersonal relationships, and the doctor is not only an object for transference but also a primary object with whom he can safely experience personal feelings that are intense and genuine. The patient often has developed social skills in an almost hypertrophied form, but these are not connected with appropriate subjective feelings. Although it rarely occurs early in treatment, the patient should be encouraged when he does make a sincere social gesture toward the doctor.

Psychopathic behavior is only partially explained by our current psychodynamic concepts. An unfortunate corollary of this is that many doctors ignore psychodynamic principles in interviewing these patients, and instead utilize a style that is more appropriate in a law officer or an experimental psychologist. The interview with the psychopathic patient affords an opportunity to explore aspects of behavior that are often concealed for many years in neurotics and that may be too fragmented or disorganized to be understood in psychotic patients. The nuclear psychopathology is difficult to treat, but the patient often experiences considerable gain from psychotherapy. If the interview is conducted with an awareness of the basic outlines of the patient's psychodynamics, it can be a rewarding experience for both patient and therapist.

References

Aichorn, A.: Wayward Youth. New York, Viking Press, 1947.

Bergler, E.: Psychopathic personality . . . Malignant Masochism. Selected Papers of Edmund Bergler. New York, Grune & Stratton, 1969, pp. 818–831.

Bromberg, W.: Psychopathic personality concept. Arch. Gen. Psychiat., *17*:641, 1967.

Cleckley, H.: The Mask of Sanity. St. Louis, C. V. Mosby, 1950.

Eissler, K. R. (ed.): Searchlights on Delinquency. New Psychoanalytic Studies. New York, International Universities Press, 1949.

Freud, S.: Some character types met within psychoanalytic work. Standard Edition of Complete Psychological Works of Sigmund Freud, Vol. XIV. London, Hogarth Press, 1958, pp. 309–333.

Johnson, A., and Szurek, S.: The genesis of antisocial acting out in children and adults. Psychoanal. Quart., *21*:323, 1952.

Rado, S.: The psychoanalysis of pharmacothymia (drug addiction). Psychoanal. Quart., *2*:1, 1933.

10 THE ORGANIC BRAIN SYNDROME PATIENT

Psychopathology and Psychodynamics

There is a wide variation in the phenomenology and severity of organic brain syndromes. The basic picture is one of cognitive impairment, memory disturbance, and affective changes, with alterations of consciousness, perception, and personality occurring in some cases. It is a convenient oversimplification to differentiate primary symptoms, which are a direct result of the brain deficit, from secondary symptoms, which constitute the ego's reactions to that deficit. However, it is not always possible to determine which symptoms are the direct result of the cerebral deficit or the release of cortical inhibitory mechanisms, and which ones reflect the organism's attempt to compensate for brain damage. Furthermore, psychic stress can precipitate the symptoms of brain impairment. The interplay of organic and psychological factors determines the form of the illness in a given patient.

Organic brain syndromes have traditionally been classified on clinical criteria into acute and chronic forms. Interviews with these patients make it apparent that such states overlap, and the diagnosis cannot always be made until it is clear whether or not the illness is reversible. It is also useful to separate the non-psychotic from the psychotic conditions, since these two groups offer different problems for the interviewer.

339

It was long hoped that a rational classification of organic syndromes could be based on their pathological anatomy. However, autopsy studies have not resolved the problems in diagnosis and classification because the degree or form of the psychiatric disturbance and the amount or location of the brain damage is not precisely correlated. The clinical picture, particularly of the chronic brain syndrome, is strongly influenced by the patient's basic personality structure. A majority of the patients suffering from chronic brain malfunction are beyond the age of 65, and therefore the symptoms of these conditions are intertwined with the problems of the elderly.

Many textbooks describe specific syndromes associated with certain diseases such as general paresis, Alzheimer's disease, senile psychosis, cerebral arteriosclerosis and many others. However, some controversy remains concerning the specificity of these organic brain syndromes, and the matter is of little significance for clinical interviewing.

This chapter will not consider the pathological syndromes associated with seizure disorders or mental deficiency.

ACUTE BRAIN SYNDROME (DELIRIUM)

Delirium is a manifestation of cerebral insufficiency that has an acute onset and is reversible. Despite the variation from one case to another, alterations of consciousness and cognitive impairment are found in this group. In addition, affective changes occur in most cases. The syndrome can be initiated by any type of insult to the brain including trauma, infection, neoplasm, toxic or chemical agents, and metabolic changes. Social isolation, perceptual distortion, and sensory monotony or deprivation are important contributing factors, as is a possible disturbance of biological circadian rhythms. This may explain why these patients are worse at night. The human organism is dependent upon sensory input for the smooth functioning of central regulatory mechanisms. As sensory and perceptual systems are impaired, the patient reacts with confusion and fear. In addition, most of these patients are seriously ill medically, and the patient's fear concerning his physical health further intensifies the anxiety that accompanies the disorder. Acute brain syndromes generally have a favorable prognosis if the associated physical illness is itself reversible Mild acute brain syndromes are extremely common in the general hospital and are often overlooked by physicians, particularly when the patient is quiet and cooperative.

NON-PSYCHOTIC DISORDERS

The patient's disturbance of consciousness is first revealed by his difficulty in concentration, diminished attention span, and tendency to be easily distracted. His awareness of self and environment is altered, so that he may fail to notice or to respond to more subtle actions and feelings of those around him. This is not necessarily accompanied by drowsiness, and on occasion the patient seems hypersensitive to environmental stimuli. The speed with which he recognizes others can be slowed, and he often appears to be perplexed or confused, even though he is able to respond appropriately when asked specific questions. Recent memory is often impaired.

The loss of cognitive powers is reflected by the heightened effort required to perform routine intellectual chores. The patient has particular difficulty with abstract thought, performing better with concrete problems. Symbolic operations are the latest brain function to be acquired, both ontogenetically and phylogenetically, and are the most sensitive to organic impairment. Mild degrees of perseveration reflect the patient's slowness and inability to shift easily from one topic to another.

Orientation for time and place refers to the patient's awareness of the temporal and spatial relationships between himself and his environment. Orientation for person involves the patient's awareness of the identity and significance of persons around him and their relationship to him. Disorientation usually first appears as the patient is awakening and it remains longer as his condition worsens. He first loses awareness of time, then place, and finally person. In some patients disorientation for time and place can occur simultaneously. The patient not only is unsure of the date, but also loses his ability to sense the duration of time intervals. With improvement, he recovers his orientation in the reverse order.

Affective changes are often a prominent early feature. Most frequently the patient complains of anxiety, although depression may occur. Often the patient shows marked lability and is easily provoked to anger or tears. Pressure to perform intellectual tasks is a common stimulus for these reactions. Some patients may complain that noises seem too loud or that other sensory stimuli are annoying.

Psychotic Disorders

The patient is considered psychotic when his contact with the world is sufficiently distorted that he no longer is capable of testing reality. There is a severe disorganization of his personality that disrupts his relationships with persons around him. The same areas of impairment that were described in the non-psychotic patient are involved, but to a much greater degree.

Typically, there are shifting levels in the patient's state of consciousness, with fluctuations sometimes occurring from hour to hour. The patient is difficult to arouse and to interview. His awareness of his environment is decidedly dulled. Memory impairment is marked, with the greatest impairment for immediate recall, then for recent memory, and finally for remote memory. In the most severe state, he is comatose.

Severe cognitive impairment appears in the psychotic patient. He is bewildered, confused, and disoriented. He has lost all sense of time. When the interviewer asks for the date, he appears perplexed, and he may even have to peer at the window in order to decide if it is night or day. His sense of place is also disturbed, and he seems oblivious to the ward personnel and is unable to identify them. This state changes in severity in proportion to his general clinical condition.

The affective component in the delirious patient is pronounced, and exaggerated responses of fear, anger, or depression are common. Screaming or crying occur, as well as extreme states of excitement. As the patient becomes more comatose, this is replaced by dullness and unresponsiveness.

Perceptual disturbances are frequently part of the picture. At first the patient has illusory distortions and misidentifies other persons and objects. Some clinicians offer the distinction that the organic usually misperceives in the direction of making the unfamiliar more familiar, whereas the schizophrenic expresses a feeling of alienation during his hallucinatory experiences. The organic patient often sees hospital personnel as relatives; the schizophrenic is more likely to see them as Communists or some other "enemy." The organic patient thinks that he is at home rather than in a hospital. This clinical point has some validity; however in acute drug psychoses and delirium tremens, the perceptual distortions are bizarre and subjective feelings of alienation from the environment are prominent. Visual and tactile hallucinations are much more common in the organic patient than in the schizophrenic. Auditory hallucinations can occur and may be accompanied by poorly organized delusions of persecution. Hallucinations may be formed images and voices or simply chaotic patterns of light or sound. The acute confusional schizophrenic is more apt to be disoriented for person before he loses his sense of time.

CHRONIC BRAIN SYNDROME (DEMENTIA)

The most common chronic syndromes are those associated with senile brain disease or with vascular disease. The basic picture consists of impaired memory and cognition with affective and personality changes. There is no disturbance of consciousness, in contrast with the acute brain syndrome patient. Chronic brain syndromes tend to be progressive. Although the basic anatomical pathology is irreversible, the brain has a remarkable ability to utilize alternate pathways and to develop compensatory mechanisms, so that the patient shows clinical remissions and exacerbations. Some of these result from the development of superimposed acute brain syndromes. For example, the senile patient may develop delirium during a febrile illness. In some cases, an acute brain syndrome may proceed to a chronic process, for example, head trauma with irreversible changes. More often, the illness is first detected as a mild chronic condition. This points to the confusion in the use of the terms "acute" and "chronic."

Psychosocial factors in the patient's life exert a direct influence on the form and prognosis of the chronic brain syndrome. The anatomical area of the brain and the mass of the lesion also play a significant role in the total clinical phenomenology. Most syndromes due to localized lesions have accompanying neurological changes that aid in establishing the diagnosis. However, the psychiatric interview is of little value in localizing the lesion. Chronic brain syndromes exist on a continuum from mild senescence to severe psychotic conditions.

As with the acute brain syndrome, the capacity for abstract

thinking is the first conceptual process to suffer, and the patient frequently expresses himself in concrete terms. Early changes are subtle and may be demonstrable only with psychological tests.

The first clinical symptom is usually memory impairment, manifested by difficulty recalling the names of persons or places. The traditional view that recent memory becomes impaired before remote memory warrants re-examination. Remote memory is also altered early in the chronic syndromes, but certain remote memories are retained as a result of constant reinforcement through repetition.

The patient attempts to compensate for his memory deficit by using descriptive phrases as substitutes for names or words he cannot recall. This leads to circumstantiality; for example, a hospitalized patient was asked to name the hospital. He replied, "Well, you know it's at 168th Street . . . that big hospital up near the George Washington Bridge." Many patients automatically attempt to conceal their memory deficit through confabulation. This process involves almost any area of cognitive functioning. For example, the patient may conceal his lack of orientation with confabulatory material much in the same way as a small child who goes to visit a strange home with his parents. When someone asks the child if he knows whose house he is visiting, he replies, "It's Grandma's house." This child has not yet developed the cognitive capacity to understand the significance of his strange environment. The idea of not knowing his location is anxiety-provoking; consequently he fabricates that he is at a familiar place. The choice of "Grandma's house" could be determined by any number of reasons, including the psychological significance of "Grandma" or the similarity of physical surroundings. In the organic patient, confabulation represents the return of these same adaptive mechanisms that are normal in a young child. The material that the patient selects to fill his memory gaps has psychological significance and can be understood like a fantasy or dream. It has meaning in terms of both past events and current conflicts. For example, a patient confabulated that one of the staff members was a childhood friend. He was lonely, confined to a hospital many miles from home, and had always seen his childhood with its social successes as the happiest period of his life.

The patient's complaints of excessive fatigue, strain, or over-work are a reflection of his heightened effort in coping with intellectual tasks. The ability to perform simple calculations is impaired, as well as the repetition of digits forward and backward. The backward repetition of digits is a more sensitive indicator. The patient responds to his primary intellectual deficit by perseveration, attempting to conceal his disability by remaining with familiar topics. Circumstantiality, or talking around the point, also has defensive significance. A defective capacity for abstraction and logical thinking is concealed by long chains of related, but unnecessary, comments that refer to a central theme. There are episodes of disorientation for time, place, and person that occur at first, during the transition between sleep and waking, particularly if the patient is in a strange environment. Later the episodes grow longer, occur during the day, and can be triggered by almost any stress.

Emotional changes are more likely to be associated with personality changes in the chronic brain syndrome patient than in organic delirium, in which the affective symptoms are more impressive. Depression is a frequent reaction to the loss of physical and social function. This may be accompanied by irritability and angry outbursts in some persons and by apathy in others. As the overall integration of brain function is impaired, there may be emotional perseveration, flattening of affect, or lability. Extreme lability may be confused with the sudden outbursts of laughing and/or crying found in persons who have pseudobulbar palsy without chronic brain syndromes.

In contrast to the cognitive impairment, the specific symptoms of personality change are affected more by the patient's basic character structure. Usually the patient adopts more rigid attitudes, partially as a compensatory device for his impairment. He often withdraws from social contact and becomes ritualistic about his daily activities, relying on obsessive devices to conceal his loss of capacity. The defenses that he utilized in his earlier life may reappear in an exaggerated form. Thus, the patient who had many neurotic defenses will appear to be more neurotic, whereas the patient who utilized psychopathic mechanisms will resort to those modes of adaptation again.

The complex conceptual and emotional function termed "judgement" is impaired, resulting in socially inappropriate behavior. Hypersexuality, often directed toward inappropriate objects, is not uncommon. The patient tends to conserve his remaining resources, both personal and financial, and may hoard useless items or become miserly, with great concern about his future economic prospects. Paranoid attitudes are common and are initially manifested by irritability, querulousness, and somatic preoccupation. Hypochondriasis is frequent. Mild organic brain syndromes without psychosis are common in the aged. Such impairment may go undetected, since it would only be diagnosed by careful examination.

PSYCHOTIC DISORDERS

The chronic brain syndrome patient is considered psychotic when there is an intensification of the basic syndrome of impaired orientation, memory, and intellectual functioning, with accompanying affective and personality changes. Psychotic distortions in the form of delusions and hallucinations may be superimposed on organic deficits. This process is usually gradual, although in some cases an acute organic brain syndrome initiates the process.

Memory impairment is a prominent feature. The patient has great difficulty recalling recent events. Remote memories remain intact, provided they have been preserved through frequent repetition. Even these fail in the more advanced case, and the patient may rely on confabulation.

As dementia progresses, intellectual functions are increasingly disabled. The patient's disorientation is no longer limited to the periods when he is awakening or falling asleep; it is permanent, although it may become temporarily worse as a result of stress. Most patients utilize confabulation in an attempt to conceal their lack of orientation. Even simple calculation is impaired. If there is no physical impairment, the ability to perform an uncomplicated mechanical task may remain for some time. Spontaneous ideation and communication are impoverished, and the patient relies on stereotyped phrases in his contact with others.

The psychotic patient commonly has emotional outbursts, and he is no longer able to control his aggressive or sexual impulses. More advanced personality changes are seen as the patient becomes withdrawn, hostile, critical, and complaining. He is often preoccupied with physical symptoms and may show paranoid hypersensitivities to those around him. Judgement is grossly impaired.

Delusions are common and often persecutory in nature. They

frequently involve real people in the environment, such as hospital personnel or other patients. Misidentification of others is a complex symptom involving impaired memory, confabulation, and illusions. Hallucinations occur as the patient reports visits from deceased or absent relatives. There are usually both visual and auditory components to these experiences. The patient has increasing difficulty in distinguishing dreams from reality. He shifts back and forth between reality, daydreams, and dreams, with less critical distinction among these states. Often a patient reports that he has not slept recently, although others have seen him sleep at frequent intervals.

PROBLEMS OF THE AGED

Environmental, social, and psychological factors in the elderly are of importance in understanding the syndromes associated with organic brain disease. We live in a society that values youth and all that accompanies it—physical beauty, strength, competitive success, and self-sufficiency. However, the emotional needs of the young continue into later life. The older person still needs sexual gratification, a sense of usefulness, recreation, and close relationships with family and friends. The relative importance of these needs varies from person to person, much as it does in earlier years. To some degree, losses in one area may be compensated for by gains in another. For example, a retired lawyer continued his painting and golf when he no longer participated in professional activities. Although these recreational outlets had been of minor importance in his earlier years, they now assumed a major role in enhancing his self-esteem. Education and maintaining an active mental, physical, and community life appears to have a protective effect in warding off dementia.

There is no direct correlation between the maladaptive psychopathological patterns in the aged and the causal factors of role change, loss of loved ones, loss of physical energy, and so on. These pressures are experienced by every older person, yet many are able to maintain their emotional health. Therefore, other factors must play a role in shaping the patient's reactions to the inevitable changes of his later years.

Major psychodynamic aspects of aging stem from issues and conflicts of the first years of life. The child is forced to relinquish

his desires for constant gratification of his impulses and to substitute productive work with the resulting approval, first of his
parents, and later of their internal representations in his conscience. In the retirement years, man is permitted to return to the
childhood gratifications with relative freedom from responsibility.
He no longer must arise at a designated hour and he may come
and go as he pleases, without constantly having to follow a
schedule. In part, the new role is the result of diminishing physical and intellectual resources. However, retirement also represents a reward for having led a productive and useful life. The
latter aspect is prominent in those persons who never fully internalized the values of work as compared with play. For instance,
some men always pursued boyhood hobbies as a source of
pleasure and derived little satisfaction from their work. They are
prone to retire early and adjust well to the new routine. On the
other hand, the person who has largely inhibited the pleasures
of childhood in favor of adult values may have difficulty in retirement if he is no longer able to maintain the approval of his
internalized objects. In some instances the patient responds
regressively to his decreasing ability to control his current environment as well as his loss of ego assets. Such patients become overly
dependent and demanding. This pattern is more likely to occur in
those who have relied on regressive patterns for coping with stress
throughout their life. These basic principles determine the direction of the therapeutic interventions.

In general, the more one has lived life with gratification and
fulfillment, the less one approaches old age with fear of physical,
social, and economic helplessness and hopelessness.

PHYSICAL FACTORS

The nature of the physical insult to the brain determines
whether the symptoms are acute or chronic. However, other
factors are important in determining whether the condition
assumes psychotic proportions. Almost every person who lives
long enough eventually develops slowing of intellectual processes
and loss of ego flexibility.

After the sixth decade, there is a sharp increase in the incidence of physical illness, particularly arteriosclerosis, diabetes,
prostatic hypertrophy, osteoporosis, emphysema, cataracts, and

deafness. The individual has lost some of his physical strength and resiliency and relatively minor illness can tip the balance toward incapacitation. A new medication, metabolic change, fracture, or a febrile episode resulting in hospitalization may serve to decompensate an already compromised cerebral vascular system. Defective sensory input occurs as the patient's hearing, sight, taste, and smell no longer function at their previous level.

Psycho-social Factors

Some patients rely on denial and attempt to conceal their deficits from themselves as well as their associates. Others become preoccupied with their physical deficiencies and exploit them to gain attention and sympathy. This is associated with anxiety about helplessness, uselessness, abandonment, and death. For some, the physical decline symbolically reawakens unresolved castration anxiety. Depression is probably the most common reaction to the loss of physical capacity.

There is a popular myth that older persons no longer desire sexual gratification. Not only is sexual fulfillment still important for the elderly, but many brain-damaged persons experience a resurgence of sexual drive resulting from the release from cortical inhibition. The patient's prior sexual attitudes and prejudices will determine whether he is able to obtain gratification with an appropriate partner or whether his drives will be transformed into symptomatic expression. The reduction of biological drive combined with a loss of opportunity for sexual pleasure leads to diminished interest in sex for some elderly persons.

Retirement is one of the major factors leading to role changes in the elderly. The patient relinquishes the gratification obtained through his work. The person who has not prepared for this suddenly finds that he has few resources. Hobbies and avocational interests can provide an important source of self-esteem.

Loss of income and financial insecurities are a serious threat to many older people who fear outliving their resources with resulting forced dependency. However, the older person sometimes places himself in a financially dependent position as a regressive defense against threatening sexual or aggressive impulses, or as a manifestation of the helpless and despondent feelings that accompany his depression. There is frequently a role reversal, with the patient becoming dependent upon his children. An example would be the elderly man with adequate financial status who lived alone and visited the emergency room of a general hospital with multiple somatic complaints whenever his children did not invite him to their homes. He was angry with them for not spending enough time with him and he sought to manipulate their guilt through this maneuver. Another man who had recently retired and was fully capable of managing for himself suggested giving all his funds to his son, who would then support him with a monthly check. Both of these patients illustrate the use of regressive defenses to gain a subjective sense of security in order to cope with threatened loss of function. Rather than accepting a dependent adaptation, other patients react to their increasing helplessness with fear or hostility. For instance, the older man who cannot find his things might claim that someone is stealing his possessions. An old lady reacted to her increasing weakness with the delusion that her food was being poisoned.

Perhaps the single most important environmental factor for the older person is the attitude of his relatives. If they are sympathetic to his needs and help to provide for them, his adjustment will benefit accordingly. In the case of the patient with an acute brain syndrome, the patient and family may both benefit from the doctor's reassurance that the patient with mild residual disorganization will frequently reorganize upon returning to his home environment.

Unfortunately, dormant family conflicts sometimes emerge when the patient makes increased demands on his children's time and patience as his friends and contemporaries die. Children who have unresolved hostility to their parents will deprive them of the opportunity to play an important and useful role and will, instead, favor institutionalization when mild physical and emotional deficits appear.

On the other hand, hospitalization is constructive when a family comes to the realization that they are unable to properly care for a sick parent at home without sacrificing the physical or mental health of all persons concerned. Excessive guilt feelings often prevent families from institutionalizing relatives who can obtain better care than could be offered at home. Reassurance from the physician helps the relatives feel better about their decision and thereby benefits the patient as well.

Management of the Interview

It is difficult to describe a typical interview with the organic patient, as has been done with several other syndromes. The various clinical pictures create differing problems for the interviewer. In general, both the degree of organicity and the predominant symptom constellations determine the nature of the interview.

THE OPENING PHASE

If the patient has an acute organic reaction, the interview most often occurs in a general hospital at the request of another physician (see Chapter 12). The interviewer begins by identifying himself and exploring the patient's understanding of the reason for the consultation. "I am Dr. X. Did your doctor explain that I would be coming?" The physician guides his next response by the patient's reply to this introduction. If the patient understands that he is being interviewed by a psychiatrist, the interviewer may proceed. If not, the interviewer must explain his presence. He tactfully explains why he was consulted, saying, "I understand that you have been upset," or, "Dr. Jones tells me that you have had some periods of confusion," or, "Your doctor thought I could help with your nightmares." The non-psychotic patient will then begin to discuss his problems and the interviewer will follow the patient's lead. Often his basic medical illness is the matter of greatest concern to the patient. The psychotic patient will be more difficult to interview and the physician must be prepared to provide more structure.

The interview with the chronic brain syndrome patient begins in a similar fashion, except that the patient is not as likely to be seriously medically ill. Again, someone other than the patient has usually requested help. Most often the patient is elderly and has been accompanied by a relative, friend, or even a policeman, if the patient was found wandering aimlessly and was brought to the hospital. After hearing the chief complaint from the other person, the interviewer asks him to wait while the patient is interviewed first. If the patient is psychotic, it is usually apparent quickly and the interviewer modifies his approach accordingly.

RELATIONSHIP WITH THE PATIENT

ATTITUDE OF THE INTERVIEWER

The physician is often inclined to concentrate on the formal mental status when interviewing the organic patient. Prejudices are prevalent even among psychiatrists as to the therapeutic value of the interview, particularly with the psychotic patient who appears to be "out of it." The patient senses this attitude and responds accordingly.

The organic patient is quick to detect the interviewer's personal interest, and he responds to the doctor's respect as does anyone else—by being more cooperative. This patient requires considerable support and he will not react favorably to the physician who is aloof, distant, or overly neutral. Although a warm, interested, and friendly attitude is generally desirable, in specific situations, the interviewer may become critical or disapproving. This may be necessary in order to modify socially unacceptable behavior that is ultimately self-destructive for the patient.

TRANSFERENCE AND COUNTERTRANSFERENCE

Patients with mild organic impairment develop a transference that is primarily determined by their basic personality type. Patients with more severe disorders usually relate to the doctor in a dependent manner. The transference attitudes of these patients are not interpreted and they will not be worked through. However, if the transference is perceived correctly by the doctor, it can be utilized constructively in the interview. If older patients relate to the physician as to a parent, it may be difficult for a young physician to accept this role. Some older patients may respond to the physician as to a son or daughter.

Countertransference problems are common with the elderly chronic brain syndrome patient. The doctor's reluctance to treat this group of patients often reflects unresolved feelings toward his parents. He may feel that older persons are set in their ways and unable to change or that their problems are realistic and therefore not amenable to treatment. Here, the physician inwardly agrees with the patient's own view that he is useless and helpless, that he has lost his friends, his financial resources, and his physical health, and that he has no reason to continue living. The doctor's anxiety about his own later years may reawaken dormant castration anxiety or fears of helplessness and enforced dependency. Some physicians may overly idealize older people and may be unable to perceive the patient's diminished capacities, damaged self-esteem, and consequent suffering.

The physician usually experiences a greater psychological distance with older patients as he is less able to see the world through their eyes. In most instances, his own grandparents were viewed as members of an older generation who may have been revered, but who rarely were understood in terms of their own problems. For instance, the physician of 25 may feel that there is relatively little difference between a person of 60 and one of 75.

The physician is often particularly blind to the continuing sexual feelings of the older person and may avoid this topic during the interview. For example, a young male physician did not immediately realize why an older woman patient dressed up and put on lipstick prior to her interview with the doctor. She did not behave in this way prior to interviews with female social workers in the home for the aged in which she lived. The therapist may tend to under- or overemphasize the psychological significance of organic complaints or he may under- or overemphasize the organic significance of functional complaints. The difficulty in distinguishing the relative significance of the psychological versus the organic factors in the patient's illness may cause the physician to feel frustrated or helpless. Actually, the answer to this question is often unimportant in conducting the interview.

SPECIFIC TECHNIQUES

BRIEF INTERVIEWS. A shorter interview is helpful if the patient fatigues easily. It may even be better to see a patient several times in one day or on several successive days for 15-minute interviews.

RECOGNIZING THE PATIENT AS A PERSON. After the patient's initial spontaneous remarks, the doctor determines the chief complaint and a brief history of the present illness and then directs his attention to the patient's personal background and current life situation. The patient with chronic brain impairment is particularly dependent upon recollections of past achievements and capabilities in order to maintain his self-esteem. Therefore, a review of the patient's earlier life is not only informative for the interviewer, but therapeutic for the patient as well. For example, a senile woman became acutely psychotic following her confinement to bed with a broken leg. She was quite disorganized during the initial portion of the interview, but her mental processes improved considerably as she related stories of her past success as a trial lawyer. She sensed the doctor's interest and was again able to feel that she was a socially valued person.

ALLOWING THE PATIENT TIME.   The interviewer can appreciate the heightened effort involved for the patient to communicate with the doctor and allow more time for responses. The patient's circumstantiality and perseveration reflect both his organic pathology and his attempts to compensate for it. The patient should be allowed to tell his story in his own way, provided he can offer some structure. If, however, the patient is too disorganized to provide his own structure, the interviewer can help by providing concrete questions that the patient can understand and answer. In providing a structural framework for the disorganized patient, it is easy to take over completely and become impatient, an approach that further increases the patient's disorganization.

STIMULATING MEMORY CHAINS.   The organic patient has a tendency to substitute descriptions for proper names that he is unable to recall. The interviewer attempts to stimulate associative patterns that will improve the patient's recall. This is particularly important in interviews subsequent to the initial meeting. The doctor adjusts the amount of refreshing of the patient's memory to the degree of impairment. With patients whose organic deficit is serious, the physician might repeat his own name and summarize the previous interview.

AIDING REALITY TESTING.   Frequently, when a physician discovers that a patient is disoriented or confused, he permits the patient to give "wrong" answers without any attempt to provide the correct information. It is sometimes helpful to say, "No, it is not August, it is December, and next week is Christmas." However, the doctor can use the incorrect response as a suggestion that he inquire about the possibility of some defensive denial in the patient's lack of orientation. For example, he might inquire about the patient's most recent Christmas holiday and whether it was a period of social isolation instead of a time of closeness.

TAKING INTEREST IN PHYSICAL COMPLAINTS.   The patient's preoccupation with his body often reflects his psychological condition. Information about the patient's interaction with his environment can be obtained from careful attention to his description of his attempts to gain help for his physical complaints.

THE MENTAL STATUS

The physician is frequently expected to write a description of the mental status after completing the interview with the organic brain syndrome patient. The unsophisticated interviewer anticipates this requirement by following a predetermined formal outline during the interview. With experience, most of the needed inquiry can be integrated into the natural flow of the interview. On some occasions when formal mental status questions seem indicated, it is possible to incorporate them into the interview in a way that makes them more meaningful for both the patient and the doctor. The specific timing of these questions as well as the wording depends on the type and degree of impairment that the patient suffers. The beginning interviewer shifts the focus to the mental status earlier if the patient shows serious organic dysfunction. This communicates his feeling of hopelessness about attempting to establish a relationship and his retreat to gathering data for the record.

When organic syndromes are suspected, but the diagnosis is not clear-cut, the interviewer can employ stress in order to evaluate the patient's clinical impairment. For example, when a patient seems uncertain in his orientation for time and date but gives an approximately correct answer, the interviewer might reply, "Are you sure?" If the patient looks quizzically out the window and then replies, "Well, the leaves have started to turn, so it must be autumn; yes, I am sure it is September," the interviewer has demonstrated a loss of function. After using stress to demonstrate a problem, the sensitive interviewer will provide support and reassurance. The patient may attempt to hide his deficit, becoming evasive and circumstantial when the interviewer asks questions that expose his problem. A sympathetic recognition of this process may be helpful. For instance, the doctor could say, "Every time I ask a question that taxes your memory, you change the subject. Have you been having some problems remembering things?" When the deficit is readily apparent, there is no need to apply stress in the interview.

The organic patient may perform much worse during the psychiatric interview than in his daily life. Asking the patient to describe the events of the last 24 hours will provide an additional evaluation of his cerebral functioning and will offer psychodynamic data as well. The patient's response will reflect his memory and orientation as well as his feelings about his illness and his present life situation. The interviewer can explore related areas by such questions as "Have you had any visitors?" or, "Have you received any mail or telephone calls?", or by inquiring about the patient's appetite and sleep patterns.

It is important to determine whether the patient's organic mental disturbance is improving or worsening. Often, one cannot learn this in one interview, and prolonged observation or data provided by relatives or the referring persons may be required. These sources can be quite unreliable, particularly when legal action that may prove beneficial to the relatives is contemplated. Psychological tests such as the Wechsler Adult Intelligence Scale or the Bender Gestalt are also helpful in delineating signs of organicity.

SUICIDAL PROBLEMS

The incidence of suicide is particularly high in elderly patients with organic brain syndromes. The evaluation of suicide is especially difficult in this group; many older people openly state that they would be better off dead or wish they were dead, but are not suicidal. Other factors such as living alone, discouragement over ill health, and mental confusion also contribute to the patient's potential for self-destruction. Most commonly, the depressed patient is actively suicidal. The depth of the patient's despair may be masked by somatic preoccupation, agitation, or mental confusion. Physicians frequently overlook the suicidal potential of the organically confused medical patient until he impulsively jumps out the window of the general hospital. This suicide represents both an impairment of reality testing and a loss of control over impulses. No interview with the organic patient is complete unless the physician inquires about self-destructive plans, impulses, or wishes.

THE PHYSICAL EXAMINATION

A thorough physical and neurological examination is necessary in the evaluation of a patient with organic brain disease. In the case of the institutionalized patient, such examinations usually are performed by the psychiatrist and constitute an important part of his contact with the patient.

INTERVIEWING THE RELATIVES

It is important for the interviewer to have contact with the patient's relatives early in the evaluation. Some relatives have difficulty recognizing and accepting the degree of impairment in their loved one and feel guilty about and fearful of institutional care. Others resent the patient and look for any opportunity to get him out of the home.

A picture of the family pattern can be obtained by asking what the patient has been told concerning the interview with the psychiatrist. For example, one of the authors interviewed an 80-year-old woman with an advanced senile psychosis. She had been brought by her daughter to arrange a state hospital commitment. She was confused, disoriented, and disorganized, and she misidentified the daughter as her sister. The daughter was asked what she had told her mother concerning the interview with the psychiatrist. She replied, "Oh, I didn't tell her anything; she really doesn't know what is going on around her. I just said we're going to the doctor." The interviewer inquired, "What was your mother's response?" The daughter paused and then added, "Now that you mention it, she said a strange thing. She said that she felt she would never come home again." The daughter had no idea how her mother, who was so confused, could have such insightful awareness. This interchange provided an opportunity to discuss the daughter's sadness and guilt concerning institutionalization. The psychiatrist explored the mother's feelings about institutional care in a second interview.

In making therapeutic recommendations, the physician must consider the entire family and not exclusively the member who is brought as the patient. Urging a family to continue caring for a relative at home, when to do so would drain the emotional resources of all concerned, is of dubious value to anyone, including the patient. It is important to help relatives understand the indication for hospitalization and the benefits for the patient. In so doing, the physician may help them resolve their own feelings of guilt or failure in not being able to care for their loved one at home.

The psychiatrist who plans to maintain a seriously disturbed organic patient in the home must obtain the cooperation and help of those living with the patient. He must be prepared to modify his plan if it seems not to be working for the best interests of the total family.

THE THERAPEUTIC PLAN

The psychiatrist may have a number of practical therapeutic recommendations to make at the end of the interview. The physician who realizes that his job is not to cure the patient's condition will be less likely to feel overwhelmed by the realistic limitations of the patient's disability or life situation. In many cases psychiatric hospitalization is not indicated and the patient may be cared for in a general hospital or at home.

OBTAINING THE PATIENT'S COOPERATION

This obvious step is frequently overlooked in the care of the patient with organic brain disease. Unless the patient is brought into the treatment plan, he can hardly be expected to cooperate. With the elderly chronic patient, it is one of the few remaining ways in which he can be helped to feel useful once again.

Many patients with organic brain syndromes are intensely ashamed of their deficits and fear becoming crazy. They are frequently reassured by an explanation of their illness in nontechnical terms. For example, the interviewer might say, "Your thought processes seem to be functioning slowly, but otherwise quite well."

If the patient is to be cared for at home, he should have his own chores and responsibilities in the house. These can be geared to his current capacities. Creative talents, avocational interests, and hobbies should be explored, and the interviewer can ask to see examples of work the patient has produced. This is also of concern with the hospitalized patient whose opportunities to feel useful are more restricted. The patient may gain self-esteem by being helpful to others in the same predicament as himself. The interviewer can discuss the patient's feeling of helplessness and vulnerability directly. The doctor's recognition and respect for the patient's premorbid accomplishments has a substantial therapeutic effect. In these ways the therapist offers himself as a substitute for the patient's lost love objects.

In one case, an 80-year-old man, who had retired 15 years earlier, moved in with his daughter and son-in-law after his wife died. He soon began to have periods of confusion, irritability, and memory loss. His main source of self-esteem during the preceding 15 years had come from dominating his wife. He attempted this same technique in his new home, but he met constant rebuff and failure. When he was able to direct his domineering behavior toward his psychiatrist, who accepted it without critical comment or interpretation, he soon improved. The physician's acceptance of hostile, critical feelings as well as dependent feelings is essential in working with these patients. The organic patient's opportunities for mastery are limited. Exercising some mastery over the therapist provides important gratification for the patient.

MEDICATION AND SPECIFIC PROCEDURES

The person who has lost his ability to work, whose friends have died, and who is physically ill may be grateful for small favors. His expectations of life have diminished so that the healthy young doctor has difficulty seeing the world through the patient's eyes or imagining himself in the patient's position. A sleeping pill or laxative or merely a sympathetic ear may be a substantial gain for the person who has so little. A clear formulation of the patient's problem can give him the feeling of being loved and protected, thereby providing gratification for his dependent needs.

The hospitalized patient with an acute organic brain syndrome may be helped by tranquilizing medication, protection from sensory monotony, a light in his room at night, and early ambulation after he has been confined to bed. The patient's contacts with his pre-hospital life can be fostered by visits from friends and family, pictures at his bedside, telephone contact with his home, copies of his favorite newspaper, and any possible reminder that there is a continuity to his past, present, and future.

REFERENCES

Aronson, N. J.: Psychotherapy in a home for the aged. Arch. Neuro. Psychiat., *79:*671, 1958.

Blessed, G., Tomlinson, B. E., and Roth, M.: The association between quantitative measures of dementia and of senile change in the cerebral grey matter of elderly subjects. Brit. J. Psychiat., *114:*797, 1968.

Engel, G. L., and Romano, J.: Delirium, a syndrome of cerebral insufficiency. J. Chron. Dis. *9:*260, 1959.

Fisch, M., Goldfarb, A. I., Shahinian, S. P., and Turner, H.: Chronic brain syndrome in the community aged. Arch. Gen. Psychiat., *18:*739, 1968.

Goldfarb, A. I.: Psychotherapy of aged persons: One aspect of the psychodynamics of the therapeutic situation with aged patients. Psychoanal. Rev., *42:*180, 1955.

Goldfarb, A. I.: Minor maladjustments of the aged. In Arieti, S. (ed.): American Handbook of Psychiatry, Vol. 1. New York, Basic Books, 1959, Chap. 20.

Goldfarb, A. I., and Sheps, J.: Psychotherapy of the aged: Brief therapy of inter-related psychological and somatic disorders. Psychosom. Med., *16:*209, 1954.

Goldfarb, A. I., and Turner, H.: Psychotherapy of aged persons: Utilization and effectiveness of "brief" therapy. Amer. J. Psychiat., *109:*916, 1953.

Goldstein, K.: Functional disturbances in brain damage. In Arieti, S. (ed.): American Handbook of Psychiatry, Vol. 1. New York, Basic Books, 1959, Chap. 39, pp. 770–794.

Grotjahn, M.: Analytic psychotherapy with the elderly. Psychoanal. Rev., *42:*419, 1955.

Hollender, M. H.: Early psychologic reactions associated with organic brain disease in the aged. N.Y. State J. Med., *69:*802, 1969.

Meerloo, J. A. M.: Transference and resistance in geriatric psychotherapy. Psychoanal. Rev., *42:*72, 1955.

Peck, A.: Psychotherapy of the aged. J. Amer. Geriat. Soc., *14:*748, 1966.

Zimberg, N. E., and Kaufman, I. (eds.): Normal Psychology of the Aging Process. New York, International Universities Press, 1963.

Section two:

SPECIAL CLINICAL SITUATIONS

In this section, specific clinical situations are described that may involve any of the major syndromes described in Section One. Here the emphasis is placed on a description of the situation and how it affects the patient and, in turn, how the problems inherent in these clinical situations take precedence in determining the conduct of the interview.

// THE PSYCHOSOMATIC
PATIENT

Psychopathology and Psychodynamics

Everyone has "psychosomatic" aspects of his emotional life.
It is impossible to separate mind and body. Emotional reactions
such as rage, guilt, fear, and love have physiological components
mediated through the neuro-endocrine system. Such responses
may, in time, lead to anatomical or pathophysiological changes
as well. This chapter will consider the interview with the patient whose symptomatology is primarily physical. Included are
patients who have the classic psychophysiological disorders such
as ulcerative colitis, asthma, neurodermatitis, peptic ulcer, essential hypertension, rheumatoid arthritis, and hyperthyroidism. It
also considers the patient who has a physical difficulty—such as
cerebral vascular accidents, myocardial infarctions, and cancer—
with secondary emotional complications. Included are patients
who do not have a specific psychophysiological disorder, but for
whom no positive organic disease can be diagnosed. The psychosomatic patient is not a single clinical entity, since both his symptoms and his psychodynamics are so varied.

DESCRIPTION OF THE PROBLEM

The patient who suffers from physical symptoms has already consulted another medical specialist prior to the psychiatrist. The task of the psychiatrist will depend in part on how the referring physician has prepared the patient for the consultation. This preparation varies with the attitude of the referring physician and his conscious and unconscious reasons for the referral. The conscious reasons include requests for assistance in diagnosis and for advice concerning the managment of emotional conflicts in a patient with physical illness. Unconscious reasons include the doctor's feelings of helplessness, hopelessness, or despair in treating a difficult and perhaps frustrating patient. At times, the referring physician may be angry with the patient and hope that the psychiatrist will take over management of the case.

Evaluating the functional component of a physical symptom is a complicated task. Traditional questions to be answered in making this determination include: (1) Were emotional or interpersonal stresses prominent in the patient's life at the onset of the condition or clearly related to remissions and exacerbations? (2) Does the patient's symptomatology not fit into a known pattern of organic disease? (3) Can the physical symptoms be explained in terms of the patient's emotional conflicts? (4) Does the patient attach unusual psychological meaning to his symptoms? (5) Can a psychiatric condition be diagnosed on the basis of positive clinical findings, and are the physical symptoms consistent with this diagnosis? (6) Does the patient obtain secondary gain from his illness?

An affirmative answer to all of these questions is suggestive of a functional disorder; however, there are many organic illnesses that take atypical forms and in which the illness and the symptoms assume a special meaning for the patient and provide secondary gains. In some patients, organic illness precipitates a latent psychological conflict. The psychiatrist's contribution will be more valuable if it contains a description of the clinical facts rather than postulating etiological connections between physical symptoms and emotional conflicts.

PSYCHODYNAMIC ISSUES

Specific psychodynamic constellations have been proposed for each of the major psychophysiological disorders. However, attempts to predict psychosomatic symptoms from dynamic formulations have been largely unsuccessful. Not only are the psychological conflicts nonspecific, but their importance in the etiology of each condition is unknown and probably varies considerably.

The fear of loss of dependent relationships is often an important factor. Chronic resentment over unfulfilled, frustrated dependency needs cannot be expressed openly by such persons without risking further loss of dependent care; therefore, they inhibit angry, resentful responses, which are then discharged physiologically.

Additional psychodynamic features develop as the patient experiences unconscious reactions to his physical illness. One common unconscious reaction is for the patient to experience the illness as a punishment for prior misdeeds. He may obtain considerable secondary gain from his illness, for example, by receiving additional dependent care or punishing his relatives through the imposition of his suffering upon them. At the conscious level, however, the patient most often is fearful concerning the impact of his illness upon his future. He dreads becoming dependent, helpless, or a financial burden upon relatives.

Physical illness initiates strong regressive tendencies in every individual. Depending upon basic character structure, one patient may submit to these regressive tendencies and lapse into a helpless and dependent state, whereas another may deny the illness and insist on maintaining his usual activities. Some patients may become depressed as a result of their inability to continue their customary routines.

Denial is the central mechanism of defense that operates throughout this entire chain of psychological events. Since the patient does not think in psychological terms, he tends to deny the existence of conflicts and their resulting emotions. When the acknowledgment of emotional conflict is inescapable, he denies the relationship of the conflict to his symptoms.

Physical symptoms frequently have an overlay of neurotic complaints built upon a minimal degree of organic pathology. Physicians sometimes feel that these neurotic complaints will disappear if the physical basis is identified for the patient. Unfortunately, this is rarely the case, and the patient will instead become even more preoccupied with his symptoms.

Management of the Interview

This group of patients usually relates to the physician in a passive, dependent manner. Since they are suffering, they are quite willing to follow the physician's advice and look to him for guidance. The patient wants to feel that his doctor is interested, concerned, and sympathetic to his suffering. Some psychiatrists find the psychophysiological patient difficult to interview because the patient prefers to discuss physical symptoms rather than psychological conflicts. However, as time passes, many of these patients are willing to give up the discussion of symptoms and reveal long-repressed emotional problems.

If the psychiatrist does not perform a physical examination himself, he must obtain the resulting information from a competent physician before he can evaluate the significance of physical disease. The patient who feels that his difficulty is primarily physical will trust his doctor only if the doctor has acquainted himself with the physical problems. It is through the interviewer's taking an interest in the physical problems that the patient will allow the psychiatrist to know him as a person.

EXPLORING THE PRESENTING SYMPTOMS

This patient is more uncomfortable than many others in coming to see a psychiatrist. Rather than perceiving the psychiatrist as a source of help, the patient fears that his doctor considers his complaints imaginary or that he may be crazy. Therefore, it is helpful if the interviewer will spend time at the beginning of the interview to put the patient at ease.

After the discussion of the chief complaint, the interviewer asks what the patient was told concerning the purpose of the consultation. This will allow an early clarification of any misunderstanding. If the patient is very ill physically, a shorter than usual interview will avoid tiring the patient. Psychosomatic patients do not respond well to long silences and the interviewer should not permit them to develop. The patient responds more quickly if the initial portion of the interview follows the traditional medical model. After exploring the chief complaint and present illness, a brief family and personal history and a description of the patient's current life situation is obtained. It is not unusual for the patient to begin the interview by saying, "Doctor, I have an ulcer so I must have emotional problems," and then systematically deny all problems and describe all of his relatives as wonderful.

As the interviewer conducts his survey of the patient's life, he is alert for clues concerning psychological stresses that may be related to the patient's difficulties. These clues include physiological or motor responses during the interview, such as blushing, perspiring, or restlessness. Other illustrations are the neurodermatitis patient who scratches himself when discussing his frustration with his employer, the migraine patient who gets a headache after describing his mother-in-law, and the ulcer patient who develops stomach pain while describing his problems at school.

Frequently, it is useful to ask the patient if he has known anyone with an illness similar to his own. The answer may reveal unconscious attitudes about his illness and clues concerning its origin. Although psychosomatic patients frequently resist attempts to correlate symptoms with specific psychological situations, they will often indicate that their symptoms occur when they are nervous. At this point the interviewer inquires, "What kind of situation makes you nervous?" Other questions include, "What did you notice first?", "Where did it all begin?", or, "When do you last recall feeling completely well?" On some occasions, asking the patient to describe a typical day in detail, or to describe all of the events of the past week, will successfully circumvent the patient's defenses.

As the interview progresses, the physician directs the patient's attention to emotional responses that occur at the time the physical symptoms begin. Although the patient initially may not be aware of these responses, he may eventually be able to develop a greater awareness and heightened sensitivity to his feelings. The patient may deny the role of anxiety, fear, or anger in the production of his physical symptoms, but may readily acknowledge the existence of psychological symptoms such as tension, depression, insomnia, anorexia, fatigue, nightmares, or sexual disturbances. He will often claim that his physical illness is making him nervous or upset. The interviewer is advised not to challenge this patient, nor the one who totally denies nervousness, too early in the interview. Instead, he waits until the patient has displayed anxiety during the interview, and then suggests that the patient may not have recognized that this behavior is evidence of nervousness. The patient who does not admit to nervousness but states, "It's just my nerves, Doc," presents a similar challenge. He does not consider himself to have a psychological problem but views his difficulty as a vague neurological condition.

The physician might inquire, "What does your illness keep you from doing?" or, "What would you do if you were well that you are not able to do now?" The patient's answers will provide material concerning the psychodynamic significance of the symptoms as well as the secondary gain involved.

The psychiatrist is often asked to evaluate a patient's complaint of pain. The interviewer can begin his evaluation by obtaining a careful description of the pain, when it began, what seems to bring it on, and what seems to help it, as well as the patient's understanding of its cause and significance. A determination of who in the patient's life is hurt by the pain will help in determining its role in family dynamics. Pain is a complex subjective phenomenon that is always experienced by the patient as real. The interviewer should never suggest that the patient's pain is not real or that he is exaggerating. Patients whose complaint of pain or preoccupation with physical symptoms is a manifestation of depression often deny awareness of depressed feelings when questioned directly. However, if the interviewer refers to the pain and other symptoms by saying to the patient, "It must be terribly depressing to suffer like this," the patient will readily acknowledge the existence of these feelings. It is more difficult to show the patient that the pain is a manifestation of his depression, rather than the depression being a reaction to the pain. It may not be necessary for the patient to develop this insight, since he can still be treated for the depression with a relief of his pain. The management of these problems is further discussed in Chapters 6 and 8. The management of the patient with acute anxiety symptoms is discussed in Chapter 14.

In exploring both the central meaning and the secondary gain of the symptoms, it is important to question the patient concerning the reactions of key relatives to his illness. A woman patient may say, "My husband doesn't realize how much I suffer with these terrible backaches." The interviewer could reply, "What does he think about them?" As the patient proceeds to discuss her husband's feelings about the illness and his lack of sympathetic understanding, the connections between the meaning of her symptoms and his disapproving, rejecting attitude will gradually emerge.

The interviewer is often unable to discover any specific precipitating stress in the patient's life, but instead the illness seems to arise as a result of the cumulative effects of life stress. This is particularly true of the individuals who live under the constant pressure of their compulsive personalities. The physician should refrain from offering well-meaning advice such as, "Stop worrying," or, "Try to relax." Instead, he might explain that the degree of physical disability is out of proportion to the patient's physical disease, or, if it is appropriate, that some disturbance in the patient's emotional life may be responsible for or aggravating his symptoms. The patient can be invited to share his worries with the physician rather than keeping them to himself.

EXPLORING THE PSYCHOLOGICAL PROBLEMS

As the interview progresses, the interviewer gradually switches from symptoms to personal affairs. Questions concerning previous medical treatment and hospitalization are particularly important. Such inquiries give the patient the feeling that the interviewer is interested in him. A detailed cross-sectional survey of the patient's life at the time the illness began should be elicited in association with the longitudinal developmental history. Beginning psychiatrists ask the patient questions such as, "What was going on in your life when your ulcer symptoms first started?" or, "Was there something emotionally upsetting at that time in your life?" Such questions pose too direct an assault on this patient's defenses, and often they not only are unproductive, but also discourage the doctor from making further inquiry.

Instead, the interviewer can take two separate histories, the first of which covers the physical problems. He then obtains a parallel history that focuses on the patient's emotional life. Often the connections that the interviewer seeks will be quite apparent to him, although not to the patient.

The patient's understanding of and feeling about his illness are important. This includes the patient's ideas concerning the cause of the illness, the prognosis, and the limitations it imposes upon his life. Patients often obtain real gains from illness; for some it is the best answer to their problems. Such people have lived the greater portion of their lives suffering from one disease or another, particularly when faced with major situational problems. For those patients, the realization of the shortcomings and dissatisfactions in their marriage or family business might prove disastrous. They are better off if their defenses are not disturbed by efforts to demonstrate a relationship between their symptoms and their life situation. Reassurance and supportive treatment based upon the interviewer's psychodynamic understanding of their problems are far more effective.

It is an error for the psychiatrist to limit his interest to the psychosomatic patient's emotional problems, leaving it to the medical specialist to worry about the physical illness. The patient will invariably experience this attitude as a rejection and a lack of interest on the part of the psychiatrist. The physical symptoms are a major source of information and provide an important barometer concerning progress with the emotional aspects of the patient's treatment. With more seriously sick patients, it is necessary to be cautious in interpreting unconscious conflicts, particularly when a patient is acutely ill.

THE PATIENT'S
EXPECTATIONS OF THE CONSULTANT

The psychosomatic patient expects to ask questions and to receive answers from his psychiatric consultant. Frequently the patient will ask the doctor, "How is talking going to help me?" The physician might explain that emotions have an important effect upon the body and offer a brief explanation of how emotional factors in the patient's life could produce or intensify his symptoms. The interviewer can then suggest that talking will lead to an understanding of what specific emotional conflicts are responsible for the patient's tension and, finally, that as a result of such understanding, the patient can be helped to resolve his conflict in some other way. Long and complicated explanations give the interview the quality of a lecture and are best avoided.

On some occasions the patient will ask, "Do you think I'm crazy, Doctor?" or, "Is it all in my mind?" The physician could reply that the patient's symptoms are real, not imaginary, and then explain the disorder. If the patient's symptoms are out of proportion to his physical disease, then this could be discussed.

In another situation the patient may surprise the interviewer by asking him, "What is my diagnosis, Doctor?" or, "What is really wrong with me?" The interviewer can respond by exploring the patient's fears concerning his illness and contrasting these with the information he has been given by his physician. The interviewer does not stop when he learns that the patient is fearful that he has cancer or some other serious illness. Instead, he proceeds to determine what consequences the patient imagines would accompany such a diagnosis. He may then assure the patient concerning his specific fears, indicating that such consequences are not necessarily to be expected in his case. For example, to have cancer no longer means that one is incurably ill.

The interviewer can best determine how much to tell the patient by evaluating the patient's response to what he has already learned and the degree of rational logic that the patient has utilized in reaching his conclusions. The patient who has used gross denial in the presence of severe physical illness should probably not be confronted with the true nature of his condition. The patient who asks, "Doctor, do I have cancer?" and then adds, "If I do, I will kill myself," does not want to be told the truth. Another instance is the physician patient who suffers from an obvious malignancy and has rationalized that it is really tuberculosis or some other benign condition.

It is common for the psychosomatic patient to open up, disclosing information of considerable psychological significance, only then to deny it with a statement such as, "All that was really silly," or, "Oh, I didn't really mean that." At this point, the physician can provide reassurance that the patient was not silly and that he should continue.

THE CLOSING PHASE

As the interview is drawing to a close, it is helpful if the physician makes a brief statement to the patient explaining what he has learned. In this way, the physician not only has an opportunity to clarify any misunderstanding of what the patient has said, but he also can obtain some measure of the patient's receptivity to psychological insights concerning his illness. For example, the physician might say to a young woman who has asthma attacks, "It seems that you only get attacks when you go to visit your sister, and that you feel it is her dog that is responsible; however, you have been exposed to similar dogs without having any trouble." The physician can then wait and see how the patient reacts to this gentle confrontation before attempting to further challenge her understanding of her condition.

The patient's expectations of magical relief place additional pressure on the inexperienced psychiatrist. The young doctor feels that he must impress not only the patient but the referring physician as well. It is preferable to schedule more than one appointment for the consultation and to resist the urge to demonstrate all of one's knowledge in the first interview.

The physician might direct the patient to observe his emotional reactions just prior to the onset of physiological symptoms. As the patient becomes more practiced at this, he may develop an awareness of feelings he had previously denied. The physician is advised to proceed slowly in attempting to explain the origin of such feelings. After a number of interviews, when he has obtained a full description of the patient's symptoms and emotional conflicts, he may then attempt to tie them all together, relating them to the symptomatology and to the patient's life stresses.

Before ending the interview, the therapist should allow the patient sufficient time to ask questions. If the patient's questions go back to the physical symptoms and leave the subject of personal relations, emotional conflicts, and feelings, the physician may conclude that the patient has not changed his view of his problem and that he will progress very slowly in any insight-oriented psychotherapy. If, on the other hand, the patient proceeds to inquire about matters related to his emotional life, he will be more responsive to an uncovering psychotherapy. It is frequently necessary for the physician to prescribe some tranquilizing or antidepressant medication for psychosomatic patients. Adequate time should be allowed to explain the medicine, how it is to be taken, and what the patient should expect it to do for him.

This patient will probably be unfamiliar with psychotherapeutic treatment. If such treatment is recommended, the interviewer will have to provide information concerning what is expected of both the patient and the doctor.

REFERENCES

Bellak, L.: Psychology of Physical Illness. New York, Grune & Stratton, 1952.

Hackett, T., and Weisman, A.: Psychiatric management of operative syndromes. I. The therapeutic consultation and the effect of noninterpretive intervention. II. Psychodynamic factors in formulation and management. Psychosom. Med., 22:267, 1960; 22:356, 1960.

Lipowski, Z. J.: Review of consultation psychiatry and psychosomatic medicine. Psychosom. Med., 29:201, 1967.

Mendelson, M., and Meyer, E.: Countertransference problems of the liaison Psychiatrist. Psychosom. Med., 23:115, 1961.

Meyer, E.: Disturbed behavior on medical and surgical wards: A training and research opportunity. Sci. Psychoanal., 5:181, 1962.

Meyer, E., and Mendelson, M.: Psychiatric consultations with patients on medical and surgical wards: Patterns and processes. Psychiatry, 24:197, 1961.

Weisman, A. D.: The doctor-patient relationship: Its role in therapy. Amer. Pract. Dig. Treatment, 1:1144, 1950.

12 THE WARD CONSULTATION

Psychopathology and Psychodynamics

Psychiatric consultations in the general hospital present many problems. One of the most significant is also the most unique. The consultation is rarely requested by the patient; in fact, it is often not directly for the patient's benefit. The patient may not have been informed of the psychiatrist's visit and may not be able to participate when the psychiatrist arrives to see him. For example, he might be at the radiology department or might be exhausted from some lengthy procedure so that the interview must be postponed. The patient may have visitors who will have to be dismissed before the interview can begin. The psychiatrist has become a participating observer in a group that includes the patient, the referring doctor, the ward staff, the other patients, and the patient's family. Frequently the problem is compounded by disagreement between different members of the staff in ordering the psychiatric consultation. Although the term "ward" is used in this chapter, the discussion applies to private patients as well.

DESCRIPTION OF THE PROBLEM

Psychiatric consultations on hospitalized patients may be requested for various reasons. The number of consultations requested by different services is largely dependent upon differing attitudes toward psychiatry and upon the personal relations between psychiatrists and other specialists.

The clinical conditions for which the psychiatrist is consulted include organic brain syndromes, postpartum and postoperative syndromes, preoperative syndromes, psychophysiological reactions, intractable pain problems, physical symptoms that are disproportionate to organic pathology, depressive or anxiety reactions, alcoholism or drug dependence, concurrent functional psychoses, conversion reactions, non-cooperation with ward routine or medical procedures, and malingering in order to obtain hospital treatment.

PSYCHODYNAMIC FACTORS IN THE STAFF

The consultant must understand the psychodynamic factors in the person requesting the consultation, since it is often more in response to that person's needs than to the patient's. The timing of the consultation in the course of the patient's hospitalization provides a good clue concerning the motivation of the referring physician and his expectations of the consultation. If the psychiatrist is asked to see a patient quickly and "get a note on the chart" because the patient is due to be discharged that day, it may be assumed that the physician requesting the consultation does not plan to make any serious use of the recommendations. A different attitude is reflected by the physician who asks for a psychiatric evaluation of a patient with ulcerative colitis at the time the patient is first admitted to the hospital. Further clues concerning the attitude of the physician requesting the consultation will be understood when the psychiatrist determines the way in which the patient has been prepared for the consultation and what the patient understands from his physician concerning the reasons for this request.

An inexperienced referring physician may ask the consultant how to inform the patient of the psychiatric consultation. Before offering a routine approach, the consultant might inquire about specific problems anticipated with this patient.

The hospital staff will often be divided over the decision to request psychiatric consultation; some members will feel that it is a useless or even dangerous undertaking. The motivations of those for and those against consultation must be understood, since on occasion, the staff members who are opposed to psychiatric consultation may be most allied with the patient. For example, the referring physician who wants the psychiatrist to transfer the drug addict off the ward may not allow him to interview the nice old lady who has carcinoma of the breast and is moderately depressed. Some physicians even hesitate to obtain psychiatric consultation for the patient who has made a serious suicide attempt.

PSYCHODYNAMIC FACTORS IN THE PATIENT

THE DIRECT IMPACT OF ILLNESS OR SURGERY ON AUTONOMOUS EGO FUNCTIONS

The direct effect of illness or surgery on the mental apparatus would be exemplified by the patient who develops a psychotic episode following open heart surgery. This delirium represents the interaction of great anxiety, physiological changes in the brain produced by illness and surgery, sensory monotony, and sleep deprivation in the intensive care unit. In the majority of postoperative syndromes, the precipitating stress involves threats to autonomous ego functions. Another example is the toxic psychosis in which there is direct impairment of brain function, as in renal or hepatic failure. Impairments of perception, performance, memory, communication, and so on threaten the integrity of the ego, with resulting transient psychosis.

PSYCHODYNAMIC REACTIONS TO ILLNESS OR SURGERY

A wide variety of emotional reactions are accompanied by anxiety or depression. Symptoms of psychogenic pain, dependency reactions, prolonged convalescence, drug dependence, or psychophysiological reactions may occur. A patient with a myocardial infarction might develop a depression as a result of his fear that he will become a chronic invalid, never to work again. This could be accompanied by fears that the least exertion might lead to death, or by a deep-seated conflict concerning the dependency gratification that is secondary to illness.

Preoperative syndromes occur most frequently as a result of the patient's fears, fantasies, or memories from the past that lead to certain anxiety-filled anticipations in relationship to surgery. Anxiety in this patient is intense and fails to respond to the usual reassurance, explanations, and sympathetic management. It is often related to family attitudes toward hospitals, physicians, and medical and surgical treatment. The patient's childhood experiences may have included frightening stories of doctors and hospitals as well as traumatic experiences.

On some occasions the loss of an important organ with symbolic significance can be sufficiently stressful to precipitate a postoperative syndrome. Examples would be a depression following a prostatectomy or a hysterectomy.

Serious illness poses a direct threat to infantile narcissism. It is this narcissistic injury that underlies many pathological reactions to sickness.

PSYCHODYNAMIC REACTIONS TO THE HOSPITAL ENVIRONMENT

These reactions are typified by the patient who threatens to sign out against medical advice or who refuses some medical or surgical procedure despite its obvious necessity. Another example is the patient who is uncooperative or disruptive of the ward routine. In attempting to understand this reaction, it is necessary to explore the interaction between the patient and staff. Not infrequently, some rigidity or hostility in a staff member that has been directed toward the patient will serve to trigger latent psychopathology in the patient, so that he becomes a management problem.

At times the patient may react to a doctor or nurse with behavior that is based upon his relation to an important figure in his past life. These reactions are facilitated by the regression that occurs in the hospital setting.

There are some patients who cannot tolerate confinement or restriction, and latent psychopathology will blossom under these circumstances. This process is further accelerated by the presence of physical disease, discomfort, unpleasant procedures, and other indignities associated with hospitalization.

Most patients accept hospitalization while they feel sick. However, as their illness improves, certain patients reach a point where they feel well but still must remain in the hospital. It is then that conflicts with authority or dependency problems are manifested. An example is the corporate executive with hepatitis who attempts to run his office from the hospital room. On the ward service, a similar patient might upset the staff with his overactivity.

In convalescent syndromes, the patient's symptoms continue to impair his functioning longer than is explicable on a purely physiological basis. These patients tend to regress and assume dependent-helpless postures while in the hospital. They are often seen as ideal patients by the hospital staff, cooperating in every way until it is time for them to begin doing more for themselves.

One of the most difficult convalescent syndromes is the patient whose dependency is manifested by addiction. This may involve not only narcotic medications, but other medications and nursing procedures as well. The patient's dramatization of his incapacity often provokes and alienates the staff as the process becomes more apparent. When the psychiatrist is called at this point, he finds the staff frustrated by the patient's unwillingness to cooperate with the treatment program. The patient, however, feels totally misunderstood and is overwhelmed by feelings of helplessness and resentment. The psychiatrist recognizes the patient's need to manipulate the hospital staff as he did his parents, playing one off against the other. The consultant can utilize his psychodynamic understanding of the origins of this behavior to enable the staff to adopt a more accepting attitude.

NORMAL RESPONSES TO ILLNESS

Hospitalization leads to regression, helplessness, and a dependent level of adaptation in almost all patients. With some it may further lead to depression if the patient is unable to allow his dependent needs to be gratified. Mild depression is a normal response to illness. In the confines of the hospital, the patient is not only deprived of close contact with loved ones and friends, but he loses the ego-enhancing effects of his normal life activities as well. In such situations, the consultant does not rush to recommend specific treatment for the depressive symptoms, but offers reassurance to both patient and doctor The most adaptive solution for the hospitalized patient is to maintain a desirable equilibrium between regression in the service of adaptation and continuing efforts at mastery. This patient cooperates with the doctor out of a desire to improve himself as quickly as possible, rather than complying with the physician in order to obtain further dependent care.

Management of the Interview

The ward consultation is particularly challenging because the psychiatrist is often unable to utilize one of his principle techniques: the interpretation of unconscious material. Many consultations are requested for the needs of the referring physician rather than those of the patient. It is inappropriate for the consultant to interpret these needs to the referring physician, even though the psychiatrist may quickly understand them. A discussion with the physician requesting the consultation is necessary prior to the interview with the patient. A review of the patient's chart with particular attention devoted to the nursing notes will provide valuable insights concerning the psychiatric problem. The consultant's relationship with the referring doctor is of crucial significance. The patient is his patient, and he is the person requesting help. The consultant may have to assume a therapeutic role in the patient's management, but only after discussion and agreement with the patient's primary physician. The insecure consultant may attempt to win the patient's allegiance away from the referring doctor.

The hospitalized patient is not receptive to interpretation of unconscious material during a time of physical illness. Even the healthiest patient regresses when he is incapacitated with a physical illness. This is not the time to attack already overburdened defenses; therefore, the psychiatrist must utilize his understanding of patient and staff problems to make non-interpretive interventions that are guided by psychodynamic principles.

In order to accomplish this, it is important that the psychiatrist establish his individual identity rather than adopt the role of a passive observer. His willingness to take an active role will permit the patient and the primary physician to perceive him as a helpful ally. One interview is rarely sufficient, and the psychiatrist should plan to see the patient two or more times. Some psychiatrists make a brief three- to five-minute visit prior to the consultation in order to introduce themselves to the patient.

THE OPENING PHASE

THE LACK OF PRIVACY

There are a number of situations in which the psychiatrist must conduct his interview without optimal conditions of privacy. Although this discussion concerns the lack of privacy when conducting an interview on a medical ward, the general principles apply to all situations in which privacy is not possible. The psychiatrist should make every attempt to provide as much privacy as is practical. He can move the patient into a visiting room, porch, or other area adjacent to the ward where it is possible to conduct a private interview. However, if the patient is not ambulatory or cannot be moved, it might be possible to ask the patient in the adjacent bed to move. In any event, by pulling the curtains around the bed, at least visual privacy will be achieved. The interviewer should sit close to the patient and speak softly so that as few people as possible will be able to overhear the conversation. If the patient seems reluctant to speak, the interviewer might comment on the lack of privacy and indicate that certain very personal topics can be postponed for a more opportune time.

The interviewer can prevent interruptions by introducing himself to the head nurse and explaining his request for privacy. Both the psychiatrist and the patient will reap dividends from the attention and consideration that the psychiatrist extends to the nursing staff. The nurses can provide the consultant with useful information and also give the patient additional nursing care.

ENGAGEMENT WITH THE INTERVIEWER

After reviewing the patient's chart and obtaining the maximal conditions of privacy for the interview, the psychiatrist may identify himself and then inquire whether the patient was expecting a psychiatrist and what the patient understood concerning the reason for the consultation. If the patient has been adequately and accurately informed of the reasons for the consultation, it is possible to continue with the interview. If not, the psychiatrist must inform the patient of the reason. The exact choice of words is particularly important when speaking to the patient who is a management problem. Tact is required on the part of the consultant so that he does not stimulate feelings of antagonism toward the patient's primary physician. For example, if the psychiatrist was called because the patient would not consent to a certain medical treatment or procedure, the psychiatrist would not say, "Your doctor called me because you refused to agree to a lumbar puncture." Instead, he would say, "Your doctor asked me to see you because you were concerned and upset about a lumbar puncture. He did not understand what was troubling you and thought that I might be able to help." In most situations the patient has faith and confidence in the referring doctor. If the consultant remembers that the patient is not his own patient, he will exercise particular care not to demonstrate his superior knowledge or make belittling implications concerning the referring physician.

A different situation is illustrated by the psychiatrist who was called to see a patient, a nurse, who suffered from a bizarre hemorrhagic illness secondary to deliberate ingestion of an anticoagulant. When the psychiatrist introduced himself, the patient promptly focused on her physical illness and resentfully protested that her internist had implied that she might be causing the condition herself. In this case, the laboratory evidence was conclusive so that the psychiatrist replied, "It is probably very difficult for Dr. Jones to discuss this situation with you calmly, since he is so intimately and personally involved. However, the laboratory studies have revealed that your condition has been produced through the ingestion of an anticoagulant." It is important in this special situation that the psychiatrist side with the patient and not with the hospital or the referring physician, thus allowing the patient to save face. He might continue by saying, "The fact that you treat yourself in this way means that there must be some serious difficulty in your life, and rather than get into a discussion about the medical details, let us try to understand what is really troubling you." The psychiatrist, furthermore, could emphasize the patient's right to be sick, but indicate that the illness must solve a problem in the patient's life.

The psychiatrist should attempt to determine the reason that the consultation was requested at this time during the patient's hospital course. In some cases he may find that there is no immediate precipitant, but that the hospital staff has noticed that the patient really has two concurrent illnesses: the medical illness and, in addition, schizophrenia or a serious character disorder. Often the patient's psychiatric illness has in no way interfered with the patient's medical or surgical management and the psychiatrist was merely called because of apprehension on the part of the referring physician when he recognized the psychiatric problem. If this patient has previously managed quite well without psychiatric assistance and is causing no problem in the hospital, it may be assumed that further psychiatric help is not indicated. The psychiatrist should not, at this time, attempt to convince the patient that he has a psychiatric problem and must seek treatment. He might, instead, support the patient by emphasizing the patient's ability to manage his own affairs quite well and then indicate that he will reassure the patient's physician that there is no cause for alarm. If the psychiatrist does feel that further help is indicated, he may suggest to the referring doctor that additional interviews be scheduled after the patient has recovered from his acute illness.

DEFENSIVE MANEUVERS MANIFESTED IN THE INTERVIEW

Most often the patient is relieved and pleased finally to find someone with whom he can discuss personal matters. He feels that everyone else is too busy or that his concerns are irrelevant to his physical problems. This eagerness to talk is sometimes confused with motivation to pursue psychotherapy following discharge from the hospital. The neophyte is surprised to learn that his "well-motivated" patient no longer wishes to see a psychiatrist after he has recovered.

Some hospitalized patients are more difficult to interview. The major defense mechanisms utilized by these patients are denial and regression. The patient who uses denial is characterized by his lack of motivation in seeking psychiatric consultation. He is unaware of any psychiatric problem. His regressive attitudes are most often manifested by helplessness and passive compliance with the medical staff. His approach to the psychiatric interviewer is essentially the same. He is willing to participate as a passive, compliant individual, although he really lacks motivation for such an interview. The willingness to participate without motivation conceals the defensive denial and the lack of awareness of emotional disturbance. If the psychiatrist appreciates that such attitudes are common, he is less likely to feel annoyed or impatient when confronted with an unmotivated patient.

Still another group of patients greet the psychiatrist angrily. Typically, this patient begins the interview with a statement such as, "I suppose Dr. Jones thinks the problem is all in my mind," or "I guess Dr. Jones thinks I'm just imagining these headaches." These responses indicate that the patient is not properly prepared for the consultation, which is not to say that the referring doctor neglected his duty. There are patients who are so fearful of psychiatry that even extraordinary efforts may be unsuccessful. Nevertheless, the psychiatrist has no choice but to make another attempt to alleviate these fears. In order to be more effective than the referring doctor, the psychiatrist must have a deeper understanding of the problem. In a sense, the patient is correct; he is a bit crazy, but not in the way he fears. This person has prominent paranoid character traits and consequently always anticipates rejection or criticism. Being referred to a psychiatrist is, in his mind, an indication of disapproval on the part of his physician. To the patient, the referral means that his doctor has given up on him. Reassurances that are directed to these issues are the most effective. The consultant could reply, "Oh, no! As a matter of fact, when Dr. Jones called me, I had the feeling that he is quite sympathetic toward you."

MODIFICATIONS OF THE INTERVIEW

THE DEFENSES AGAINST EXPOSURE OF THE CONFLICT

After the initial concentration on the reasons for consultation and a discussion of the patient's immediate experience in the hospital, his feelings about the ward, and so forth, the doctor can pursue some other aspects of the patient's functioning. This will begin with the patient's present illness, and then might shift to some neutral topic in which the patient has a particular interest or has had particular success in life. This support enhances the patient's self-esteem and will make it easier for the patient to then explore some of his less acceptable feelings concerning his illness and hospitalization. The psychiatrist can feel free to enter into such discussions with the patient and share his own knowledge and understanding of the areas in which the patient has particular interest and competence.

The psychiatrist may then discuss the patient's feelings about his illness and hospitalization and how these things have altered his life and will affect his future. He can also examine the effects of the patient's hospitalization on his family, as hospitalized patients frequently worry about how their relatives are managing at home. The psychiatrist should not challenge the denial and projection encountered at this time. The exploration of the patient's past history includes a detailed study of the patient's relationship with family and other important figures. For example, a patient whose usual attitude toward people is one of fear and mistrust will certainly manifest such attitudes toward other patients, hospital personnel, and the psychiatrist as well. The psychiatrist may also inquire about the supportive relationships in the patient's life, so that appropriate efforts may be made to re-establish them and to provide similar relationships during the hospitalization.

Patients with chronic disabling illnesses rarely express overt anxiety. They reveal discouraged feelings indirectly, such as expressing sympathy for the doctor who works so hard with such poor results. Such patients have protected themselves from the true psychological impact of illness through the use of denial and other defenses. The doctor, on the other hand, may feel overwhelmed by the helplessness and futility of the patient's severe organic disease or the possible threat of death. The patient may be reacting to a family conflict or other less serious problem with which the doctor can provide assistance rather than reacting to what the doctor imagines to be the most upsetting aspect of the patient's life. This provides the doctor with an opportunity to be useful to the patient and offer a sense of hope and a feeling that people are helping him to cope with his problems.

Some specific psychiatric syndromes may be recognized during hospital consultations. The patient with a passive-dependent or passive-aggressive character structure may initially appear to be unmotivated for help, but with persistence he may be engaged in a psychotherapeutic relationship. Severe family and social pathology, as characterized by complicated problems involving the courts or social agencies, a destructive or alcoholic husband or father, and so on, may overwhelm the psychiatrist with a feeling of helplessness and inability to contribute to the patient's management and welfare. The patient may have many mechanisms for coping with such situations that are not initially appreciated by the psychiatrist, and a minimal amount of intervention may allow the patient's precarious adaptive balance to readjust in the direction of adequate adaptation. The patient who has had a psychotic episode during a previous hospital experience may have difficulty remembering what happened or may seem confused concerning the past hospitalization. The consultant may utilize his awareness of this possibility to better understand the patient's present fears and adopt prophylactic measures against a recurrence.

Maintaining the Therapeutic Alliance

The psychiatrist attempts to establish the most appropriate doctor-patient relationship within the framework of the ward consultation. He will answer this patient's questions while he attempts to understand their deeper meaning. When the patient asks him about the nature of the illness or reveals confusion concerning the meaning of certain tests or procedures, he will attempt to clarify the patient's understanding of these issues. He may provide general information about medical procedures, but will direct questions concerning specific test results to the referring physician. He can suggest that the patient ask such questions of his doctor or may himself volunteer to communicate the patient's lack of understanding of these issues to the patient's other physician. In this way, the psychiatrist serves to facilitate communication between the patient and his primary doctor. In other situations, the psychiatrist might indicate that he will intervene in order to obtain appropriate social service assistance.

In instances in which the patient is angry with his physician and the hospital staff, it is important that the psychiatrist offer himself as the patient's ally and friend. This is accomplished by sympathizing with the patient's immediate and anticipated problems. A positive transference is encouraged by the consultant's recognition of areas of successful achievement in the patient's past life and discovery of healthy elements in the patient's present adaptation to the hospital. The psychiatrist increases the patient's hopes concerning the benefits of hospitalization and diminishes his fears and despair concerning his illness. Once the psychiatrist has obtained the patient's trust and confidence, he will attempt to repair the damaged relationship between the patient and the medical staff. The psychiatrist can feel free to do things for the patient which the patient is unable to do for himself. This might include arranging for a social worker to meet with the patient's spouse or handing the patient a glass of water. In helping the depressed patient, he may provide substitute gratification during the patient's time of critical need in the hospital. However, the psychiatrist must beware of promising more than he can realistically deliver, as he will ultimately disappoint the patient.

INTERPRETATION OF THE DEFENSIVE PATTERN

The psychiatrist will utilize his knowledge of psychodynamics in conducting the ward consultation as much as with any other patient; however, he will use it in a different way. The basic technique of the ward consultation is non-interpretive, psychodynamically oriented intervention. For example, the psychiatrist may recommend additional attention from a female figure of authority such as a ward nurse for a patient who is responding to a feeling of maternal deprivation. On some occasions, the psychiatrist may interpret an obvious conflict that is interfering with the patient's ability to cooperate with the treatment program.

Under special circumstances, humor provides a mode of gentle interpretation of otherwise painful material. Most opportunities for the utilization of humor arise from some factor that the psychiatrist and patient have in common, such as a similar ethnic background, or shared interest.

Sometimes it is possible to help the patient achieve more insight into his problem through the use of some anecdote or story that does not directly involve the patient but allows the patient to extract the principle and apply it to himself.

At times it is necessary for the physician to interpret the patient's emotional response as inappropriate to the current situation. This is best done when the source of the patient's inappropriate emotional reaction is quite clear to the psychiatrist and can be interpreted to the patient.

On some occasions the psychiatrist is required to take a very firm stand, based upon his understanding of the patient's defensive behavior, but without interpreting the defenses to the patient. This occurred with a phobic woman of 50 who had an advanced carcinoma of the breast and refused surgery. The surgeon was aware that the patient dreaded cancer and had phobicly avoided treatment for two years following the discovery of the lump in her breast. Sensing the patient's terror of death, he had not told the patient the diagnosis. The psychiatrist, half-way through the initial interview, advised the patient that her lesion could turn to cancer at any time and that it was imperative that she have surgery immediately if her life were to be saved. A similar example concerned an older man with severe congestive heart failure. This patient wished to sign out of the hospital although he was advised that he would most likely die. The psychiatrist interpreted the patient's suicidal intentions to him and to his closest relatives and then worked with this patient just as he would with any other suicidal patient.

The patient who becomes depressed following a hysterectomy should be reassured that the operation has in no way impaired her femininity and that her monthly cycles, ovulation, and ovarian function will continue unchanged until her natural menopause. She may be given direct reassurance concerning fears of weight gain, loss of libido, and so forth. In treating the man who develops a depression following a permanent colostomy, the psychiatrist understands that early experiences concerning the control of the bowels are contributory to such a reaction, and uses this knowledge in his interventions. Rather than pointing out the patient's fear of the consequences of loss of control of bowel function, he emphasizes the patient's ability to control the bowel function through the colostomy, and stresses that the patient can regulate his bowels himself. He may liken the patient's feeling of social unacceptability to other situations from the patient's past when the patient initially felt unacceptable but later learned to overcome these feelings.

In working with the patient who expresses exaggerated feelings of helplessness and dependency, the psychiatrist should search for the patient's desire to do more things for himself. The patient may be praised and rewarded for this desire rather than criticized for his inability to strengthen such desires on his own. Indicating to the patient that everyone experiences feelings of helplessness may reduce his unconscious guilt and actually strengthen his sense of independence. If the patient has had a protracted hospital course, the psychiatrist will, of necessity, interpret the patient's fears concerning his return home. It may be necessary to intervene with the patient's relatives, thereby assisting the patient in coping with the home environment following his discharge from the hospital. The psychiatrist can help the patient distinguish remote or unlikely fears from the more plausible and factual aspects of the situation.

THE CLOSING PHASE

The goals of psychiatric intervention during the patient's hospitalization are limited. Ambitious plans concerning personality reconstruction are not appropriate at this time. A psychodynamically oriented plan of intervention can facilitate medical or surgical management. The psychiatrist may communicate to the patient in general terms what he has learned as a result of his consultation. Before terminating the interview, he could indicate to the patient that there will be another meeting and make a definite appointment if possible. If indicated, he should obtain the patient's permission to speak with a relative who is involved. When inappropriate behavior on the part of the medical staff has contributed to the patient's problem, the psychiatrist can indicate his awareness of these factors to the patient before terminating the interview. The patient's physical condition may necessitate a briefer interview than is the customary practice of the psychiatrist. Several short interviews at frequent intervals may be preferable in helping this patient.

The ward psychiatrist is often asked to arrange the involuntary hospitalization of a patient. Forced hospitalization is to the psychiatrist as litigation is to the attorney—a course of action to be pursued after all other means of negotiation have failed. It is the psychiatrists' court of last resort. However, other measures for dealing with seriously disturbed patients require a considerable amount of time and human resources. It is far easier to sign the papers and have the patient "shipped off" to a state hospital. When this action is unavoidable, the consulting psychiatrist can be helpful not only to the referring physician but to the patient and his family as well. The psychiatrist can make commitment a much less traumatic procedure by spending some extra time and showing sensitivity to the patient's and his relatives' fears.

Finally, the consultation cannot be considered complete until the psychiatrist has written a chart note and met with the referring physician to discuss his findings. The note should be brief and should include observations, conclusions, and treatment recommendations. The personal conversation could include an elucidation of the patient's problems, a description of the immediate precipitants, and further discussion of therapeutic recommendations to help the referring physician and the patient cope with the situation. A more detailed formulation of the patient's life-long developmental psychodynamics might be included, depending on the degree of interest shown by the referring physician.

REFERENCES

See reference list following Chapter 11.

13 THE PSYCHOLOGICALLY UNSOPHISTICATED PATIENT

Psychopathology and Psychodynamics

Certain patients seem to be psychologically constricted and uninteresting. The beginning interviewer prefers patients who think introspectively, describe themselves and others in terms of motives and feelings, and display insight. The constricted patients may have nothing at all to say, and, if they do, they talk in terms of actions or events. When they describe a person, it is chiefly by his physical or occupational characteristics. Denial, projection, externalization, and inhibition of assertion and curiosity are major defenses.

In some of these patients, a genuine constriction of personality is a manifestation of individual psychopathology. This patient is inhibited, even if viewed in the framework of his social and cultural background. In others, an apparent constriction of the personality is the product of social distance between the doctor and the patient. This person would not be viewed as constricted by the standards of those from his own environment. This group includes many from the lower socioeconomic group as well as others who are middle class by economic standards. For example, many skilled laborers or independent farmers, in spite of their middle class incomes, do not think in psychological terms and rarely consult a psychiatrist.

DESCRIPTION OF THE PROBLEM

It is important that the interviewer differentiate between patients who are really constricted and those whose cultural background makes it difficult to relate in the manner to which the psychiatrist is accustomed.

The truly constricted patient will have difficulty relating and expressing himself on any topic, including those with which he has the greatest familiarity. He has few interests and generates little enthusiasm. Diagnostically, these patients are predominantly schizophrenic or have severe character disorders.

The culturally constricted patient will not seem constricted when he is discussing subjects with which he is familiar and comfortable. He will express enthusiasm in his areas of individual interest, although these may be foreign to the interviewer. It is this difference in background that creates the illusion of constriction. There are, of course, a number of lower class patients who are constricted on the basis of both their deprived cultural background and their individual psychodynamics.

The interviewer often reacts to the unsophisticated patient with boredom or disinterest. This response is surprising in an individual who is interested in people and has an opportunity to study someone different from himself. It stems from a defensive withdrawal secondary to the social distance between the doctor and the patient. This response changes with an increased knowledge of psychodynamics and interviewing skill. The patient's lack of familiarity with introspection often provides a unique opportunity for the testing of psychodynamic hypotheses without the contamination produced by educational exposure to psychological information. Dramatic responses to specific interpretations with accompanying relief of symptoms may occur. The psychodynamic derivatives of normal development—e.g., dependency conflicts, sibling rivalry, castration anxiety, and Oedipal conflicts—are often revealed with great clarity during the interview.

In recent years, the psychiatric literature has contained an increasing number of articles concerning problems of interviewing lower class patients. The observation has been made that these patients often drop out of therapy after one or perhaps two initial interviews. This is sometimes a response to their dissatisfaction with the traditionally conducted psychiatric interview. Not only is the model of the traditional psychiatric interview poorly suited to the lower class patient, but the inexperienced interviewer is frequently unfamiliar with the vastly different background of his patient. Other patients feel that their difficulties have been alleviated after one or two interviews that the doctor considered diagnostic. The opportunity to ventilate their feelings provides dramatic relief.

The most common forms of psychopathology leading to a request for psychiatric intervention include psychotic disturbances, psychophysiological disorders, and characterological problems such as alcoholism, drug addiction, and sexual disturbances. Psychoneurotic reactions are common; however, they seldom motivate these patients to seek psychiatric help. For the person who is poor, unhappiness seems to stem from physical hardship directly relating to his poverty. Often it is only after a person becomes more affluent that he discovers the existence of personal problems within himself that are not solved by the acquisition of more material goods.

The moral and social values of this patient's society differ from those of the middle class patient. This leads to the development of styles of thinking different from those of the middle and upper classes. There is less value placed on intellectualization and intellectual achievement, which sometimes causes the interviewer to grossly misjudge the patient's intelligence. He is not introspective and does not consider the subtleties of his emotional life important. He does not think that talk can be helpful in the solution of his problems, but is more concerned with action, and therefore desires direct advice as to what he should *do*. His anti-intellectual attitudes are reflected in his lack of interest and knowledge concerning world and national affairs. He avoids philosophical discussions and he is interested in ideas only for their practical value. He is not accustomed to describing his feelings about others, particularly to strangers, nor is he inclined to reveal highly personal material about himself. Physical activity is an important aspect of his life. Success in his job requires strength and endurance, and his recreational interests center around sports in which, again, physical prowess is the chief evidence of masculinity. Gambling is another frequent pastime.

Women from the lower classes tend to assume a more maternal attitude toward their husbands. Much of their time is taken up having children and taking them to clinics as well as visiting a variety of service agencies. The wife manages the home, raises the children, handles the finances and, if she is able, holds a part-time job. In contrast to the middle class stereotype of sexual freedom among the poor, many of the women tend toward rigid sexual morality and are often inhibited in their sexual behavior.

Patients from this group tend to blame the outside world rather than themselves for their misfortunes and unhappiness. The tendency to externalize responsibility frequently influences the interviewer to consider this patient a poor candidate for insight-oriented psychotherapy. The patient whose constriction is based upon severe psychopathology, such as a borderline mental defective with schizophrenia, may require a different psychotherapeutic approach.

The differences between the various ethnic groups in the lower classes are often more prominent than the similarities.* For example, the typical Italian family is strongly cohesive. The Negro family often consists of a woman living with her children and possibly her own mother, as her husband has responded to the frustrations and humiliations of the white world by a pattern of wandering and irresponsibility.

THE SPANISH-SPEAKING LOWER CLASS PATIENT

There is a subgroup of people who, in addition to the usual problems of the lower classes, have unique problems of their own. This group includes a large number of persons who have migrated to the United States from Puerto Rico, Cuba, and Mexico. The majority live in the ghettos of large cities and suffer from cultural isolation, deprivation, and rejection as well as

---

* This work was done by Dr. Gladys Egri of the staff of the Vanderbilt Clinic, Department of Psychiatry, Columbia University.

poverty. Although many have been in the United States for substantial periods of time, they often have not learned to speak English.

In Puerto Rico, English is a mandatory subject in the schools from the first grade through high school. Since this is not the case in Cuba and Mexico, it is less indicative of pathology if individuals from those countries do not speak English after a brief period in the United States. The inability to master a new language is often due to a learning difficulty in a person whose personality constriction and poor psychological integration impair his adaptive capacity.

Family psychodynamics also influence the migrants' refusal to learn the new language. The children learn English in school and quickly assimilate the new cultural values. A power struggle soon develops between the generations as the parents seek to shape the development of their offspring. Their unwillingness to learn English is only part of the parents' greater struggle to maintain their identity through the preservation of their traditional ways. One study of patients who showed an unwillingness to learn English revealed that many have difficulty communicating adequately in their native language. They were mistrustful, not only of English-speaking doctors, but of Spanish-speaking doctors as well. Paranoid tendencies were common. Another group initially claimed to speak only Spanish, but later, when a trusting relationship with the doctor developed, revealed that they were also able to speak some English. Certain patients utilized their alleged inability to speak English as a passive-aggressive technique in dealing with the establishment. This was particularly prominent in dealing with welfare investigators, truant officers, and officials of that sort.

The predominant psychopathology of lower class Puerto Rican migrants includes narcotic addiction, sexual disturbances, paranoid schizophrenia, severe depressive and phobic reactions, conversion reactions, and hypochondriasis.

In order to understand the psychodynamics of the individual, one must first understand his cultural situation. The Cuban or Mexican patient has often lived in a rural culture and is poorly educated. The Puerto Rican patient is more likely to have had an urban background. The migrant quickly learns that he is unwanted in the new city. He has beliefs and values that were

accepted and normal in his old country, but that create difficulties in the new environment. For example, it is common for
the lower class Puerto Rican, Cuban, or Mexican patient to feel
that his trouble has been caused by evil spirits. Such a belief
not only complicates the problem of diagnosis, but also colors
the patient's expectations and motivations in seeking help. The
interviewer should not dispute the patient's belief in evil spirits
in general, but should advise him instead that his immediate
problem is not caused by evil spirits. The patient may already
have consulted a spiritualist practitioner who has given the patient conflicting advice. The interviewer should not attempt to
debunk this practitioner, but merely indicate the disagreement
and support any evidence the patient has offered that corroborates
the physician's opinion. If the patient had been satisfied with the
spiritualist consultation, he would not be seeing the physician.

In the new environment, the patient's traditional beliefs
emphasize his difference and increase his social isolation. Slowly,
he adopts some of the goals and values of the new culture. Many
of these are in conflict with his background, and this leads to
confusion. Despite his shift toward the new values, he learns
that he is still excluded from equal participation in important
areas of life. He is sent to inferior schools; he is treated unfairly
in seeking employment or joining a labor union; and he is even
discriminated against in clinics and by the professional staffs of
hospitals. This rejection is based both on his lower class status
and his inability to speak English. An examination of the clinic
waiting lists in New York reveals an inordinately high proportion of Spanish-speaking patients. Most physicians require the
services of an interpreter in interviewing these patients. Chapter
16 discusses the techniques involved in this situation. In the
preparation of that chapter, the authors failed to uncover a single
article in the American psychiatric literature on the subject of
interviewing through an interpreter. This is further evidence of
the rejection of this group of patients by the medical profession.

Not only does the patient suffer the direct effects of rejection
by important social institutions, but his attempts to measure himself by the standards of his new culture further dramatize his
sense of inadequacy and adaptive failure. Although he experiences
an internal pressure to conform to the social and moral codes of
this culture, he soon finds that such conformity does not bring
the desired rewards. In his frustration, he is likely to resort to

behavior patterns that are considered disturbed and deviant by the dominant culture. Some persons withdraw into themselves, abandoning all hope of gratification, but others direct their resentment outward through defiance of prevalent community standards, hoping to obtain immediate gratification of impulses. They have learned that the development and pursuit of long-range goals only leads to increased frustration.

The more fortunate person, who is successful in his new identity, moves up in the culture only to encounter different problems. He is likely to feel rejection and contempt toward the characteristics of his group of origin, i.e., skin color, dress, mannerisms, and speech patterns. For example, he is likely to develop disdain for those with a skin color darker than his own. Unconsciously, he experiences a deep sense of guilt and alienation from his family, and even from himself, for leaving behind the others who were less successful.

Management of the Interview

The psychologically unsophisticated patient is not a single clinical entity. The methods of interviewing discussed in this chapter will be applicable to many, but not all, of this group of patients. If the interviewer develops a stereotyped approach to lower class patients, he will grossly mismanage interviews with those who have developed middle class values and attitudes. There are also a number of middle or upper class patients who should be interviewed in a manner that is ordinarily associated with the lower class patient. The criteria discussed earlier in this chapter together with the patient's socioeconomic status will determine which approach is appropriate.

Much of the material from Chapter 14 has application in the interview with the unsophisticated patient.

THE OPENING PHASE

As with most other patients, the interview begins with an exploration of the patient's chief complaint; however, this patient will often say that he has no complaint, or that he came to the hospital because someone sent him. The interviewer can respond by asking who sent the patient and why this person felt that psychiatric help was indicated. The interview should proceed with a discussion of whatever material the patient offers, whether or not it seems immediately relevant to the patient's major problem. For example, the patient may refer to previous episodes of emotional difficulty or may indicate that he has recently quit his job, dropped out of school, separated from his spouse, or made some other change in his pattern of living. At an appropriate point, the interviewer can ask if such experiences have made the patient nervous. The term "nervous" is particularly useful as it circumvents the patient's denial of emotional problems.

The interview with this patient is characterized by its sparseness. The patient volunteers little and his answers to the physician's questions are very brief. The interviewer feels that he is doing all the work and soon resents the patient for being so difficult to interview. The physician expresses his resentment by becoming less interested in the patient as the interview progresses, and he is inclined to dismiss the patient early. On the other hand, too great a show of warmth or too much personal interest will cause some of these patients to discontinue treatment. This is particularly true when the psychological constriction occurs in a schizophrenic patient.

The patient is not accustomed to discussing his feelings about friends and relatives with anyone, and particularly not with a stranger. Therefore, in the initial portion of the interview, concrete questions will usually produce more material than open-ended ones. For example, the interviewer should not say, "Describe your parents," but should instead ask, "What kind of work does your father do?" The interviewer might then inquire whether the patient's mother works as well. He could ask practical questions concerning their interests and hobbies and what they do for recreation rather than asking, "What are they like?"

Early in the interview, some approximate determination should be made concerning the patient's intelligence. The interviewer should be careful that he neither talks down to the patient nor talks above his capacity to understand. Any comments offered by the patient that emphasize the social distance between the patient and the interviewer should immediately be explored in an open manner.

Inexperienced interviewers mistakenly assume that their interview is going badly when this patient fails to produce material containing psychological insights. They become frustrated and annoyed with the patient, as though he were deliberately interfering with the conduct of the interview. This response is less probable if the physician realizes that he is working with a constricted patient who is unable to participate in an introspective discussion. Prolonged silences tend to become awkward, increasing the distance between patient and interviewer. They are to be avoided, particularly in the initial interview, although brief pauses are to be expected while the patient or interviewer collects his thoughts.

MODIFICATION OF THE INTERVIEW

Mutuality of the expectations of patient and therapist is the crucial factor determining the success or failure of the interview. When the interviewer directs the discussion toward the patient's expectations, this patient responds by discussing the basis for his suffering in terms of external reality. For example, he may even inform the doctor that he has come to the clinic to enlist the physician's help so that he might obtain a larger apartment through the welfare department. Because the lower class patient's expectations of therapy are incongruous with those of the physician, it is essential that the interviewer adopt a flexible and active approach in conducting the initial interview.

Treatment must be modified in order to meet the patient's expectations. Direct answers to the patient's questions, practical help with environmental problems, and medication all facilitate the development of a trusting relationship. The physician can gradually explain the manner in which the patient is expected to participate and at the same time define his own role. He should point out that the patient can be helped but that change requires time and that he has no magical cures. He can introduce the concept that talk constitutes work in psychotherapy, particularly talk that is accompanied by an expression of the patient's emotions. The patient needs help with his belief that having critical feelings about his family indicates that he does not love and respect them. As the therapy progresses, the patient will be able to accept a less structured interview.

If the therapist adjusts his conceptual framework to that of his patient, he will avoid the use of analogies that would be foreign to the patient's experience. He may expect less fantasy material, since this patient does not allow himself much freedom of imagination. The therapist will be more responsive to the patient's needs if he does not concentrate on past developmental material in the first interview, but instead aims for simple insights related to the patient's current life situation.

The beginning therapist is generally reluctant to interview the person who initially indicates no desire to be a patient. This individual may have a great desire to receive treatment. Since the therapist tends to avoid the constricted patient, he is only too eager to accept a verbal denial of motivation. It is only natural for someone unfamiliar with introspective thinking, unaccustomed to close interpersonal relations, and burdened with many reality problems to resist asking for psychotherapy. His initial demand may concern drugs or environmental manipulation. The physician can offer a considerable degree of help in these areas, and by so doing can make a substantial contribution. He will have to assume a directive role and may have to give practical advice. Early in treatment, intellectual interpretations based upon psychodynamic reconstructions of the past offer little help. They generally lead to frustration in the therapist and alienation from the patient.

It is important that the physician assume an authoritative and self-confident position. The patient must feel that the physician has answers to his problem rather than that the patient is expected to provide his own answers. Praise, disapproval, and direct reassurance should be used whenever appropriate in helping the patient to better cope with his environment. The longer the physician works with this patient, the more the patient can gradually accept increased responsibility for his involvement in treatment.

The tendency to reject such patients is not entirely the fault of the physician. Most training programs offer little individual supervision on the management of this type of patient and instead concentrate teaching on more analytically oriented psychotherapy. When the constricted patient is mentioned to a supervisor, it is likely that the supervisor will accept the student's statement that the patient cannot be helped.

THE CLOSING PHASE

Before terminating the interview, the therapist should establish definite arrangements for a second appointment, rather than asking the patient when he wants to return or saying that he will contact him. By now the patient has revealed his conscious doubts and reservations concerning treatment; he has discussed his expectations, his own view of his problem, and the help he is hoping to receive. A few minutes should be allowed for the patient to raise additional questions. Finally, the physician can make a brief statement to the patient, formulating the problems in simple terms as the physician understands them and, at the same time, outlining a practical approach to treatment.

The therapist assumes an active role in reaching out to the unsophisticated patient so that understanding may be achieved at whatever level the patient's capabilities permit. This does not mean that he limits his interventions to advising, reassuring, cajoling, lecturing, and so on. The therapist utilizes his knowledge of the role of unconscious processes in the formation of symptoms just as much with this patient as with any other. Ultimately, the same unconscious psychodynamic conflicts must be worked through in order to resolve the patient's symptoms. The preliminary active interventions strengthen the patient's ego and coping mechanisms and enable him to accept interpretations of inner conflicts.

REFERENCES

Baum, O. E., and Felzer, S. B.: Activity in initial interviews with lower-class patients. Arch. Gen. Psychiat., *10:*345, 1964.
Behrens, M. I.: Brief home visits by the clinic therapist in the treatment of lower class patients. Amer. J. Psychiat., *124:*371, 1967.
Glazer, N., and Moynihan, D. P.: Beyond the Melting Pot; the Negroes, Puerto Ricans, Jews, Italians, and Irish of New York City. Cambridge, Mass., M.I.T. Press, 1963.
Hollingshead, A. B., and Redlich, F. C.: Social Class and Mental Illness. New York, John Wiley & Sons, Inc., 1958.
Sifneos, P. E.: Two different kinds of psychotherapy of short duration. Amer. J. Psychiat., *123:*1069, 1967.

14 THE EMERGENCY PATIENT

Psychopathology and Psychodynamics

A psychiatric problem becomes an emergency when some person's anxiety has increased to the point that immediate aid is requested. The phrase "psychiatric emergency" does not define a single clinical situation, as many different types of patients may be interviewed under emergency conditions. A person may experience anxiety himself and seek help, or he may elicit anxiety in a partner who labels the situation an emergency and seeks assistance for the patient.

Previous chapters have emphasized the artificiality of boundaries between initial diagnostic and later treatment interviews. This is particularly true in emergency situations, in which therapy begins with the patient's awareness of the availability of treatment.

In all emergency situations—psychiatric, civil, military, and others—people do not know what to do. The doctor's most important function is to project the feeling that he knows what *he* can do, and to assist the patient and those who accompany him in developing a clear notion of what *they* can do. These role definitions convert the emergency into a problem, and allow the individuals involved to employ their own adaptive skills in

401

mobilizing the resources of their environment. The patient is not always the doctor's ally in this endeavor. If he is convinced that he is helpless and unable to cope with his problems, he may actually conceal his own resources in an attempt to make the doctor take care of him. After the emergency has subsided, it is not uncommon to find that the patient failed to mention a close relative, a supply of funds, or a contingency plan that could have been invoked if the doctor had failed him.

The sense of urgency that permeates every emergency is analogous to pathological anxiety in other situations: It impairs effective adaptive behavior and efficient utilization of resources. The physician's task is to avoid being overwhelmed by this urgency, thereby reducing its impact upon his patient. His most important tool is the aura of competent self-assurance that he maintains throughout the interview. The doctor should convey the feeling that he is interested and is capable of assisting the patient with his problem. This professional approach together with the early definition of roles reduces the disorganizing effects of the crisis and establishes a firm basis for treatment.

Psychiatric emergencies can best be understood by first classifying them according to three basic categories of presenting symptoms: intra-psychic, somatic, and interpersonal. A classification based on these three modes of presentation is initially more useful than the traditional diagnostic categories, since emergencies frequently require decisions and action before a diagnostic evaluation can be completed.

A central question in the psychodynamic evaluation of any crisis is, "Why did it occur now?" What has happened in the patient's life to disrupt his previous functioning? An understanding of the stress that altered the patient's psychological equilibrium and led to the presenting symptom is a critical step in managing the emergency. The precipitating stress may activate psychological conflicts directly, or it may operate at a physiological level, impairing the autonomous and executive functions of the ego. In either case, the individual will respond with characteristic patterns determined by his basic personality structure. Some individuals are crisis-prone and frequently respond to stress with an emergency syndrome; others bind their anxiety more effectively and rarely experience crises.

The patient arrives not only with (1) a presenting symptom

and (2) a precipitating stress, but also with (3) certain expectations concerning the treatment he will receive. These three factors determine the physician's approach to the emergency interview.

INTRA-PSYCHIC PROBLEMS

The most common intra-psychic problems are depression, anxiety, and confusion.

DEPRESSION

The patient's depression may stimulate anxiety either in himself or in a friend or loved one. The psychodynamics of depression have been discussed previously. It commonly results from the real or imagined loss of love and the lowering of self-confidence and self-esteem. The emergency aspects of depression frequently develop from the possibility of suicide. This danger must be explored with every depressed individual, whether or not the patient introduces the subject himself. The discussion of suicidal thoughts and feelings as a route to increased understanding of the depressed person is dealt with in Chapter 6. The evaluation of suicidal risk in the emergency interview is described below.

An acute grief reaction, the normal response to the death of a loved one, may present a picture that is quite similar to depression. The sadness and pain of grief, together with crying spells and insomnia, also bring individuals to seek emergency psychiatric help. The grief-stricken patient should be supported and given an opportunity for ventilation of his feelings. He should be encouraged to accept help from others, to take medication if he has difficulty sleeping, and to rely upon friends and loved ones. Above all, the interviewer makes it clear that the patient's response is normal and healthy, that it will end in a short time, and that he will then be able to resume his normal role. Regressive desires and dependent needs are supported and gratified during the acute stress, and the patient is helped to work through the grieving process by being allowed to discuss his loss and express his sadness.

ANXIETY

Anxiety, the emotional response to danger, is a cardinal feature of any psychiatric emergency. When it occurs in the patient, it may be the major presenting complaint. In emergency situations, this usually occurs when: (1) an event in the patient's current life reawakens fears that have lain dormant in his unconscious, or (2) the patient feels that his ability to control sexual or aggressive impulses is threatened and he fears the consequences. He is rarely aware of the specific fear that has been aroused; instead, he feels an overwhelming sense of dread or panic. A common clinical example is the adolescent boy who leaves home for college and is asked to share a room with another boy for the first time in his life. Homosexual feelings become increasingly difficult to repress, and when he is under the influence of alcohol, his defenses are further weakened and he begins to panic. Another typical emergency room problem is the woman who becomes increasingly resentful of the burden of caring for her newborn infant. She becomes terrified that she will accidentally injure the baby, stick him with a pin, or drown him in the bath. Some patients will become aware of the feared impulses, as the adolescent in sexual panic, but more often these impulses are denied, as in the postpartum woman, or projected, as in the boy who responds to his homosexual feelings by fearing that his roommate will attack him. In each of these situations, the balance between the patient's drives and his ego defenses has been disturbed, resulting in an acute increase in anxiety, which may be accompanied by new defenses.

Anxiety over the possible loss of control may disturb either the patient or significant figures in his environment, depending upon (1) whether the impulses involved are primarily transgressions against his inner standards or social mores, and (2) whether it is he himself or others who feel that it is likely he will act upon them. Both of the examples given above are of patients who fear that they will act on impulses that they themselves consider repugnant. The parents of the adolescent girl who bring her to the hospital because she has threatened to run away with her boyfriend, and the woman who brings her alcoholic husband because she fears that he may injure their children in one of his drunken rages are examples of emerging impulses that disturb the patient's partner rather than the patient himself.

Surgical procedures and other physical threats to the body are a common precipitant of exaggerated anxiety because they symbolically reactivate primitive fears of bodily damage. Academic examinations may represent more abstract symbols of the same type of danger. The therapist must understand the relationship of the anxiety to the unconscious imagined danger, since the patient will focus on the realistic threat to his safety and simple reassurances directed to this end will have little effect.

Anxiety leads to neurotic symptom formation in some patients. They may present with acute anxiety attacks, phobic or conversion reactions, or the hyperventilation syndrome. These patients usually request help themselves, although others may be involved before they reach the physician. The psychotic individual may respond to anxiety by fears of ego disintegration and of gross disorganization. This patient is often unable to seek aid himself, and he may provoke others to define the situation as a psychiatric emergency.

Confusion

The confused patient may not know where he is or how he got there. He has difficulty communicating intelligibly and his thought processes are fragmented and disorganized. He feels that his senses are unreliable and may misinterpret sights and sounds in strange ways. Anxiety and depression usually result from stresses that threaten the psychological defenses of the ego. They indicate difficulty in resolving conflicts, controlling impulses, and maintaining dependency gratification. Confusion, on the other hand, relates to those areas of ego functioning that are usually immune from psychological conflicts. These autonomous or conflict-free functions of the ego include memory, perception, and learning. They are impaired in organic mental syndromes and some acute functional psychoses. The patient is confused and bewildered. He is either frightened or so helpless that others are concerned about him and often he passes through these two stages sequentially.

The acute precipitant of the emergency may be an event that did not directly impair autonomous ego functioning, but that instead placed new or increased demands upon an already damaged ego. The move to a new apartment, with the many adaptive tasks it entails, can precipitate an acute psychiatric crisis in an old and slightly brain damaged person. He is unable to find the bathroom, forgets the location of the phone, misses his familiar neighbors, and becomes agitated and frightened. His poor memory and impaired spatial thinking were adequate for a familiar environment, but are not for a new one. The interviewer must seek information pertaining to practical aspects of the patient's current life in order to evaluate what skills he needs and what type of assistance would allow him to utilize his remaining abilities most effectively. It may be quite unimportant whether an elderly man living alone knows the month and year or the name of the President, but it is crucial whether he remembers to turn off the gas or is able to find the grocery store.

This patient will usually be brought to the doctor by another person who is anxious to prevent the patient from acting irrationally or harming himself. Although the psychopathology is intra-psychic, the definition of the emergency and the plans for treatment involve interpersonal dynamics. A common error is to accurately diagnose the underlying illness (usually an organic psychosis) and to make appropriate recommendations, only to have the treatment plan fail because the needs and expectations of the emergency partner have been ignored.

SOMATIC PROBLEMS

Somatic symptoms that are based on psychological causes are easier to treat when the patient is aware of this relationship, or at least is aware of concomitant psychological problems. Unfortunately, in emergency situations this is seldom the case. The interviewer may quickly determine that the somatic complaint is only a symptomatic manifestation of an underlying psychological difficulty, and he may focus the interview on the patient's emotional conflicts. However, at the end of what he thought was a successful interview, the patient may surprise him by asking, "But what about the pain in my chest?" Such experiences demonstrate that somatic symptoms must be treated as seriously and explored as thoroughly as any other psychological symptoms.

The patient whose symptoms include the somatic manifestations of anxiety, hyperventilation syndrome, or depression is most likely to acknowledge the existence of emotional problems.

Other psychiatric patients who complain of somatic problems will resist the suggestion of psychological conflict. Hypochondriasis, somatic delusions, conversion reactions, hysterical elaboration of physical symptoms, and psychophysiological reactions are usually not perceived by the patient as stemming from psychological conflicts. They are only seen as psychiatric emergencies when some other person feels that the problem is urgent and defines it as psychiatric.

Somatic symptoms are often associated with extensive denial of emotional problems, and therefore the patient is resistant to seeing a psychiatrist. He fears that the doctor will tell him that the problem is in his mind and will ignore his serious physical symptom. This is further complicated if the referring individual or emergency partner is a physician or member of the health profession. Again, the symptom must be taken seriously, discussed in detail, and explored with the patient. It is not sufficient to ascertain from a hospital chart that the referring physician performed a complete physical examination. Usually, if such an examination reassures the patient, he is not referred to the psychiatrist. Furthermore, the precise details of the physical symptoms and their course are an important source of information about the psychological problems.

INTERPERSONAL PROBLEMS

Interpersonal problems frequently involve one individual complaining about the behavior of another—the wife whose husband is alcoholic, the adolescent boy who threatens to leave home, or the psychotically excited man who is brought by the police. These situations are furthest removed from the traditional medical doctor-patient model, and therefore are often difficult for beginning physicians. It is important to search for appropriate psychodynamic points of intervention rather than to become a judge or referee. When the patient is psychotic, this may be easier, but when the major pathology is a character disorder, it may take some time to identify what the psychiatric problem is and which person (or persons) is best considered the patient.

A patient may be brought to the psychiatrist by someone

else because he is unable to recognize his own problems. The most obvious examples would be the very young or the very old—the child with uncontrolled temper tantrums whose parents frantically ask for guidance, or the elderly confused man, brought by his family because he has been wandering aimlessly in the streets.

Whenever one person brings another—that is, whenever an emergency partner is involved—there is an interpersonal problem in the emergency situation, even if the basic psychopathology is intra-psychic.

THE FOCUS ON THE PRESENT

Psychodynamic formulations rely heavily on developmental material, understanding the patient's conflicts through relating them to his early experiences and his habitual modes of coping and relating. In an emergency, the patient's attention is directed to his current crisis, and time is usually limited. Therefore, it is necessary to focus on his means of coping with *this* stress, his feelings and conflicts *now*. One must construct a formulation of the acute crisis rather than of the lifelong personality pattern. After the emergency has subsided, more developmental material can be obtained and a more complete psychodynamic explanation attempted. It is an error to concentrate on obtaining childhood historical material from a person in panic—the focus of inquiry must always be on that which is immediately emotionally meaningful to the patient.

It is important to determine early in the interview which symptoms are acute and which have been present for a considerable time. More recent symptoms are more easily understood and provide clues to the problems and conflicts involved in converting a chronic problem or life style into an acute crisis.

Management of the Interview

Emergencies seldom occur at convenient times or in convenient places. In spite of this, the traditional amenities of the interview should be maintained as far as possible. These include a quiet, comfortable place to sit and talk without a sense of rush, a cigarette and ashtray if the patient smokes, and a minimal number of interruptions.

The emergency interview invariably requires more time than the beginner anticipates. He should realize that the most experienced psychiatrist often devotes several hours to such problems. Otherwise, he will become dissatisfied with his own performance and annoyed with the patient. Furthermore, these patients are often unable to express appreciation for the physician's efforts, and he must obtain satisfaction independent of the patient's gratitude.

The exploration of the patient's problems follows the major outlines that have been discussed for non-emergency situations. A special characteristic is the increased emphasis on the precipitating stress and on the expectations of all persons concerned. In addition, the interviewer must structure the interview to include areas that are crucial for immediate therapeutic decisions.

WHO IS TO BE INTERVIEWED?

If someone has accompanied the patient, the interviewer must decide who will be taken into the consultation room. The customary procedure is to begin an interview by speaking to the patient alone. There are situations in which it is preferable to begin by jointly interviewing both the patient and the person accompanying him. The decision to include the partner in the interview is made when both the patient and the partner either verbally or non-verbally indicate their desire for a joint interview. If the patient seems reluctant to leave the partner, then both should be invited into the consultation room. This usually indicates that the person accompanying the patient is emotionally involved in the emergency and therefore must be considered in its management. If the initial portion of the joint interview reveals that the companion inhibits the patient's communication, he can then be excused. If, on the other hand, the patient leaves his partner in the waiting room and then seems unable to describe his problem, the partner could be invited to join the group.

Sometimes the person accompanying the patient will ask to speak with the doctor first, alone. It is a mistake to allow this, as the patient may no longer perceive the doctor as his ally.

The physician can indicate that he is interested in what the companion has to say, but that he first wants to see both the patient and companion together. If the patient objects to this, the interviewer should see the patient alone. If the companion insists on a private interview, the interviewer should still see the patient first. Later in the interview, the patient usually agrees to a separate interview with his companion.

In a family or group crisis, there are actually multiple patients, and the entire family may be interviewed and given emergency treatment. One individual may become the focus of pathological interactions in a family, the scapegoat for family conflict. It is important to broaden this family's notion of who is in trouble, so that appropriate help may be made available to others.

The selection of the initial interview group is important, but it does not limit the doctor's freedom to change the membership of this group as the interview progresses. It is customary to ask the partner to wait outside after he has related his views of the problem. It may be useful to ask the various persons concerned to enter or leave the consultation room during the interview. This enables the physician to obtain new information, while mobilizing the interest and involvement of others. The establishment of direct relations with anxious family members is vital for the effectiveness of the treatment plan.

If the patient's companion is not included in the initial consultation, he should be asked to remain nearby in case the physician should wish to speak to him later. This will also facilitate the patient's transportation home or, if necessary, to a hospital. The failure to make this request explicit may result in the doctor spending an hour or two attempting to reach the patient's husband, who has returned to his night job at a hard-to-locate factory, or otherwise struggling to make practical arrangements that the companion could have handled with little difficulty.

THE OPENING PHASE

The more formal portion of the interview begins, as always, with a discussion of the issue of greatest concern to the patient, his chief complaint. While exploring this presenting problem, the doctor attempts to determine: (1) Who felt the need for help?

(2) How was the problem identified as psychiatric? and (3) What was the precipitating stress? The first two questions are of crucial significance in assessing the patient's awareness that his problem is psychiatric: Unless he has at least partially accepted this idea, it is unlikely that he will follow the doctor's treatment plan.

(1) WHO FELT THE NEED FOR HELP? The need for help may have been felt by the patient, his family, friends, a social worker, another physician, or some other person. Psychiatrists tend to be more accepting of self-referred patients, since they are more likely to have intrapsychic symptoms and to express emotional suffering in psychological terms. Beginning psychiatrists find them easier to engage psychotherapeutically, and generally prefer them. Patients with somatic symptoms may be preferred by the general physician, but he becomes discouraged if their symptoms have no organic basis and the patient's complaints are not relieved by his therapeutic efforts. Such patients often antagonize the physician with their clinging dependence and a psychiatric referral may be as much an attempt to dispose of a problem as to solve it. Patients with interpersonal complaints may be self-referred, but are more often accompanied by a family member or referred by a social agency. Such patients may quickly sense that the psychiatrist prefers patients who are self-referred and who seek psychotherapy. In order to please the doctor the patient may alter his history. It then becomes necessary to carefully explore the details of the search for help in order to identify the actual referring source.

On occasion the psychiatrist is called to see a patient when there is no valid indication for a psychiatric referral. For example, a surgeon requests a consultation after repairing the lacerations of a young man who was involved in a bar room brawl. The patient greets the psychiatrist with protests that he was "only having a fight" and that he has no need to see a psychiatrist. If the doctor persists, asking if such incidents have occurred previously, the patient may answer, "Yes; so what!" The inexperienced doctor attempts to convince the patient that he must have emotional problems. However, the real problem concerns the interviewer, who is unsure of himself, reluctant to discharge the patient without completing a formal examination, and also reluctant to tell his surgical colleague that no consultation is indicated, since the patient has no awareness of a psychiatric problem and will not profit from the interview. This patient should be told, "There is no need for you to talk with me if you don't want to," and then should be given an opportunity to respond to this statement. The doctor's willingness to terminate the interview may stimulate the patient's desire to continue. If not, the therapist merely advises the patient of the availability of future psychiatric help if he changes his mind.

(2) How Was the Problem Identified as Psychiatric? The patient may be certain that his problem is psychiatric, he may tentatively consider the possibility, or he may be certain that it is not psychiatric. Often he has made some effort to obtain help prior to the interview, consulting another doctor, a minister, teacher, or social worker. He may have studied books on psychology, or turned to prayer. His description of these attempts and their meaning to him will reveal his initial view of his problem and the way in which it was defined as psychiatric.

If the patient himself did not define the problem as psychiatric, he may have been referred to the psychiatrist for varying reasons. The referring physician may not have been able to fit the somatic complaints into a classical clinical syndrome, or he may have sensed underlying emotional problems. Occasionally, factors extraneous to the immediate emergency, such as past history of emotional illness, will determine the psychiatric referral. Understanding the reason for the referral and the patient's feeling about it will help in evaluating his attitude toward psychiatry and toward treatment.

For example, a college student was referred to a psychiatrist by the family physician, who was also a close personal friend of his parents. The parents were devoutly religious, and were greatly disturbed by their son's rejection of the church and its teaching. They were unable to see this as other than a symptom of illness, and had enlisted the aid of the family doctor, a member of the same church, in reviving their son's faith. The boy was well aware of their feelings, and saw the psychiatrist as just another agent of parental control. In fact, he was acutely troubled, but not over religion. His girlfriend had recently told him that she was pregnant, and he had become panicky and depressed, contemplating suicide. He felt unable to discuss this with his family, and kept them at an emotional distance with the religious issue. He was able to tell the story only after the doctor had clarified his role, explaining that he had no preconceived idea of what the problem was or of how it could be resolved, but was willing to discuss whatever the boy thought was disturbing him and see if he could help.

(3) WHAT IS THE PRECIPITATING STRESS?   The "why now" question considers what has happened in the patient's life that has disrupted his previously operating system of defenses. The changes may be in the intra-psychic, physiological, interpersonal, or external environment. Such information is usually not volunteered, and often not even conscious, but it is essential that it be elicited and understood early in the initial interview.

A direct question of, "What brought you here today?" is often met with, "Things just got to be too much for me," or, "I couldn't take it any more." The interviewer should pursue the matter further. He might ask, "How did you select this hospital?", "Have you sought help from anyone else?" or, "Did something happen that was the last straw?"

A detailed description of the events of the past week and particularly the past twenty-four hours is often illuminating. Important events in the patient's life or changes in his role are considered. Anniversaries and holidays lead to emotional reactions based on their symbolic meaning—for example, depressions can regularly recur on the anniversary of the loss of a loved one. The week before Christmas is also a common time for acute depressive reactions.

The physician must ask questions based on knowledge of the psychodynamics involved in specific symptom complexes. For example, if a depressed patient does not spontaneously report a loss, the interviewer might inquire in this area. Similarly, if a patient is anxious about becoming psychotic, one can investigate recent experiences in which he feared losing control. One of the authors has had several emergency consultations with college students fearing impending psychosis without apparent cause. In response to specific inquiry, they revealed that the recent use of LSD or marijuana had triggered their panic. Such an episode will lead a patient to seek help, but his shame or fear of its significance may make him reluctant to reveal the crucial features of the history. He seeks reassurance but wants to avoid exposure. The doctor's direct questions not only elicit the specific information, but also reduce the patient's anxiety by assuring him that the doctor is familiar with this kind of problem and knows how to deal with it.

SPECIFIC SYNDROMES

In this chapter, only the emergency aspects of the specific syndromes will be considered. For a discussion of these interviews in greater depth, the reader is referred to the appropriate chapter.

DEPRESSION AND SUICIDE.   When interviewing depressed patients in emergency situations, the most obvious area of structured inquiry is the exploration of suicidal risk. The patient may be asked about this directly. If the doctor is anxious about the topic or employs euphemisms such as "doing something to yourself," the patient might feel inhibited. The interviewer determines the patient's thoughts and impulses, his attitude toward them, and the actions that have resulted. For example, if the doctor asked, "Have you had thoughts of suicide?" or, "Have you wished to be dead?", the patient may reply, "Yes, I've felt that I should just end it all." An appropriate response from the doctor would be, "Did you go so far as to plan how you would do it?" If the patient replied, "No, the thought was too upsetting," and further inquiry revealed that he had not acted on impulses in the past, the risk would seem small. Another patient might reply to the initial question, "I had some thoughts of suicide last week, but not today." The alert physician could inquire further, "Did you think of how you would do it?" The reply, "I wondered about shooting myself. In fact, I bought a gun and some ammunition a few days ago," would suggest a serious risk. If the doctor then asked, "Were you frightened?" and the patient replied, "Oh, I don't know, I think everyone would be better off if I were dead," immediate protective measures would be indicated.

Communications relating to suicidal impulses are frequently non-verbal or indirect. If a depressed patient arrives in the emergency room with his bag packed, he is asking to be hospitalized; if he has left the door of his home unlocked, spent his last few dollars on a good meal or a phone call to a distant friend, or is unconcerned about the time or place of the next visit, he may not expect to be alive very long. These messages indicate his ambivalence about living or dying. If someone cares enough about him, that person may succeed in tilting this ambivalence in the direction of life. Persons who have had a close relative or friend who committed suicide present a greater risk, as do patients with a personal history of previous attempts at suicide. If the patient has recently made a will, or straightened out his financial affairs, he may plan to die. A belief in life after death or the fantasy of reunion with a dead person that he loved is another important piece of information. A variety of demographic, ethnic, and social factors have a demonstrable relation to suicidal risk.

The interviewer inquires who would remain behind if the patient killed himself. He may save the patient's life by convincing him that suicide would inflict great pain and suffering upon someone the patient loves. In the case of the suicidal patient who is physically ill, is elderly, and has no loved ones and no money, the physician could say, "I can understand how badly you feel and how little you have to live for, but I have seen others who felt just as you do, who were then helped by treatment and recovered. You have nothing to lose by giving yourself a chance to get well." Beginning residents often attempt to reassure the patient with statements such as, "Don't worry—we won't let you kill yourself." This invites the patient to relinquish his own controls and to rely upon the physician to arrest his self-destructive drive, and it is a promise that the physician can rarely keep. The doctor may instead ask the suicidal patient if he would like to come into the hospital, where he may feel greater ability to resist his suicidal urge, until he is better. If hospitalization is not indicated, the physician should let the patient know exactly where he can be reached, day or night, and whom he might call if the physician is unavailable. Obviously, the person whom the patient can call must be told about the patient in advance.

Anxiety Attacks.   The patient with acute anxiety and hyperventilation syndrome may respond dramatically to direct explanation of his symptoms. This must, of course, be geared to his capacity to understand. An unsophisticated patient can be told, "When someone is frightened, they breathe very rapidly without knowing it. Fast breathing can cause many of your symptoms." The patient might be further convinced by asking him to hyperventilate deliberately and then showing him how to control his symptoms by regulating his respiratory rate.

Patients with overwhelming anxiety have already been told by others to relax. If this had been helpful, the patient would not be seeking further assistance. The doctor should avoid repeating such advice, and should instead reassure the patient that his problem will at last be understood rather than simply suppressed.

Simple reassurance is of little value to the patient who is afraid of going crazy. Rather than telling him that he is not going crazy, the doctor finds out what the word "crazy" means to him. This reveals the significance of his fears and allows exploration of the sources of his anxiety. The doctor can inquire, "What do you mean by 'crazy'?" or, "What do you think it would be like to go crazy?" The patient can then be asked if he has ever seen anyone who was considered crazy, and what he observed at that time. Finally, the doctor finds out how the patient thinks people will respond to his craziness. Frequently the patient with an acute anxiety attack expresses fears concerning aggressive or sexual impulses. Having uncovered the specific fears, the doctor's reassurance will have much greater impact.

THE CONFUSED PATIENT.   The doctor is sometimes asked to see a patient who at first appears to be completely out of contact with his surroundings. The scene is the emergency room of a general hospital; the patient is lying on a cot, difficult to arouse, and disheveled. He does not respond to questions or mumbles incoherently without looking at the examiner. The first impression suggests the aftermath of a major neurological catastrophe. Patients with confusional syndromes need a constant input of sensory stimuli and orienting information in order to maintain their attention and contact with the outside world. The physician should introduce himself and briefly assess the situation. He may then encourage the patient to sit up and, if possible, conduct the interview with the patient in a chair. The interviewer can initially structure the discussion by focusing the patient's attention on his immediate life situation. The response may be dramatic; on occasion it is possible to obtain a history and make a detailed evaluation of the patient's problem.

THE INTOXICATED PATIENT.   One of the most difficult of the organic syndromes is the alcoholic who is acutely intoxicated. This condition has many potential complications, some with a significant mortality. In addition to the medical complications of delirium tremens, hallucinosis, or pathological intoxication, the patient's emotional controls are weakened and he is often depressed. Suicide or other impulsive behavior is a problem. The physician must determine why the patient is drinking, and whether this episode is different from previous ones. The interviewer will have little success in attempting to conduct an interview while the patient is acutely intoxicated, as the alcohol provides a chemical barrier that impairs effective communication. The patient has usually lost his emotional controls and is either belligerent and uncooperative or morose and depressed. If he can be observed for a few hours, a bewildering clinical picture often clears considerably and a more careful evaluation is possible.

THE "PSEUDO-CORONARY." The patient who is convinced that he is having a heart attack is a common emergency room problem. As with any patient with somatic symptoms, a careful medical history is indicated. The interviewer uses his questions in order to demonstrate the connection between symptoms and emotions. Someone who would be annoyed at a question like, "Did you think the chest pain might have been because you were frightened?" will respond quite comfortably to, "You must have worried a great deal about your chest pain." It is often useful to perform the physical examination personally; it provides an air of authenticity for later assurances about physical illness. Certainly if this patient proffers the affected portion of his body for examination, an examination should be performed. He wants to show his problem, and if this doctor appears disinterested he will seek another.

When the somatic symptom is pain, the physician never challenges its being real. Pain is a subjective sensation, and only the person experiencing it can tell whether it is present. This does not mean, however, that the physician must accept the patient's explanation of its cause, for this is a medical matter. The doctor can say, "What you describe is certainly painful, but we need more information to determine the cause of the problem."

One of the most difficult differential diagnostic problems in emergency psychiatry is the patient suspected of malingering pain in order to obtain narcotic drugs. Although most patients with pain want medical treatment for their underlying condition, the patient with severe pain may initially seek only relief from his symptom. He will rarely specify how this is to be given, whereas the addict who is malingering may have a specific drug and dose in mind. The problem cannot be discussed in detail here, but it is well established that the malingerer is psychiatrically disturbed. The physician is less likely to cause damage by administering these drugs when they are not indicated than by denying appropriate relief to a person in distress.

INTERPERSONAL CRISIS.   The patient with an interpersonal crisis will initially tend to blame someone else for his difficulties and may indicate that he wants only environmental manipulation. As the physician would not tell the patient with psychogenic pain that it is all in his mind, similarly, he would not make massive assaults on this pattern of defenses. The doctor who asks, "Why do you continually need to get into such messy situations?" may feel that he is searching for the origins of a psychological problem, but the patient will experience it as an accusation. Consider the adolescent girl who is brought to the emergency room by her distraught parents after she has ingested 10 aspirin in a dramatic suicidal gesture. She has been fighting with her mother about her late hours and her current boyfriend. The mother is obviously controlling her rage as she asks the doctor whether the girl is all right. She then adds, "We have tried to bring her up right, but we can't do anything with her."

The doctor finds himself torn between the girl's plea for sympathy and independence and the parents' frustrated helplessness. He is tempted to interpret either her manipulative coercion or their overcontrolling domination, thereby taking one side or the other. Instead, he can explore the events that precipitated the emergency. The process of discussion will provide the family with an alternative to the pattern of dramatic scenes and uproar that has been their characteristic mode of interaction.

THE ASSAULTIVE PATIENT.   The management of an interview with an assaultive patient is always a problem. If the scene is a hospital emergency room, by the time the doctor arrives he may find the patient lying on the floor, forcibly restrained by several attendants. Usually this demonstration of force will suffice to help the patient regain control over his aggressive impulses. The physician can kneel beside the patient and ask him, "What is all the commotion about?" As the restrainers relax their grip, the physician can quickly ascertain whether the patient plans to renew the struggle. If not (and this is usually the case), the physician can ask, "Wouldn't you rather sit in a chair and talk with me?", and then help the patient to rise while the other personnel are dismissed. The interview continues with an immediate inquiry, "What happened?", and a discussion of the patient's loss of control. On rare occasions, usually with organic psychoses, the patient must be kept in restraint while the physician administers tranquilizers parenterally. When the medication becomes effective, the interview continues as it would under other circumstances.

Beginning interviewers are concerned that if they ask the wrong thing the patient will again become violent. Usually the patient is even more concerned about this than the doctor, and he should be asked to tell the interviewer if he feels his assaultive impulses recurring.

Some patients have not actually assaulted anyone, but they are on the verge. They may seem to be unaffected by the doctor's calm manner and continue to pace the floor in a state of great agitation. These patients are offered tranquilizers before continuing the interview. The therapist can remain with the patient while the medication takes effect and should not increase the patient's fear of being trapped by placing himself between the patient and the door. Such fears may provoke either aggression or flight.

If the physician arrives to see the severely agitated patient just a few minutes too late he may find himself trying to interview someone who is heading out the front door. He should firmly, but gently, say, "Just a minute," and if the patient stops, continue the interview wherever they are located, even if it's outdoors on the sidewalk. Rapport can be best established by exploring the patient's great haste to get away. Once this step is accomplished, the doctor suggests that the interview be continued in a more comfortable setting and proceeds as with other cases.

The assaultive patient is reassured by the confidence that the experienced clinician feels and exhibits. The same patient is quick to detect simulated confidence concealing fear, and he may react to the doctor's fear with assaultive behavior. If an inexperienced physician continues to fear the patient, he should administer tranquilizers or utilize auxiliary personnel to control the patient so that he can conduct the interview more comfortably.

HANDLING THE PATIENT'S EXPECTATIONS

The patient comes to the doctor with expectations about the outcome of his visit. Such expectations are both conscious and unconscious, both positive and negative. They must be considered by the physician early in the interview and re-evaluated at its termination. Frequently, it is possible to help a patient modify his expectations during the course of the interview, after he has first gained an awareness of them The psychiatrist can demonstrate the inappropriateness of certain expectations, while strengthening and supporting others that he can reasonably hope to satisfy. If the patient has not been able to formulate any realistic expectations, the doctor must do this for him. If the physician fails to do so, the patient will be dissatisfied by the interview and will seek help elsewhere.

The patient should not be directly asked what kind of help he hopes to receive too early in the interview. He may interpret this as the doctor's refusal to accept responsibility for ascertaining his difficulties, or as a hostile rebuff. Nevertheless, once rapport has been established, this question can reveal a great deal. Inquiry regarding previous attempts at finding help is also useful. A patient who has sought the police before arriving at the emergency room often expects controls to be imposed. With patients who have sought help from religious advisors, one should inquire into the specific kind of help requested. The patient who sought the name of a psychiatrist has different expectations from the one who sought help through prayer. A difference even exists between the patient who prayed for strength in coping with a situation and the one who prayed for a solution through omnipotent intervention.

When there is an individual in the patient's life who would have been an obvious source of help, but whom the patient avoided, questions concerning the avoidance may reveal some of the fearful expectations he has brought to the interview. The interviewer might also inquire directly concerning negative expectations. Such inquiry is not always successful, but the patient's feelings may be revealed indirectly through stories of his family's and friends' experiences with psychiatrists, anecdotes about the hospital, jokes, and so on. If a patient starts the interview by joking, "Where are the men in the little white coats that cart you off to the booby hatch?", this not only reveals some ability to maintain a sense of humor, but also fear of being seen as crazy, with all of the many possible unconscious implications.

The emergency partner will also have expectations, and these may be similar to or different from those of the patient. When the partner has initiated the request for help, his expectations must also be considered, otherwise the search will continue, regardless of the effectiveness of the interview with the patient.

UNCONSCIOUS EXPECTATIONS.   The unconscious expectations of the patient are closely related to the psychodynamics of the precipitating stress. The most common unconscious expectation is that the doctor will directly resolve the patient's conflict. For example, the depressed patient wants his loss replaced, and an important early task is to shift this desire to a hope that his pain will be comforted and his diminished self-esteem restored. In the case of a man who is depressed following the loss of his job, the doctor inquires why the patient blames himself. By pointing out the discrepancy between the patient's critical attitude toward himself and his successful functioning in other areas of his life, the doctor focuses on his current adaptive skills and his desire to find a new job rather than his lost hopes and his fantasy that the doctor will somehow get his old position back for him.

Another situation is illustrated by the depressed woman who is angry with her husband but is fearful that he will leave her if she ventilates her rage. She feels that she is a martyr, but is afraid to rebel. When she asks, "Do you think it is fair that I have to live like this?" she is seeking permission to act. This patient may become depressed if the doctor does not grant this permission, but she may be even more threatened if he does. It is important first to establish a trusting alliance and then to search for alternate patterns of behavior that may allow some gratification of her impulses without dire consequences.

CONSCIOUS EXPECTATIONS.   The conscious expectations of emergency patients include hospitalization, medical treatment, medication, environmental manipulation, psychotherapy, reassurance, no effect at all, and actual physical or psychological harm.

Hospitalization may be seen as a protection from the threat of inner impulses or as a means of influencing the environment. For example, a woman seeks help a few weeks after giving birth to a child because of obsessive fears that she might drop the infant or use salt rather than sugar in his formula. When the doctor inquires further, she says, "I hoped you would put me in the hospital or take my baby away before I kill him." She is seeking control. The very act of seeking control implies that some inner controls are working, and these must be found and strengthened. The patient herself will be the best ally.

If the patient views treatment as a means of controlling

others, he may first insist that he be hospitalized and then be equally insistent that he be discharged one or two days later. A patient who loudly protests against hospitalization, while at the same time acting crazy, may actually be requesting hospitalization but refusing to accept responsibility for it. His expectation is that he will be forced into a hospital against his will, and he may become more upset if his expectation is not met.

A patient may fear that the doctor will select the wrong alternative in treating an impulse problem. Thus a religious patient who is concerned about sexual feelings may wish to remove or suppress them, and may fear that the psychiatrist will encourage sexuality. If his hopes and fears are made explicit, the patient can be helped. The doctor might say, "I have the feeling that you'd like to eliminate your sexual feelings and that you fear I may only make things worse by encouraging them."

Patients with little psychological sophistication and those with somatic symptoms will want medication from the doctor. These patients may request medication early in the interview, and beginning therapists often comply much too quickly. The problem may appear different at the end of the interview, and advice concerning medication can wait until that time, even when the doctor feels confident that drugs will be necessary. If the patient feels that all the doctor can do is to prescribe medication, he loses interest in the interview once he receives his prescription, and what follows is anticlimactic. In an emergency situation, the prescription should be for only enough medication to last until the next visit. If the physician reassures the patient that things will soon be better and then provides a three-month supply of medicine, the patient may not trust the doctor's words. A starter dose of medicine, supplied directly by the doctor and perhaps taken in his presence, has special value. It carries the magical power of the doctor's personal tool of therapy. A patient with whom the doctor is not thoroughly familiar should never be given a potentially dangerous quantity of medication. Even if the patient is not suicidal, he may feel that the doctor is either careless or unconcerned about his welfare.

The psychiatrist often makes recommendations that involve manipulating the patient's environment. He may recommend a homemaker, or a leave of absence from school or his job. In doing this, he distinguishes between the patient who must be encouraged to relinquish his pathological sense of obligation and the patient whose tenuously maintained self-esteem is dependent upon his continued functioning. For example, the suggestion of a homemaker could upset a mother who, despite her depression, takes pride in her continuing ability to care for her children. The patient with interpersonal problems will often want the doctor to alter the environment and therefore remove the problem. Thus, a woman might complain that her husband beats her, and want the physician to remove him from the home. The psychiatrist might reply, "Only the police can do that, and you have told me that you have been to them many times. However, I might be able to help with the troubles that lead to his drinking, or your uncertainty about leaving him, if you are also bothered by those problems." The patient may already have some awareness of these considerations, and this can sometimes be elicited by comments such as, "If you only wanted someone to straighten out your husband, you would not have come to a psychiatrist." In this way the physician is reinforcing the patient's more realistic expectations.

Psychotherapy is more likely to be expected by patients who are better educated or are from a higher social class, and whose symptoms are psychological in nature. However, a patient's awareness of psychological problems does not mean that he will not need medication, direct guidance, or hospitalization. This patient's distress, like that of the patient with somatic symptoms, may require the initial adjunct of medication. Indeed, an acutely heightened awareness of inner conflicts is often indicative of the too rapid breakdown of defenses.

NEGATIVE EXPECTATIONS AND THE UNWILLING PATIENT. The patient with negative expectations anticipates no help, and may expect further injury and humiliation. When depressed, he is likely to be suicidal; when paranoid, he will probably be belligerent and combative. He does not accept psychiatric intervention. These negative expectations must be openly discussed if there is to be any hope of engaging the patient's cooperation. When discussing this patient's unconscious expectations, it is crucial that the psychiatrist ally himself with the patient's unconscious hope rather than his unconscious fear.

It may be necessary to force treatment against a patient's will in order to protect him or others around him. This must be done openly. It is better to tell a patient, "I will have to send you to the hospital even if you don't agree to go," than to conceal this by saying, "We'll have to arrange for another consultation in the building across the street." The patient will ultimately appreciate the physician's honesty and directness and his attitude toward other doctors will be favorably influenced.

Before forcing hospitalization on a patient, the interviewer should exhaust every possible means of convincing him to go voluntarily. This process begins by explaining the therapeutic rationale behind hospitalization at this time—usually the need to supply the patient with external assistance in controlling suicidal or assaultive impulses. If the patient did not wish to have these impulses curbed, he would not have allowed himself to be interviewed, and would have kept their existence a secret until he was free to act upon them. This should be explicitly pointed out to the patient.

Few judges will force a commitment against the wishes of the patient's relatives unless he has committed a crime. Patients have been hospitalized repeatedly only to be signed out, against medical advice, by a relative on the following day. Therefore, it is necessary to gain the relatives' support when the doctor is recommending hospitalization. Frequently a relative, friend, priest, or someone else whom the patient trusts can exercise greater influence in helping the patient to accept hospitalization than can the physician.

A careful discussion of the patient's fears of hospitalization is essential. He may think that he cannot obtain his own release when he no longer feels the need for hospitalization, or there may have been previous unpleasant experiences with a psychiatric hospital. Discuss his alternate plans that would provide assistance in controlling his impulses. Sometimes this may convince the doctor that hospitalization is not the only way to cope with the emergency. The physician may then feel free to alter his recommendation. Finally, when a patient indicates reluctance about accepting hospitalization, he should not be left unsupervised after the subject has been mentioned, and especially not after a positive decision has been made.

TREATMENT PLAN

As the interview draws to a close, the doctor begins to formulate his suggestions and plans for further treatment. These must be conveyed to the patient in a way that will help him to accept them. The patient's own treatment plans are to be explored first. How has he handled similar problems in the past, and what were the results? If his plan differs radically from the doctor's, has he considered alternatives? If he indicates that he has already rejected the doctor's plan, one can point out that he thought of it himself, and at least considered it as a possibility. The interviewer finds the patient's own reasons for and against it, and deals with his arguments rather than with those of the physician. If he has not considered the specific alternative that the doctor has in mind, it is suggested to him and he is asked to consider it during the interview. If he reaches the same plan as the doctor, he is far more likely to follow it than if he is simply informed of the doctor's thoughts.

As an example, let us consider an acutely depressed college student who sought help in the week of his final exams. He had never had a similar episode in the past. He described his problems, and the physician inquired as to his plans. He replied that he expected to take his exams, but that, in his current state, he was sure that he would fail. The physician asked, "Have you considered any alternatives?" The patient said, "Yes, I thought of asking to be excused from the exam, but the professor would probably say no, and anyway, it wouldn't be fair." The doctor asked, "Could you tell the professor that you weren't feeling well, and ask if you could make up the exam when you were better?" The patient had not considered this because, like most depressed people, he did not feel that he would get better. He replied, "Well, I don't know, I don't want the professor to know I've seen a psychiatrist. He would never understand." The doctor was then able to explore his reaction and to demonstrate that the patient's fear had no foundation in reality, but was instead based upon his diminished self-esteem and consequent assumption that others would be intolerant of him. This sort of discussion will help the patient to employ the doctor's recommendation, although initially he was quite resistant to it.

If the emergency partner has initiated the consultation, he too must be considered in the treatment plan. If the physician does not reduce his anxiety, he will continue to pursue other avenues of help. It is not sufficient to merely acquaint him with the treatment plan if he was not present during its formulation. His expectations must also be made explicit, and any discrepancies between these and the actual treatment must be discussed.

Closing the Interview

Since the emergency patient does not know the length of the appointment, the doctor should always indicate that time is drawing to a close when there are still a few minutes of the interview remaining. He can say, "We will have stop in a few minutes," or, "Our time is almost up now." This provides the patient an opportunity to add more material or, more important, to ask questions. The doctor can ask, "Is there anything we have not talked about?" or, "Is there something else you would like to tell me, or something you would like to ask me?" The patient's choice will reveal what he considers to be a crucial problem or major anxiety. Occasionally he will reply, "There is nothing." This reply does not necessarily mean that the patient is satisfied. The interviewer does not stop at this point, but pursues discussion of an area that was not fully explored earlier. The topic can be one that, although affectively charged, was not developed because it was tangential to the emergency. The patient who has no questions to ask is provided an opportunity to reveal additional material through his trend of associations.

In closing the interview, it is preferable to give the emergency patient a specific appointment, rather than suggesting vaguely that he come back later. If the problem were severe enough to precipitate an emergency, it should be reevaluated in a second interview. If he does not have a specific appointment, the patient may have to create another emergency in order to return.

The psychodynamics of emergency behavior encompasses all of the specific clinical syndromes, but there are special considerations added by the emergency situation. An understanding of these additional dynamic issues will enable the physician to utilize his existing knowledge most effectively. His systematic approach to the problem will allay his own anxiety by protecting him from the crisis atmosphere produced by the patient and partner. This allows the physician to reduce the patient's anxiety, and, as a result, the patient can mobilize his own adaptive skills to cope with his problems.

References

Bellak, L.: The emergency psychotherapy of depression. In Bychowski, G., and Despert, L.: Specialized Techniques in Psychotherapy. New York, Basic Books, Inc., 1952.

Brill, N. Q., and Storrow, H. A.: Social class and psychiatric treatment. Arch. Gen. Psychiat., 3:340, 1960.

Coleman, D.: Methods of psychotherapy. Prog. Psychother., 5:78, 1960.

Coleman, D., and Zwerling, I.: The psychiatric emergency clinic. Amer. J. Psychiat., 115:980, 1959.

Errera, P., Wyshak, G., and Jarecki, H.: Psychiatric care in a general hospital emergency room. Arch. Gen. Psychiat., 9:105, 1963.

Gwartney, R. H., Auerback, A., Nelken, S., and Goshen, C. E.: Panel discussion on psychiatric emergencies in general practice. JAMA, 170:1022, 1959.

Kalis, B. L. et al.: Precipitating stress as a focus in psychotherapy. Arch. Gen. Psychiat., 5:219, 1961.

Lindeman, E.: Symptomatology and management of acute grief. Amer. J. Psychiat., 100:141, 1944.

Litman, R. E., Farverow, N. L., Shneidman, E. S., Heilig, S., and Kramer, J. A.: Suicide prevention telephone service. JAMA, 192:107, 1965.

MacDonald, J. M.: Homicidal threats. Amer. J. Psychiat., 124:475, 1967.

Murphy, G., and Robins, E.: Social factors in suicide. JAMA, 199:81, 1967.

Robin, E., et al.: The communication of suicidal intent. Amer. J. Psychiat., 115:724, 1959.

Schwartz, D. A., Tidd, C. W., and Waldron, R.: Use of home visits for psychiatric evaluation. Arch. Gen. Psychiat., 3:57, 1960.

Ungerleider, T.: The psychiatric emergency. Arch. Gen. Psychiat., 3:593, 1960.

Yessler, P. G., Gibbs, J. J., and Becker, H. A.: On the communication of suicidal ideas. Arch. Gen. Psychiat., 3:612, 1960.

Section three:

TECHNICAL FACTORS AFFECTING THE INTERVIEW

In the final chapters, certain specific factors that will affect the management of the interview are discussed. Some of these are mechanical in nature; others involve special artifacts of the patient or the interviewer or the circumstances under which the interview is conducted.

15 THE ROLE OF THE TELEPHONE IN THE PSYCHIATRIC INTERVIEW*

The telephone plays an important role in contemporary psychiatric practice. At first glance the topic seems too simple or straightforward to warrant careful consideration. However, it involves an area of clinical work with patients and therefore should be subject to study. Since the topic is not usually discussed in the training of psychiatrists, it is an area in which the personal style of each interviewer will emerge without self-scrutiny, and countertransference problems can easily be recognized.

Most patients make their initial contact with a psychiatrist via the telephone and often have subsequent occasions to call. Telephone calls during the interview also present a problem. Some psychiatrists accept telephone calls while interviewing a patient; others never accept telephone calls in this situation; a third group occasionally accepts telephone interruptions, with varying criteria for the decision. In addition, the telephone can be used for psychiatric interviews both in emergencies and on a long-term basis.

---

* This chapter was presented in a modified version in *Psychiatry*, Volume 33, No. 1, Feb. 1970.

THE PATIENT TELEPHONES THE DOCTOR

THE INITIAL TELEPHONE CALL

Each doctor has his own way of handling an initial call from a prospective patient. Most psychiatrists expect some information concerning the patient before making the first appointment. Often this has been provided by the referring physician, but not infrequently a person whom the psychiatrist does not know telephones requesting an appointment.

It is expected that a caller will ask for the doctor by name, will identify himself, and will make some explanatory comment pertaining to the purpose of the call. The young psychiatrist soon learns that the patient who telephones him does not always follow customary social expectations, and thus provides clues concerning his personality pattern and the degree of his illness.

Even if the psychiatrist answers his telephone by saying, "Hello," rather than by stating his name, a psychotic patient may immediately launch into a discussion of his problem. The interviewer can interrupt this recital with the inquiry, "Who is calling?" The patient will usually respond by identifying himself and indicating that he wishes to make an appointment. If he only identifies himself and then continues with a discussion of his problems, the doctor can interrupt again and ask, "Did you call in order to make an appointment?" Before actually making the appointment, it is useful to inquire, "Might I ask how you obtained my name?" If the patient obtained the physician's name from an appropriate referral source, such as a colleague or a social agency, one may then ask the prospective patient if the problem he wishes to discuss pertains to himself. The caller may reply, "No, actually the patient is my wife," or, "In fact, I want to see you about my child." Such situations require further telephone discussion before making the appointment, thus sparing the physician a possible waste of time and the patient a possible waste of money. The discussion may reveal that the caller himself has difficulty coping with the person about whom he is calling, and that it would be appropriate to arrange an appointment with the caller. If, however, the caller wants the physician to come to his home, posing as a guest, to arrange for commitment of a psychotic relative; some clarification of the psychiatrist's role is required. A brief telephone discussion will also help the psychiatrist avoid making unwanted appointments with salesmen, insurance agents, and others.

When the patient indicates that he obtained the doctor's name from the classified telephone directory, one should determine whether he wants a general practitioner or a psychiatrist, thus avoiding a misunderstanding.

Obsessive or paranoid patients will take particular care that they are speaking to the doctor before disclosing anything about themselves. These patients will frequently misunderstand a brief conversation and consider it a cue to launch into a lengthy discussion of their problem. When this occurs, the physician might say, "We can discuss this in more detail when you come to my office." Obsessive patients often attempt to control the doctor while making their first appointment by suggesting a list of times when they would be available. Rather than interpret this behavior on the telephone, the doctor might indicate an hour that is convenient for him. The obsessive patient will often inquire concerning the doctor's fee before scheduling an appointment. Such questions are best answered directly by telling the patient the fee. The patient may ask, "Is that subject to negotiation?" When the patient raises this issue during the initial telephone call, it indicates ambivalence concerning treatment. Since an immediate exploration is not practical, the therapist must confront the ambivalence directly rather than accede to it. This is done by replying that the fee is not negotiable. The patient may then vacillate indecisively about scheduling the appointment. The physician could then suggest that if the fee is too high the patient can try another doctor who might have a lower fee.

A patient calling for a first appointment may ask for directions to the doctor's office or for information concerning parking in the neighborhood. It is appropriate to offer brief, factual answers to such questions. The patient may ask for permission to bring someone else with him to the office. If this person is involved in the problem or is a close relative of the patient, the doctor can agree without hesitation. If the relationship seems unclear, it is preferable to inquire about the patient's motives before granting permission.

Between the time of the initial call and the first appointment, the patient may telephone a second time. This might be to indicate he will be late for the appointment, or, if he is already very late, he might ask, "Since only a few minutes of the hour are left, should I still come?" If the patient will have 15 minutes in the office, it is worthwhile to suggest that he come for the brief period; otherwise schedule a new appointment. Another patient may telephone the morning of his first session to say, "Doctor, I have a cold, and my temperature is about 99°; should I come this afternoon?" The doctor could ask, "Do you have any reason for hesitation about the appointment other than your cold?" or, "If you are leaving the decision up to me, does that mean you feel well enough to come?" Such comments indicate that the doctor expects to see the patient at the scheduled hour and the conversation may be promptly terminated. After the first few interviews, when the doctor is familiar with the specific dynamic issues involved, other techniques may be more appropriate. A full discussion of these problems goes beyond the scope of this chapter.

CALLS FOLLOWING THE FIRST INTERVIEW

Different issues are involved when the patient telephones the doctor following the first visit. Something discussed during the interview may have upset the patient, and if this is not explored, the patient might be frightened away from treatment. On other occasions the patient telephones because he feels that he got away with something during the session. He might say, "Oh, Doctor, I forgot to tell you," or, "I made a mistake in telling you thus and such," or, "I would like to add the following to what I reported." Such comments indicate that the patient was dissatisfied and may have felt that the doctor did not understand him or did not accept the patient's view of himself. The physician might comment to that effect and then suggest that the issue could be explored further during the next appointment. Another patient may use the telephone to "confess" some embarrassing or humiliating information that he was unable to disclose during the face to face interview.

Phobic patients frequently telephone after the first hour complaining of their symptoms and expressing a desire for reassurance. The physician could remark to the patient, "Something during the hour must have upset you; this is not unusual, and your anxiety will pass." It is essential to offer this type of reassurance to the phobic patient in the initial phase of treatment in order to help establish a working therapeutic relationship.

One example of covert hostile reactions to the therapist would be the patient who calls after the first session to say, "This is Miss Smith, the patient that you saw on Thursday morning at 10:00." The implication is clear, that so little emotional contact was made that the doctor might not remember the patient. The interviewer may choose not to respond to this aspect of the comment until the next interview. However, on occasion, he may ask, "Do you feel you made so little impression on me that I would not remember you?" A less challenging comment would be, "Yes, of course, I remember you."

At the end of the first interview, a patient may ask the physician for his home telephone number. The patient might be asked if he is anticipating an emergency, as that is usually the reason for such a request. The doctor could explore what type of emergency he expects and how he has coped with such situations in the past. It was pointed out in an earlier chapter that phobic patients require the therapist to enter into various neurotic bargains before they will establish a therapeutic relationship. It is essential that the psychiatrist tell such patients that his answering service is able to contact him in the event of an emergency. Depending on the physician, the answering service either will offer his home telephone number when the patient calls or will telephone the doctor, who will then return the patient's call.

The authors subscribe to the minority view, which favors allowing the patient to obtain the number directly. This implies to the patient that the psychiatrist is not afraid of the patient's dependent needs, nor will he feel unduly troubled or bothered if the patient has an emergency. The authors' experience has been that patients rarely abuse the doctor's privacy at home. The ability to contact the physician quickly may relieve the patient's anxiety and actually decrease the frequency of his calls.

Severely depressed or suicidal patients are often so fearful of being a burden that they need definite permission to ask for the physician's help. The psychiatrist may provide this permission by giving his home telephone number directly to the patient rather than indicating that it can be obtained from the answering service. However, if the physician gives his home telephone number because of his own insecurity and anxiety, he may actually precipitate a crisis.

Occasionally the physician may telephone the patient following the first hour to change the time of the next appointment. Such requests do not require an explanation to the patient. The patient might ask, "Why is this necessary?" or say, "I hope nothing is wrong." It is sufficient to reply, "Something has come up that makes it necessary to change the hour." During the next session, the interviewer can explore the patient's reaction to the change in time as well as the meaning of his curiosity, if this seems indicated.

Some patients interrupt the doctor with telephone calls in order to demonstrate the hostile and inconsiderate nature of their personalities. The doctor should not become angry or abrupt with such patients; it is better to show them consideration, even though they are incapable of reciprocating. This helps the patient to adopt the physician as a new ego ideal. One can say in a polite and friendly tone, "I'm busy just now, could I call you back in a little while?"

On occasion, a message from a new patient leaves some confusion as to whether to return the patient's call. Messages are frequently garbled, and the psychiatrist does not know his patient well enough after the first few interviews that he can be certain what is happening with the patient. Therefore, until the doctor is thoroughly acquainted with his patient, all telephone calls should be returned. This will forestall a number of potentially serious misunderstandings. Patients who are forced to cancel an appointment appreciate the doctor's calling to inquire about their problem.

At times the physician must decide whether or not to telephone a patient who has missed an appointment without notifying the doctor. During the initial interviews it is a good idea for the physician to telephone the patient under such circumstances. Such behavior on the patient's part indicates a problem in the transference that requires immediate therapeutic intervention.

When a patient has telephoned, it is usually helpful to refer to the call in the next session. The patient is then afforded the opportunity for discussion of his reactions to the telephone conversation and exploration of its deeper meaning to him. The therapist will gear his analysis of the unconscious meanings of the call to the patient's capacity to develop insight. With more seriously ill patients, this uncovering may be deferred until late in treatment.

TELEPHONE INTERRUPTIONS DURING THE INTERVIEW

Telephone interruptions can be considered in terms of their effect on the on-going interview rather than upon the relationship between the doctor and the patient who is calling. Many doctors feel that this problem can be circumvented by never accepting telephone calls when they are with a patient. This has both advantages and disadvantages. The interviews are never interrupted; the patient and physician are never distracted by an irrelevant conversation. However, not accepting calls during an interview caters to the infantile omnipotence of the patient, encouraging his fantasy that he is the only person of concern to the doctor. Some doctors who follow such a system permit the patient to hear their telephone ring before it is answered by a secretary or an answering service. Furthermore, they may continue with the interview, ignoring the telephone as though it had not intruded. The patient is less likely to comment on the distracting influence of the telephone if the doctor attempts to ignore it, but he may nevertheless be disturbed.

Other psychiatrists have an arrangement whereby they may turn off the bell, allowing a light to flash instead. The usual practice is for the light to be placed where it will be visible to the doctor, but not to the patient. It is then possible for the doctor to accept or not accept telephone calls, depending on the patient, the situation, and his own mood. If the physician is not accepting calls during an interview, it is preferable that the patient be unaware that the telephone is ringing. In practice, the authors do not permit more than one telephone call during any given session.

In treatment of more seriously disturbed patients, the physician's telephone conversation can help the patient to improve his reality testing and his recognition of emotions. For example, a psychotic patient may grossly misinterpret the nature of the call. The telephone interruption is useful if the doctor reconstructs the conversation and attempts to determine how the patient came to his conclusions. The physician can point out gross distortions and then disclose the true nature of the call. The doctor thereby helps the patient to cope with reality by improving his ability to communicate and to interpret the communications of others. As the patient demonstrates improvement, his speculations become more perceptive and accurate. Situations in which the patient continues to misinterpret are indications for further therapeutic work. The principles are similar to those used in working with the patient's reactions to other people in a therapeutic group.

During the first few sessions of treatment, the patient most often shows no reaction to a telephone interruption. In more advanced stages of therapy, reactions to a telephone call become obvious. These responses are manifestations of the transference and accordingly are subject to analytic study and interpretation. Hearing the doctor talk with another person on the telephone gives the patient an opportunity to experience a facet of the physician's personality different from that which is elicited by the patient's personality. This may lead to a discovery that the doctor is capable of expressing tenderness, warmth, anger, and so forth, and in the later stages of treatment may help the patient achieve a more realistic image of his therapist. For example, one patient had abandoned his career as a teacher because of his feeling that it was a passive, feminine, and hence demeaning profession. He overheard his doctor's brief telephone conversation one day, and deduced that his therapist was also a teacher and that he was able to function effectively as a man in this capacity. This helped the patient to work through his neurotic conflicts.

The effects of a telephone interruption on any given interview depend upon the problems of the patient, the personality of the psychiatrist, and the specific events at the time of the interruption. The doctor who has a thorough knowledge of all the factors can predict his patient's reactions to a given telephone interruption. When he feels that an interruption would have an unfavorable effect upon the therapy, he can turn off the telephone.

The Patient's Reactions to the Interruption

Consideration will now be given to specific reactions that patients and therapists have to telephone interruptions, as well as to ways in which the therapist might respond.

RELIEF.   Patients may experience relief after telephone interruptions for several reasons. They may discover that other people have problems similar to their own. The doctor's willingness to accept urgent phone calls from others gives permission for this patient to call the doctor in time of need. A third basis for relief is the reaction that the patient describes as "saved by the bell." This typically occurs when the patient has started to discuss or is just about to discuss some very difficult material.

In the first instance, the interviewer might explore the feelings underlying the patient's surprise at learning that others have problems similar to his own. Likewise, exploration would be indicated when the patient is relieved to learn that it is permissible to call the doctor in time of need. However, the patient who feels saved by the bell requires a different approach. He is using the telephone call as a method of resistance. Sometimes the doctor can merely direct the patient back to the comments he was making when the telephone rang. On other occasions, it is more useful to explore the patient's feelings of relief at the interruption, as a way of making the patient more aware of his resistance. If the patient continues to react in this manner to telephone calls, the psychiatrist can simply turn off the telephone, particularly when the patient is discussing difficult material. The phobic patient will typically react with this type of resistance.

DISTRACTION.   The typical distracted response is characterized by the question, "Where was I when the phone rang?" or, "What was I saying, Doctor?" Such a reaction also indicates resistance, although this patient is less likely to accept an interpretation. Compulsive talking, which superficially resembles free association, may be used as a defense against the emergence of disturbing thoughts. An unexpected interruption may bring such material to the patient's attention. After the call, the patient attempts to reconstitute his defenses by resuming his previous discussion. Rather than exploring the resistance aspect, it is more useful to ask the patient what he was doing while the telephone conversation was in progress. Often illuminating material will be obtained in response to such an inquiry.

Frequently it is appropriate for the physician to say nothing, thereby giving the patient the opportunity to pursue his own free associations. During the period of initial history taking, the doctor might completely ignore an interruption and merely help the patient to continue with what he had been saying. The therapist must exercise care in following the latter course, since the simple distraction is frequently a defense against concealed responses of anger or curiosity about the tele-phone conversation. Once this is recognized by the doctor, he may work with the deeper feelings.

ANGER.   Angry responses to the telephone interruption include direct angry statements and indirect sarcastic remarks, such as, "Can't you afford a secretary, Doctor?" or, "You owe me three minutes." It is important that the interviewer not re-spond with anger or defensive behavior. Explanatory remarks deflect the treatment from the important issue. The doctor either listens while the patient ventilates his rage and then continues with the interview, or interprets the patient's feeling that he is being cheated or deprived of the interviewer's complete at-tention. Such comments are supportive of the patient's anger and will help him feel that the doctor really does understand him. If the call lasts more than a minute, the interviewer might ask the patient if he could stay a few minutes at the end of the session. Obsessive or paranoid patients are most prone to feel overtly angry in response to interruptions.

DENIAL.   The characteristic example of denial is the pa-tient who ignores the call, seeming to remain in a state of suspended animation until the interviewer concludes his con-versation. The patient will then finish his sentence as though there had been no interruption. This response is designed to conceal either the patient's anger or his intense interest in every detail of the telephone conversation and fantasies concern-ing the call. Some patients will use fantasy formation to avoid overhearing the conversation. Such denial is a defense against expression of forbidden impulses. The denying patient also mani-fests a striking lack of distraction and it is useful for the inter-viewer to comment, "You seem not to have been distracted by the telephone call." If the patient denies having distracting thoughts, the interviewer could comment, "It is interesting that you were able to keep your mind on the very word you had started to say." This type of response may occur in the hysterical patient who was interrupted in the middle of a rehearsed drama, or with the obsessive patient who was busily following his mental notes. If the interviewer successfully uncovers the patient's re-sentment, the focus of the interview is shifted to this issue.

GUILT OR FEELINGS OF INADEQUACY.   Responses of guilt or feelings of inadequacy immediately reveal that the patient has carefully listened to the conversation. His typical remarks will be, "You have such important responsibilities," or, "Why do you bother with me when there are other people who need you so much more than I do?" The patient may even offer to step outside while the physician is in the middle of the telephone call. These responses basically stem from anger, which the patient turns inward against himself. The patient's self-esteem is very low and he does not feel entitled to ask for much in life. Underneath, he resents the necessity that he share the doctor with other people, whom he believes to have problems that are considered more important than his own. Because of his profound sense of inadequacy, he feels that he has no right to complain. Therapists are often tempted to interpret the patient's underlying resentment and usually encounter failure. Instead, it is more helpful to comment to the patient that even in his illness he seems to feel that he is a failure—that his symptoms are less interesting or that his case is less challenging than that of someone else.

The patient who reacts in this manner also suffers from hidden feelings of intense competitiveness. His response to the telephone interruption provides a ready opening for discussion of such feelings. Initially, the patient may only accept the idea that competitiveness is a mental attitude through which he is constantly making unfavorable comparisons between himself and others. Later he may acknowledge that competitiveness is associated with a feeling of resentment that he is always in the losing position. The patient may be more willing to accept this if the doctor does not immediately attempt to focus the feeling of resentment upon himself. Hostile feelings are easier to accept when they are directed toward someone not physically present. The interviewer's position as a figure of authority and a potential source of supportive care also inhibits expression of hostile feelings by such patients. The response of guilt or inadequacy is characteristic of the depressed patient or the patient with a masochistic character.

ENVY OR COMPETITION.   The openly envious or competitive response is a variation of the overtly angry reaction. After listening to the telephone conversation, the patient may ask, "Why can't you be that way with me?" The interviewer's warmth or friendliness to the caller has aroused feelings of competition and jealousy in the patient. The patient feels that the doctor does not care enough about him. Such feelings may be more subtly expressed with the comment, "That must not have been a patient!" When the patient is asked why or how he made such a determination, he replies that the interviewer sounded "so friendly." As in treating openly angry reactions, the interviewer should not attempt to defend himself or convince the patient that he is not being deprived. Instead, he might encourage the patient to further express his feelings of deprivation.

PARANOID RESPONSES.   A typical paranoid response would be, "Were you talking about me?" or, "Was the call for me?" The interviewer will learn more if he does not hasten to correct the patient's misinterpretation. First, he might explore the patient's fantasy, and then determine the process through which the patient came to his decision. This avoids provoking the patient into an angry defense of his views. Exploring the content of the fantasy will elucidate important transference feelings, and pinpointing the distortions in the thought process may be useful in helping the patient improve his reality testing. The paranoid patient does not know whom to trust. He compensates for this inability either by indiscriminately trusting everyone or by trusting no one. The physician might inquire, "Who did you think I was talking to?" and, "What did you think we were discussing?" The fantasy revealed by the patient provides useful information concerning the psychodynamics of the patient's emotional disorder. After the interviewer has fully explored the patient's ideas, it is useful to show him how he misinterpreted the conversation.

On occasion, a call may be about the patient. In this situation, it is wise for the interviewer to indicate to the patient the identity of the caller as soon as the interviewer has determined who is calling. This can be done by addressing the caller by name and then proceeding with the conversation. This gesture helps the patient to recognize that the physician is not willing to hold secret discussions.

CURIOSITY.   Curiosity, like denial, is a type of response in which the patient has no awareness of any conscious emotional reaction. He has become involved in the conversation, but he is only aware of an interest in what is going on between the doctor and the caller. Typical remarks would include, "Was that your wife who called?" or, "Is everything all right at home, Doctor?" or, "I hope that wasn't bad news." The curiosity is usually a defense against a deeper emotional reaction, such as residual childhood curiosity concerning parental bedroom activities. Remarks displaying curiosity offer the interviewer an opportunity to comment, "Let's take a look at your curiosity in this area." Rather than answer such questions, it is better to establish with the patient that he does have curiosity concerning such material. Another approach would be to explore the meaning of the patient's curiosity and to trace it back into his childhood.

SYMPATHY. The sympathetic response is elicited when it becomes apparent that the caller is in distress. The patient in the office may comment, "I hope that person will be all right," or he might volunteer to relinquish his appointment to enable the doctor to see the other person. Such reactions are frequently defenses against experiencing angry, envious, or guilty feelings. Interpreting the underlying emotion is difficult; the therapist can do very little at that time except continue the interview. Perhaps he may thank the patient for his good intentions. Responses of sympathy are more common in depressed or masochistic patients.

FRIGHT. At times when it is appropriate for the physician to express anger to the caller, the patient in the office may react with fear. An illustration of this occurred when an insurance agent interrupted a psychiatrist for the third time and seemed unwilling to accept the doctor's statement that he was not free to speak. Instead, he insisted on completing his rehearsed speech. When the doctor became angry and abruptly terminated the call, the patient appeared shocked and said, "You certainly weren't very nice to that person!" The patient feared that he also might evoke an angry response from the doctor. Patients who inhibit their own aggression often fear that as a result of therapy they might lose control of their impounded rage and cause injury to others. Any indication that the doctor can get angry will increase this fear.

A variation of such a reaction might be characterized by the patient's disappointment in the doctor. This could happen when some unattractive aspect of the physician's personality is demonstrated before the patient for the first time. The physician might cope with such reactions in different ways, for example, interpreting the patient's disappointment that the physician is not perfect, or helping the patient to recall previous experiences of disappointment in persons he admired.

PLEASURE. The patient is sometimes pleased with the

way in which the doctor conducts himself on the telephone. He may, for example, experience vicarious pleasure by hearing the doctor express his anger in a way the patient is unable to emulate. In this situation, the doctor could direct the interview toward the patient's characteristic ways of expressing anger and attempt to uncover the fears that prevent him from a more open type of emotional expression.

Another situation in which the patient might be pleased would be when the doctor has obviously received good news. This reaction would require further discussion only if it were apparent that the patient was insincere in his expression.

THE INTERVIEWER'S REACTIONS TO THE INTERRUPTION

It is important that the interviewer be aware of his own emotional reactions to telephone interruptions. He may experience relief from boredom or relief if the patient has been expressing hostility. He might be distracted and then experience guilt feelings for having lost the continuity of the interview. He could react by feeling happy or sad in response to good or bad news. He may become angry for several reasons: as a result of the interchange with the caller, merely because of the interruption, or because of the particular time at which the interruption occurred. He can recognize countertransference in some reactions, as, for example, when he has used a telephone call in order to enhance his status in the eyes of the patient in his office.

Customarily, when answering the telephone, the interviewer indicates that he is not free to converse. However, if a brief conversation is unavoidable, the physician can find useful therapeutic opportunities if he closely observes the patient's behavior during the call.

On rare occasions, the interviewer may ask the patient to leave the consultation room when he receives a telephone call. An example would be a call involving a serious emergency in the personal life of the physician. Under such circumstances, the doctor would place an undue burden upon the patient by the unnecessary disclosure of his personal problem.

Someone seeking to reach the patient may call the doctor's office. If the patient is in the office at the time, the doctor can simply hand the telephone to the patient. Should the patient not be there, he may take the message and convey it to the patient. If the matter was not sufficiently urgent to warrant the interruption, the doctor could analyze the patient's motivation for allowing such unreasonable behavior from friends or relatives.

On some occasions the patient may ask to use the doctor's telephone. If the request is made at the end of the session and would cause the doctor to be late for his next appointment, it could be suggested that the patient call elsewhere. If the request is made at the beginning of the session, the doctor might permit the call but then direct the patient's attention to his reasons for not locating a telephone before his appointment. The use of the doctor's telephone, however, can be therapeutically valuable. In one case, a patient asked to use the telephone and proceeded to phone her stock broker, placing several "buy and sell" orders in an arrogant manner. Before the interviewer could comment on this unusual behavior, she volunteered, "Doctor, you have just observed a portion of my personality of which I am very ashamed —I hope you will be able to help me."

TELEPHONE CALLS
FROM PATIENT'S RELATIVES

Relatives of the patient may occasionally telephone the interviewer and ask either for an appointment or for information concerning the patient. Information concerning the patient should not be divulged, but the relative could be told, "I would like to tell John that you called and expressed an interest in his problem." At times the relative may ask the doctor to promise not to reveal the call. If the doctor agrees to such requests, he is placed in an untenable position and therapy is inevitably damaged.

The therapist may accurately suspect that the caller wishes to interfere in the therapy. The authors consider it an error to refuse to speak to him if he is close to the patient. Frequently the caller exercises important influence over the patient's life or the patient is dependent upon him. Alienating such persons can only injure the patient. If the patient gives his consent, an interview with the relative could be arranged with or without the patient present.

TELEPHONE EMERGENCIES

A patient may telephone the doctor in a state of serious depression or acute anxiety that constitutes an emergency. It is apparent that the psychiatrist is at a disadvantage in treating a patient over the telephone. His examination is limited to auditory material and he is unable to utilize other sensory impressions of the patient. Rather than work under such a handicap, some physicians insist that the patient come for a personal examination or refuse to aid the patient.

Such rigidity seriously limits a physician's usefulness. Surely the patient is also aware that a personal interview is preferable to a telephone call. In an emergency, however, even a brief positive contact with the physician may be lifesaving for the patient. It is essential, therefore, that one respond to such a patient with the same degree of respect and dignity as is shown in a personal interview. Many doctors react to the telephone interview with annoyance and resentment, which are quickly communicated to the patient. Frequently, the telephone call is the patient's test to determine if the doctor is an accepting or rejecting individual. It is a prejudice of many therapists that all requests for telephone interviews are manifestations of resistance. This is not always valid.

The physician might begin by obtaining the patient's name, address, and telephone number, if the patient has not already identified himself. The patient may be reluctant to provide some of this information. In this situation, the patient can be asked why he feels that it is necessary to conceal his identity.

It has been our experience that the telephone patient has often had prior contact with a psychiatrist. It is therefore useful to make inquiry about such contacts early in the interview. This is particularly true of the patient who refuses to disclose his identity.

After obtaining a brief description of the presenting problem, it is useful to ask the patient if he has considered arranging for a personal interview. If it becomes apparent that the patient is psychotic, the doctor can ask if the patient fears that a personal visit might lead to hospitalization. If so, the therapist might then investigate specific symptoms that the patient feels might require hospital treatment. After such a discussion, it is frequently possible to assure the patient that these symptoms do not require hospitalization. Such a patient can be told that treatment, in order to be successful, requires the cooperation of the patient, and that treatment forced upon the patient probably will not help. The doctor may further assure the patient that he does indeed seem to have some motivation to receive help, since he has called a physician.

Patients resort to telephone interviews for various reasons. The problem of physical distance prevents some patients from coming in person. Other frequent motivations for telephone interviews are the fear of inordinate expense associated with psychiatric help or the fear of humiliation as the result of discussing embarassing material face to face. Some patients experience such intense desires to commit suicide that they fear that they may not live long enough to be interviewed in person and, therefore, are using the telephone contact as a measure of true desperation.

On rare occasions, at the conclusion of a 45-minute interview on the telephone, the doctor realizes that a patient who still refuses to come for a personal appointment is seriously in need of help. It may then be useful to make an appointment for a second telephone interview. After several such telephone interviews, the patient usually will be willing to come for an appointment in person.

If someone other than the patient is calling, it is necessary to determine the relationship between the patient and the person on the telephone. In a recent example of this, one of the authors was telephoned by a very distraught colleague. Fifteen minutes of clinical presentation had transpired before it became apparent that the patient was the colleague's wife and not a case from his practice. This was not a simple misunderstanding. It arose out of the colleague's strong need to detach himself from his own personal relationship, describing his wife merely as another patient about whom he was concerned.

It is important that the interviewer ask the age of the person to whom he is speaking early in a telephone contact. Meeting the patient in person provides visual clues about his age, making it unnecessary to inquire explicitly. Errors of many years can easily be made if estimates of the patient's age are based on the sound of his voice. Other basic identifying data that the physician routinely obtains when speaking to the patient in person are also frequently overlooked during the telephone interview.

An obvious but often neglected technique for reducing the handicaps inherent in a telephone situation is to ask the patient to describe himself physically. Although no one answers such a question objectively, certain patients tend to distort more than others. This tendency is based on how they feel about themselves. It is possible for the physician to reduce such distortion by asking the patient if the answer he has given is more a reflection of how he appears to others or how he actually feels about himself.

A doctor may decide to summon the police in response to a telephone call from a severely suicidal or homicidal patient who is on the brink of losing control of his impulses and cannot come to the hospital. This should be done openly, with the patient informed of the action. If the patient objects, the physician can increase the patient's responsibility for this decision, pointing out that he made such action possible through the disclosure of his name and address.

For example, a patient may telephone the doctor and announce that he has just ingested a full bottle of sleeping pills. Obviously, the doctor asks the patient his name, address, and telephone number at once and then asks the name of the medication and the approximate number of pills. If he has taken a dangerous dose, the physician can advise him that the police will be sent immediately and that the patient should open his door to facilitate their entry. The physician might inform the patient that he will call back as soon as he has summoned the police. He can also inquire about the name and phone number of the closest neighbor in the event that the police are not immediately available.

If the patient refuses to disclose his name and address, the doctor might comment, "You must have some uncertainty concerning your wish to die or you would not have called me. There are only a few minutes remaining in which you can change your mind. You have taken a fatal dose and it may already be too late to save your life, but we can still try." Realizing that the outcome is already uncertain, the patient may allow "fate" to intervene and may provide the identifying data. An analogous situation could occur with the patient who is on the verge of homicide.

A special problem of the telephone interview is silences, which occur as they do in conventional interviews. It often is difficult for the telephone interviewer to allow these silences to develop during the conversation. This is a reflection of the interviewer's discomfort, dissatisfaction, or impatience. Only through experience can a therapist relax and be professionally at ease while conducting a telephone interview.

In the later portion of the telephone interview, the physician may inquire if there is anyone else with whom he can converse; by obtaining another person's view of the patient's problems the therapist may gain information that would help him to assess the clinical situation.

CONDUCTING REGULAR THERAPY SESSIONS BY TELEPHONE

On rare occasions a psychiatrist may elect to treat his patient by telephone. For instance, a patient might be forced to move to some part of the country where psychotherapy is unavailable. Under these circumstances, regular treatment sessions might be continued by telephone.

Three brief vignettes illustrate some major points. In the first case, a middle-aged depressed woman who had had several years of therapy went to Nevada for six weeks to obtain a divorce. Her marriage had contributed to her depression, but she was unable to face the prospect of the divorce without the emotional support of her therapy. Her treatment was successfully conducted twice a week for six weeks on the telephone.

The second case was a 30-year-old depressed woman with anxiety and hypochondriacal trends. After one year of treatment she became pregnant and seemed likely to miscarry. Her obstetrician insisted that she remain in bed for three months. Her home situation was intolerable and she lived too far away to receive psychotherapy at home. The psychiatrist treated her twice weekly by telephone during this period.

The third case involves a situation that was in some respects more unusual. The patient was a 30-year-old phobic housewife who moved to the suburbs after several years of treatment. One day a severe snowstorm forced a cancellation. The patient waited until her appointed hour to telephone, as she had hoped to find some means of transportation. The physician sensed that she was eager to terminate the call and commented to that effect.

The patient revealed disturbing thoughts about the doctor that she had successfully suppressed while she was in the office. As the patient would have isolated her feelings if the matter had been left until the next appointment, it was discussed at that time. Subsequently, the patient deliberately sought another telephone session the next time more difficult material emerged. That time the physician refused, as it was clear that the patient's request was a form of resistance.

Admittedly these are all special situations, but nonetheless they are scarcely unique. The arrangement to continue a patient's treatment by telephone implies that the patient's dependence upon the doctor is realistic. In situations in which this would be undesirable, telephone sessions are not indicated.

As the reader has surmised, the telephone consultation presents many challenging and difficult problems. The physician who has developed skill and flexibility in this situation will be able to work more effectively with a wider variety of patients.

REFERENCES

Saul, L.: The telephone as a technical aid. Psychoanal. Quart., *20*:287, 1951.

16 INTERVIEWING THROUGH AN INTERPRETER

Special problems occur when the interviewer and patient are separated by a language barrier. Not only is direct verbal communication impossible, but the interviewer is usually unfamiliar with the cultural values and background of his patient. Conducting the interview with the assistance of an interpreter is, at best, only a partial solution to these problems. It neither overcomes the cultural barrier nor provides the interviewer with an understanding of the patient's background. This language barrier becomes an issue when a psychiatric problem develops in a newly arrived immigrant or a foreign visitor. The barrier is also present with members of ethnic groups who do not speak English. It is common for wealthy persons from other countries, where there are shortages of psychiatrists, to seek psychiatric treatment in the United States. The most frequently encountered non-English-speaking patient in this country is the lower class Puerto Rican, Cuban, or Mexican immigrant. This group was discussed in some detail in Chapter 13.

SELECTING THE INTERPRETER

The ideal interpreter would be a unique communication machine that could convert one language into another, capturing the meaning of the words and sentences and translating them instantly, including the nuances and the feelings of the interviewer. This, of course, is impossible. Often the translation of subtleties involves the loss of finer emotional tones or humor. The interpreter must have an intimate knowledge of both cultures in order to make even approximate translations in such situations. This is an exceedingly difficult task to perform rapidly and smoothly. The best example of this type of interpreting would be found at the United Nations, where a speech is translated line by line as it is being delivered.

Ideally, the interviewer would select a professional interpreter. In practice, this is usually not possible and an attempt must be made to obtain the services of a bilingual member of the staff, such as a social worker, nurse, secretary, or attendant. There are many times when such personnel are not available and the interviewer is obliged to utilize a family member or friend who accompanied the patient. If there is a choice, permit the patient to select the family member or friend with whom he feels most comfortable. Be sure that the person selected has a good command of English and seems capable of following instructions. Usually the patient will select an adult of the same sex. If he asks to utilize a child or a person of the opposite sex as an interpreter, he is probably attempting to protect himself from certain aspects of the interview. On occasion he may suggest having more than one interpreter, but this is not a good plan as the two interpreters will often disrupt the interview with disagreements about the precise meaning of a certain phrase.

INSTRUCTIONS TO THE INTERPRETER

The interpreter will be more useful if the physician instructs him concerning his role before starting the interview. It is preferable that he translate the patient's and doctor's statements rather than explain his understanding of their meaning. He should neither amplify remarks nor explore ideas of his own. The doctor can maintain better rapport with a sentence by sentence interpretation than with a summary that paraphrases the general content of the conversation. It is not desirable that the interpreter merely translate words without their accompanying feeling. His expression and voice should reflect the affective tone of each interchange. If the patient converses directly with the interpreter during the interview, it is likely that the interpreter has become involved in a defensive maneuver of the patient. A patient may seek out the interpreter after the interview in order to continue the discussion. This behavior reflects the patient's feeling that he needs direct, practical assistance, which can be better provided by a successful member of his own culture. The interviewer can support the patient's attempt to improve his social and adaptive skills. However, the patient's relationship to the interpreter can also be used as a resistance to involvement with the psychiatrist. The psychiatrist expects to learn about and supervise these extra-session contacts so that the interpreter can become an auxiliary therapist.

When the interpreter is a close relative, it may be particularly difficult for him to adhere to his role. In fact, the interviewer may find himself conducting a family interview. This is not necessarily undesirable; however, it should be remembered that family members, particularly in an initial group interview, usually tend to protect each other and keep certain pertinent information away from the interviewer.

TRANSFERENCE AND COUNTERTRANSFERENCE

The interviewer should face the patient with the interpreter at the patient's side. He should speak as though the patient could understand his words, rather than saying to the interpreter, "Ask him if he does thus and such." If the interviewer addresses the interpreter in that manner, it encourages the patient to reply, "Tell the doctor that. . . ." The inexperienced interviewer becomes anxious if he cannot "get to the patient," and his role as the physician is threatened. He responds by relating to the interpreter in a dependent way rather than utilizing the interpreter as his assistant. The patient's perception of a greater social closeness to the interpreter than to the physician may further draw him to the interpreter. A third person in the room will inhibit both patient and interviewer; however, as the interview progresses, this effect tends to diminish. The extra time required by translation and the presence of the interpreter may make the physician impatient.

When attempting to converse with someone who does not

speak the same language, there is a natural tendency to shout at the person, as if that would enable him to understand. The interviewer should resist this tendency and speak in a normal tone of voice rather than behaving as if he were conversing with a deaf person. By speaking slowly, he allows himself to express feelings with his tone of voice, gestures, and facial expressions. This facilitates the development of rapport even though the patient does not directly understand the interviewer's words. If at some point in the discussion the patient inexplicably becomes upset or does not react as the physician expects, one should go back in the conversation and determine whether something was translated incorrectly.

Under most circumstances, the patient will develop a transference to the physician just as if the interpreter were not present. On some occasions the patient may utilize the interpreter in a defensive manner to avoid relating to the doctor. The therapist must guard against feeling rejected, angry, or depressed. Competitive attitudes toward the interpreter may also interfere with the therapist's functioning.

MODIFICATIONS OF THE INTERVIEW

The non-English-speaking patient usually presents a rather polite, passive, compliant façade, frequently misleading the interviewer into believing he has achieved a greater degree of understanding and rapport than is actually the case. The patient conceals disagreement and confusion, but he later expresses it by not returning for the next interview.

In an attempt to suppress any prejudice, the interviewer frequently ignores all references to the patient's race and ethnic background. The patient, however, correctly perceives these omissions as direct evidence of prejudice on the part of the interviewer. It is, therefore, important early in the interview to make inquiry into the patient's family background, length of stay in this country, present living conditions, and experiences in the new culture. In the case of a lower class patient, the interviewer often does not want to hear data about how badly the patient has been treated by the majority group. A discussion of the patient's living conditions, economic circumstances, and unhappy experiences in the new culture may give the interviewer a more intimate understanding of the problems, as well as giving the patient a feeling that someone really cares.

If it seems that the interpreter is deviating from the instructions and is not translating every comment made by the patient, merely remind him of the nature of his task. Do not attempt to interpret his behavior. By concentrating his attention on the patient, the interviewer will enable the interpreter to feel more comfortable. This will minimize the likelihood of the interpreter's experiencing untoward emotional responses during the interview.

The patient will expect to concentrate less on past developmental material and direct attention more toward the present. It is always helpful to determine how the patient was referred for psychiatric care and who considered the problem to be psychiatric. The non-English-speaking patient is almost invariably accompanied by someone else, usually someone who speaks English. If the interview has been conducted through a hospital interpreter, it is important that the interviewer talk with the person who accompanied the patient as well. This will further help the physician in his task of attempting to understand the patient's problem.

When the interpreter is a family member or a friend, the interviewer should touch lightly on subjects that the patient may not wish to discuss in front of this person, such as sex. However, each case is evaluated individually. On some occasions, the patient may come from a culture in which this subject is less taboo.

Whenever the interviewer has difficulty understanding the data provided by the patient in terms of its cultural significance, he can be very open in admitting his ignorance of the patient's culture. He may then ask the patient directly if such behavior is considered normal, unusual or significant in terms of the patient's own background. In this manner he can greatly reduce the obvious handicap of his limited knowledge and can give the patient confidence in the interviewer's genuine interest. If the interviewer has accumulated some knowledge of the patient's culture, he can facilitate more rapid development of a trusting relationship by demonstrating this understanding.

The interviewer often learns that the patient is able to speak more English than he initially admitted. This disclosure is evidence of the patient's greater trust, and no interpretation or comment from the interviewer is required, as it will only make the patient feel criticized for his behavior.

The patient needs time at the end of the interview in order to ask questions. Arrangements must be made for an interpreter to be present when the second interview is scheduled. As with all new experiences, the interviewer's comfort and proficiency will increase substantially as he acquires more experience in conducting his interviews with the assistance of an interpreter.

17 NOTE TAKING AND THE PSYCHIATRIC INTERVIEW

A discussion of psychiatric interviewing often leads to consideration of the purpose, function, and methods of note taking. The beginning psychiatric interviewer is often distressed to learn that considerable variation in opinion exists among experienced psychiatrists concerning the quantity and the method of recording notes. The diversity of advice given the beginner is extreme. Notes are often suggested by a supervisor, thereby representing the intrusion of a third party into the interview situation. This may disturb either the patient or the interviewer. Therefore, a discussion of note taking must include the supervisory relationship. One supervisor may advise a student to make no notes whatsoever and, instead, to concentrate fully on what the patient is saying, relying on memory to reproduce the material. At the other extreme is the supervisor who recommends taking verbatim notes. Often the student is confused as to the definition of verbatim, but, in the spirit of cooperation, he writes frantically, trying to include everything said by both himself and the patient. The same supervisor may seem inconsistent, having a different approach for different students, or even a different approach for the same student with different patients. In order to understand this complex problem, it is necessary to establish some fundamental principles.

All interviewers make mental notes concerning various aspects of the interview. One of the basic tasks in improving one's skill as an interviewer is learning to listen more carefully to the patient. Simultaneously, the interviewer must observe the patient's behavior and affective reactions, and his own responses to the patient. Furthermore, he is expected to note the correlation of specific topics with particular body movements or affective responses. His teachers suggest that he learn to identify the "red thread" or the unconscious continuity that exists between the patient's associations. The interviewer is also expected to consider every remark that he will make to the patient and be able to recall his own comments, questions, interpretations, suggestions, advice, and so forth when reporting the interview. In order to accomplish all of this, the beginner feels he must be a combination of expert juggler and electronic computer.

The intense pressure on the inexperienced interviewer may be lessened by concentrating on one or more of the above-mentioned areas. Some teachers emphasize historical data concerning the patient, but others direct their attention to the interpersonal process that is taking place between physician and patient. Supervisors who emphasize historical data tend to be more insistent about note taking during the interview and usually want a precise record of the data concerning the patient. Those supervisors who emphasize the interpersonal process will encourage a detailed report of the interviewer's statements, whether the notes are recorded during or after the interview. Note taking is, thus, part of a much broader question: Which aspect of the interview will occupy the attention of the interviewer?

This chapter will concentrate on the more narrow issue of what kind of record is to be made and when it is to be done in relation to the interview. The need for keeping written records about patients is ubiquitous in medicine. There is a legal and moral responsibility to maintain an accurate record of each patient's diagnosis and treatment. Such requirements are quite broad; however, young physicians in training are subject to the policies of their particular institution. Although such policies undoubtedly influence the physician's attitudes, the manner in which the material is to be recorded in usually left to the discretion of the individual. Another important purpose of record keeping is to aid one's own memory concerning each patient. Therefore, each individual has to decide what type of information he has the most difficulty remembering and use this knowledge as a guideline in his own system of record keeping. Certainly such basic identifying data as the patient's name and address, the names of other family members, the ages of children, spouse, siblings, parents, and so forth should be written, as this information is not easily recalled. A concise description of the patient and his behavior during the initial interview often proves to be helpful later in treatment. Always include initial diagnostic impressions. Studies have suggested that students who formulate a case on paper are consistently more successful as therapists than are those who only organize the case in their mind.

The chief disadvantage in making notes during the interview is the distraction from attending to the patient. With experience, it becomes progressively easier to make notes with a minimum of distraction, giving full attention to the patient. The patient who speaks slowly or who has a diminished production of ideas makes it much easier for the interviewer to make notes during the interview. Many therapists make fairly complete notes during the first few sessions, while eliciting historical data. After that, most doctors record only new historical information, important events in the patient's life, medications prescribed, transference or countertransference trends, dreams, and general comments about the patient's progress.

The anxious or uncomfortable interviewer may find his notes a convenient refuge from emotional contact with the patient. They allow him to avert his eyes and occupy his thoughts with other matters. He may fall a sentence or two behind the conversation. The interview fades into the background and whatever was making him anxious becomes less disturbing. This is an indication that the notes should be put aside and the countertransference problems explored. As an example, a young resident told one of the authors he had been particularly impressed by an article he had read that likened the maneuvers between beginning therapists and female patients to the dating or courtship interaction. The resident readily accepted the idea that note taking helped him establish the feeling of having a professional identity and that he was relating to the patient in the proper and appropriate manner. Here, note taking clearly functioned to help establish a professional identity for the neophyte, and to help provide a distraction so that he could be more involved with the notes than with his feelings toward the patient.

There is a business-like quality to any note taking, and

this can be used therapeutically. The doctor can establish a sense of heightened intimacy by putting his pen and paper aside. This is customary in discussing material about which the patient is expected to be reticent—his sexual life, his transference comments, or his negative feelings about a previous doctor.

In presenting material to a supervisor, the obsessive resident takes comfort in bringing copious notes. He is uncertain about what material is most important and is concerned that, if left to his own judgment, he is liable to bring the wrong data. He compensates for his inability to discriminate by attempting to bring everything. Invariably, he leaves out the most important things, those that took place on the way into the office or at the end of the interview when he had already put the note pad away. Since it is more difficult to write while talking than it is to write while listening, there is a tendency for the notes to be more complete and accurate concerning the remarks made by the patient than those made by the interviewer. Often when a supervisor suggests that the student might have said such-and-such, or asked the patient about so-and-so at a certain point during the interview, the student quickly assures the supervisor that he did, in fact, say that, only he did not have a chance to write it down.

It is obvious that verbatim notes are not actually verbatim. In fact, there is no such thing as a complete record of a session. Even an audio tape is not a total report of all that transpired during the interview, as it contains only the auditory aspects. Furthermore, many of the subtle verbal innuendos may be obscured by the recording equipment or completely missed if they are separated from the visual cues that accompanied them. The crucial data of the interviewer's subjective feelings and responses cannot be directly recorded by any means. It is the quality of the relationship between the supervisor and the student that determines how much of the important material of the session is reproduced during a supervisory hour. The resident should respect and trust his supervisor, and not perceive him as someone out to damage or weaken the resident or prove his inadequacy. If the resident is frightened, the supervisor is not likely to learn many of the important things that transpired during the session, even though the student may provide copious notes.

Audio or video tapes are a kind of note taking that modern

technology has made increasingly popular. When these methods are employed, one must consider the effect they have on both the patient and the doctor. The doctor's concern about the patient's rights and privileges is revealed by the manner in which he introduces these procedures to the patient. In the author's experience, it is uncommon for a patient to object to a recording, but every patient will want the procedure explained in advance and his permission requested. The equipment should be started only after the patient knows about it and has given his permission. He is far more concerned with doctor's attitude about invading his privacy than with the content of what might be revealed.

The interviewer, on the other hand, is often quite concerned about the scrutiny of his colleagues and supervisors. This will stifle his spontaneity and lead him to conduct a "safer," more stereotyped and more intellectual interview. In addition, his responses to the recording equipment are often projected onto the patient, and the doctor may pursue the patient's anxiety about the recording when the patient is, in fact, relatively indifferent to it. One of the authors began his first interview on video tape with, "I imagine you're wondering about the television equipment," only to hear in reply, "Oh, don't you always do that?" On some occasions the doctor's exhibitionism will take over, and he will attempt dramatic maneuvers. In any event, he is responding to an unseen audience rather than to his patient.

Thus far we have considered note taking largely from the point of view of the therapist and its effects upon him. Now let us consider the effects of note taking on different types of patients.

The paranoid patient is most likely to be upset by the note taking. He feels that the records represent damaging evidence that may be later used against him. In working with such patients, it is generally wise to confine any note taking in the patient's presence to basic historical information. In the hospital setting, it is preferable to answer suspicious patients' questions about who has access to the notes. It is important to tell such patients that they may discuss issues confidentially and be assured that the interviewer will be discreet in his recording. Making notes at the end of the session will minimize some of these problems, but is often impractical.

The obsessive patient may at times feel that the doctor is

getting the goods on him, but he is more prone to view the doctor's note taking as a cue to the importance of what he has said. The patient may also indicate his awareness of the importance of the notes by pausing periodically to facilitate the recording. The patient is usually unwilling to acknowledge that this behavior is motivated by his resentment that the doctor shows more interest in the notes than in him.

Patients who are being treated by resident therapists in teaching centers often have some awareness of the teaching role of the particular institution to which they have gone for help. They often do not ask directly about supervisors or supervision, but they will very frequently couch such curiosity in questions about the note taking. A common question is, "What do you use those notes for, Doctor?" The resident often senses that the inquiry is really directed at the supervisory process and represents a potential exposé of his inexperienced status. Therefore, he is often tempted to answer the patient with mild degrees of dishonesty, offering such answers as, "The notes are an important part of your treatment record," or, "The hospital requires that treatment records are kept." Prominently concealed in such inquiries is the patient's fear that the doctor will breach his confidence. The evasiveness of the beginning therapist may also stem from guilt or discomfort at the idea of revealing his patient's confidences to a supervisor or at a conference. It is helpful to answer such inquiries by asking the patient if he has some specific idea concerning the purpose of the notes. The interviewer may uncover thoughts that the patient has concealed. Pursuing this point may lead to direct questions about the therapist's supervision. Such questions are threatening to the security system of the novice, but he is surprised to learn how frequently the patient is reassured at the idea that his young, inexperienced physician is aided by a more experienced psychiatrist. At other times the patient already knows the answer to these questions and is relieved and impressed that his therapist is open and honest about his inexperienced status.

On occasion the patient may ask, "What did you just write down?" or, "Why did you write down what I just said?" Such questions indicate either the patient's search for some magical answer to his problem or his fear and mistrust of the physician. The interviewer will gain more understanding of the underlying process if he does not answer the question. He could reply,

"What do you think I wrote?" or, "What is it that you are concerned about?" Uncovering the covert meaning of the question will shift the focus of the patient's interest from the doctor's notes to his own anxiety. Other variations of this situation occur when the patient tries to read the doctor's notes upside down while they are being written. This behavior may be accompanied by comments from the patient indicating that he has just read something. The doctor might put down his pen at this point and explore the meaning of the patient's interest as suggested above.

Obsessive and schizophrenic patients will frequently become concerned about the ownership of the notes. A common statement is, "Those notes are about me so they must be mine." The doctor replies, "No, they belong to me because I made them." Patients sometimes ask if they can read the notes or if they can have them. They may feel that the notes contain the magic answer that will immediately provide a solution to their problems, if only the doctor would share it with them. The interviewer should determine to which aspect of the note taking the patient is responding, rather than allow the patient to read the notes. Once the interviewer has identified the basis of the patient's interest, the concern with the notes is forgotten.

Ownership of the notes may also become a problem for patients who have problems with impulse control. A typical patient might ask, "What would you do if I were to run over and grab those notes?" Interpretations about the patient's concern over loss of impulse control are important. Such comments may be unsuccessful with very literal-minded patients, making it necessary for the interviewer to tell the patient that the notes belong to him, not to the patient, that the patient may not look at them, and that he will not tolerate the patient's trying to take the notes away from him.

Hysterical and depressed patients tend to resent note taking. These individuals want the undivided attention of the therapist, and any interference can only provoke their anger and make them feel deprived. Often their resentment about the notes is revealed in dreams long before they openly complain during the session. As with other patients who are disturbed by note taking, one can avoid the problem by making notes after the session. However, it may be difficult for the interviewer to relax and recall the transactions of the interview in an orderly manner. Important data are omitted and other data is distorted both in content and order. Years of experience are necessary before the interviewer is able to make an accurate and precise appraisal of the major trends of a session. Only then can this dimension of the session be recorded reasonably well following an interview.

INDEX

ISBN 0-7216-5973-X

90038

9 780721 659732